Facsimile reproduction on reduced-size of the 1804 and 1807 original editions
The Anatomy and Surgical Treatment of Inguinal and Congenital Hernia
The Anatomy and Surgical Treatment of Crural and Umbilical Hernia, &c. &c. (Part II)
By Astley Cooper, F. R. S.

Published by Jiku Publishers, Ltd.
4-18-3 Koishikawa, Bunkyo-ku, Tokyo, Japan
©2015 Jiku Publishers, Ltd.
All rights reserved

THE ANATOMY

AND

SURGICAL TREATMENT

OF

INGUINAL AND CONGENITAL HERNIA.

By ASTLEY COOPER, F.R.S.

MEMBER OF THE ROYAL MEDICAL AND PHYSICAL SOCIETIES OF EDINBURGH; LECTURER ON ANATOMY AND SURGERY, AND SURGEON TO GUY'S HOSPITAL.

ILLUSTRATED BY PLATES.

LONDON:

PRINTED FOR T. COX, ST. THOMAS'S STREET, BOROUGH;

AND SOLD BY

MESSRS. JOHNSON, ST. PAUL'S CHURCH YARD; LONGMAN AND REES, AND ROBINSONS, PATERNOSTER ROW; MURRAY, FLEET STREET; HIGHLEY, FLEET STREET; PHILLIPS, GEORGE YARD; CALLOW, SOHO; AND CREECH, EDINBURGH.

1804.

T. BENSLEY, PRINTER, BOLT COURT, FLEET STREET.

TO

HENRY CLINE, Esq.

LECTURER ON ANATOMY AND SURGERY,

AND

SURGEON TO ST. THOMAS'S HOSPITAL.

MY DEAR SIR,

Two reasons strongly impel me to dedicate the following Work to you. The one is, that many of the ideas which it contains have been derived from your public and private instructions:

The other, that it gives me an opportunity of acknowledging, with gratitude, the kind attention which I invariably experienced from you whilst an inmate of your family.

That you may long continue to enjoy an exalted professional reputation, acquired solely by merit, and unsullied by a single unworthy art, is the ardent wish of,

Your sincere friend,

And colleague,

ASTLEY COOPER.

LONDON, JAN. 10, 1804.

PREFACE.

IN the following pages I have endeavoured to describe the anatomy and surgical treatment of inguinal and congenital hernia.

No disease of the human body, belonging to the province of the surgeon, requires in its treatment a greater combination of accurate anatomical knowledge, with surgical skill, than hernia in all its varieties. Symptoms, immediately threatening the extinction of life, occur at times, and in situations, that afford but little opportunity for consulting the authority of others; and demand in the surgeon a prompt resolution and decisive practice. Accurate anatomical knowledge is frequently required to detect the presence of this disease at that period at which alone the milder process of reduction is practicable; and still more is the combination of skill and intelligence necessary to enable the surgeon to meet all the occurrences which may happen, when the use of the knife becomes the only method of saving the patient.

It has therefore been a primary object with me to trace the progress of the disease from its commencement, to explain the nature and uses of the parts contiguous to hernia, which are in any way connected with its formation and increase; and especially to describe, with sufficient minuteness, the surrounding arteries, as far as their course interferes with the operations of the surgeon.

Another object of this Work is, to lay down rules for operating, calculated to meet all the varieties of hernia hitherto discovered. These varieties are in their nature sufficiently complicated, but it is the business of the surgical teacher to simplify the practice as much as possible, prescribing general rules, of easy application, to embrace the majority of cases that are likely to occur, and distinguishing how far the anomalies of the disease are to furnish exceptions to the accustomed modes of practice. Thus prepared, the operation itself being, on the whole, easy, and attended with but little danger to the patient, the surgeon will undertake it with that decisive confidence, which is the fruit and reward of the pains employed to acquire a clear insight into the several steps to be pursued.

The mode of operating for inguinal hernia here proposed, has been taught by me since the year 1792, when I first began to give public lectures on surgery, and since that time having had several opportunities of putting it in practice myself, and of seeing it adopted by others, I can recommend it with confidence as being both safe and effectual.

Something remains to be said as to the execution of the Work. Much confusion is often created in anatomical description by a want of uniformity in the use of terms employed to express the relative situation of parts. It was my wish to have adopted the philosophical and accurate nomenclature of Dr. Barclay, of Edinburgh, which would at once have obviated every source of uncertainty; but on mature reflection, I hesitated to venture on such a total change of language in a work intended solely for practical utility in a particular branch of surgery. I have therefore endeavoured, in some degree, to supply the defect, (though imperfectly) by limiting the use of certain terms expressive of relative situation, in those cases where doubts could arise in the mind of the reader from any variety of meaning usually attached to these appellations. I am aware that in the course of an entire work, it is scarcely possible always to preserve consistency of nomenclature, where the terms are in common use, and are perpetually occurring to the mind in a sense different to that to which they have been thus artificially restricted. I hope, however, that it will be found sufficiently correct, in that part of the anatomical description, where all the relative situations of organs, with their mutual bearings, have been described. Here, I have restricted the terms, *above, below—top, bottom—up, down—superior, inferior—*

ascending, descending, to imply the direction from head to foot: the terms *before, behind—over, under—forwards, backwards—anterior, posterior,* to a direction from the surface of the abdomen and fore part of the body, to the viscera and deeper-seated parts: and the terms *inner, outer—within, without—internal, external,* imply situation nearer to, or further from, a line (perpendicular when the body is erect) drawn through the chin, navel, and pubis.

I have almost uniformly, in the following work, avoided quoting the opinions of authors on this part of surgery. This I have done, certainly not from any wish to slight or undervalue the labours of some of the most excellent physiologists and practitioners that have adorned our profession, but because it did not form a part of my plan to give a history of this branch of surgery, and because I wished to confine myself to the very wide scene of observation afforded by the two noble institutions of St. Thomas's and Guy's Hospitals, and to that portion of the practice of this metropolis, which I have been personally enabled to authenticate. I have therefore related no case, and given no remark, to the truth of which I cannot vouch; and for the same reason the subjects of all the plates annexed to this volume are from preparations, either in my own possession, or in the Anatomical Museum at St. Thomas's Hospital, which may at all times be consulted.

The Plates have been executed by Mr. Heath, from drawings of Mr. Kirtland: of their excellence, in point of art, my readers must judge, but I may add, that to insure their accuracy as faithful copies of the original preparations, all the outlines have been laid down from an exact measurement of parts.

It is my design to publish a second part of this Work in the course of a few months, describing the other species of hernia, the drawings of which are already in the hands of the engraver.

St. Mary Axe, Jan. 25, 1804.

CONTENTS.

CHAPTER 1. General Description of Hernia, ... Page 1

2. Of the Anatomy of the Parts concerned with Inguinal Hernia, ... 4

3. Of the Inguinal Hernia, ... 8

4. Of the Causes of Hernia, ... 12

5. Of the Reducible Hernia, and Use of Trusses, ... 14

6. Of the Irreducible Hernia, ... 17

7. Of the Strangulated Hernia, ... 20

8. Of the Treatment of Strangulated Hernia, ... 23

9. Circumstances to be considered previous to the Operation, ... 26

10. Of the Operation for Inguinal Hernia, ... 28

11. Mortification of the Intestine, ... 33

12. Of the Treatment after the Return of the protruded Parts, ... 41

13. Of very large Herniæ, ... 43

14. Of Small Inguinal Herniæ, ... 48

15. Of the Inguinal Hernia on the inner Side of the Epigastric Artery, ... 51

16. Of Hernia in the Female, ... 55

17. On the Congenital Hernia, or Hernia Tunicæ Vaginalis Testis, ... 57

ERRATA.

Page 7, line 4, in lieu of *instead of*, read *besides*.
10, ... 16 from the bottom, instead of *as it*, read *which*.
12, ... 8 from the bottom, read *an inch*, in lieu of *an inch and an half*.
15, ... 25 from the bottom, read *herniæ*, instead of *hernies*.
21, ... 9 from the bottom, *extremely rare occurrence*: this expression may be misunderstood. I do not mean to deny the contraction of the mouth of the sac, but only to state that it is not generally independent of, but is, on the contrary, generally occasioned, when it does exist, by the pressure of the surrounding parts, and sometimes by the pressure of a truss.
28, Operation *of Inguinal Hernia*, read *for Inguinal Hernia*.

OF INGUINAL HERNIA.

CHAPTER I.

General Description of Hernia.

A PROTRUSION of any viscus from its proper cavity is denominated a hernia. The protruded parts are generally contained in a bag, formed by the membrane with which the cavity is naturally invested. Definition.

Several parts of the body afford examples of this disease. A deficiency of the bones of the head will sometimes allow of the protrusion of part of the brain and its membranes, from the inner to the outer side of the scull, forming a hernia of this organ. Hernia of the head;

An imperfect state of the intercostal muscles may permit part of the lungs, with its pleura, to form an external tumour, or hernia of the cavity of the chest. of the chest;

But the disease most frequently occurs about the cavity of the abdomen; and on this account, as well as from the superior importance in surgery of hernia of the belly, I shall confine my observations to this species, with its several varieties. of the abdomen.

Many reasons may be assigned for the very frequent occurrence of protrusions from the abdomen. Causes of its frequent occurrence.

First: The viscera of this cavity are numerous, many of them very moveable, and but loosely connected by peritoneal attachments with the surrounding parts; and they are habitually exposed to changes of size and relative situation, from sudden or gradual distention.

Secondly: The parietes of the abdomen are composed of muscles, the action of which is to contract the dimensions of this cavity, to compress the bowels, and thus to force them from their natural situation.

Thirdly: For the passage of vessels and nerves, these muscles and their tendons have various apertures, which, though naturally only wide enough for this purpose, often become so much relaxed as to allow the viscera themselves to protrude.

Lastly: The muscles are sometimes imperfectly formed, and the viscera escape through unnatural apertures.

The following are the situations in which abdominal hernia is found: Situations of the abdominal.

It appears at the abdominal rings, passing in the same course as the spermatic cord in the male, and the round ligaments of the uterus in the female; thence it is continued down into the scrotum in the one sex, and the labium pudendi in the other. This hernia of the abdominal ring is known to surgeons under the various appellations of inguinal hernia, scrotal hernia, bubonocele, and oscheocele. Inguinal.

It also penetrates under Poupart's ligament to the upper part of the thigh, through a small aperture in a tendon formed for the passage of the femoral vessels. In this situation it is called femoral hernia, crural hernia, or merocele. Crural.

Another species is formed at the navel by the protrusion of the hernia through the opening which was left in the fœtus for the passage of the umbilical cord. This has received the name of umbilical hernia, or exomphalos. Umbilical.

Similar protrusions are also found through the tendinous covering of the anterior part of the abdomen. The linea alba and semilunaris are perforated to transmit vessels going to the common integuments: when these holes are either originally of an unusual size, or are enlarged during a relaxed state of body, herniæ will occasionally be formed in them, which are then called ventral. Ventral.

Ovularis obturatoria.   Another part at which hernia is sometimes produced is the foramen ovale of the pelvis; when it takes the name of the aperture, and is termed hernia foraminis ovalis, or ovularis obturatoria.

Perinei.
Vaginæ.   Sometimes a hernia passes between the bladder and rectum in the male, and between the rectum and uterus in the female, appearing in the perineum. It is then called hernia perinei. I have seen the vagina protruded forwards by a descent of the viscera between the rectum and uterus, and pushed backwards by the bladder, forming a considerable external tumour when the bladder was full, which disappeared as soon as it was emptied.

Ischiatocele.   Sometimes, though rarely, a hernia is produced at the ischiatic notch projecting by the side of the sciatic nerve under the glutæi muscles. This takes the name of the part, and is termed hernia of the ischiatic notch, or ischiatocele.

Diaphragmæ.   Hernia has been known to protrude through the diaphragm, sometimes by the side of the œsophagus, sometimes by the vena cava inferior, sometimes, though more rarely, by the side of the aorta, but more frequently through unnatural apertures in the muscle.

Labii pudendi.   I have met with a hernia protruding into the labium pudendi, passing under the branch of the ischium along with the internal pudendal artery, but continued into the pelvis by the side of the vagina.

Mesentery and Mesocolon.   I have two preparations in my possession, of hernia occasioned by the viscera passing between the laminæ of the peritoneum, in one case into the mesentery, in the other into a bag formed by a separation of the laminæ of the mesocolon, in which all the small intestines were contained.

Sometimes holes are left by an imperfect structure of the mesentery, through which the viscera pass and become strangulated, but these cannot be called true herniæ, as the intestine remains in the cavity of the abdomen.

Congenita.   That species of hernia, which from its appearing at the time of birth, is called congenita, takes the same course through the abdominal rings as the inguinal hernia; but instead of passing upon the fore part of the spermatic process, it is formed within the tunica vaginalis testis, and ought therefore to be named the hernia tunicæ vaginalis.

There is no part of the abdomen, excepting where the parietes are formed of bone, at which hernia may not occur; for, where the formation of the muscles is defective, it may happen even at the loins, in which case *The most frequent.* the kidney has been known to be part of the protruding substance. But of all the varieties of this disease which I have enumerated, the inguinal, femoral, and umbilical herniæ most frequently occur.

The inguinal hernia is more commonly a disease of the male sex, the femoral and umbilical of the female.

Named from contents.   The names that have been given to different kinds of hernia, have been derived from their contents, as well as their situations. If they only contain omentum, they are called omental hernia, or epiplocele; if only intestine, intestinal hernia, or enterocele; if both omentum and intestine, entero-epiplocele; if the stomach is contained in the tumour, gastrocele; if the liver, hepatocele; if the bladder, cystocele, or hernia cystica; if the uterus, hysterocele; and the same of others; for, excepting the duodenum and the pancreas, which are too closely connected with the spine easily to change their situation, all the different abdominal viscera have occasionally been found as the protruding contents of hernia.

Viscera most frequently found in them.   However, the viscera of the most usual occurrence in hernia are the omentum, and the small intestine, the ilium; the next in frequency is the colon, then the cæcum, and often the jejunum; sometimes the appendix cæci is the only part of the intestine found in the hernial sac.

Hernial Sac.   The cavity of the abdomen is every where lined by the peritoneum, which in hernia generally protrudes prior to any descent of the viscera, and thus a bag or sac is formed by this membrane, in which the protruded viscera are afterwards contained.

Its formation.   The older surgeons thought that herniæ were formed by a laceration of the peritoneum and abdominal muscles, which gave rise to the term *rupture*; but dissection has proved that such a rupture of the membrane scarcely ever happens. The peritoneum in forming a hernial sac is not dragged from its natural situation, but becomes elongated by gradual distention, and it is usually not only lengthened, but slightly thickened; for a long continued pressure of moderate force will produce an elongation and thickening of fibre, though a greater degree will bring about an entire absorption of parts. This is proved, in the first case, by the vast increase of size and thickness which the tunica vaginalis undergoes in old hydrocele; and in the second, by the entire removal of the sternum and cartilages of the ribs in aneurism. It is then by the first of these principles in the animal economy that a hernial sac is produced, and if the sac be compared with the peritoneum from which it originated, it will generally be found to be a more dense and compact membrane. But when the hernia becomes of a very considerable magnitude, the peritoneum forming the sac becomes thinner than natural; for the extension may go beyond the degree at which pressure thickens; and from this cause it is that in old and large herniæ, the peristaltic motion of the intestines may sometimes be seen through the sides of the sac. Sometimes thinner than the peritoneum.

This is also one reason why herniæ are sometimes found without sacs, for, the process of extension having ceased, the sac becomes either entirely absorbed or remains only at the orifice; and over the larger part of the tumour no covering is left for the protruded viscera but skin and cellular membrane.

On the other hand, the sac has occasionally been observed to be so much thickened as to retain nothing of its original peritoneal texture, and to be divisible into layers. But from what I have seen of this disease, I am induced to believe that this opinion has originated from the want of sufficient distinction between the covering of the sac, and the sac itself; for, as far as I can discover from dissection, it is the former which is extremely thickened in old hernia, whilst the latter is but little denser than the peritoneum. As to what has been said by surgeons of stricture being formed by a thickening of the orifice of the sac, I shall have occasion to shew in a future part of this work, that the stricture is not in the sac, as has been supposed, but in another part external to it; at the same time, however, I would not be understood to deny altogether this alteration in the mouth of the sac, but to state my belief, founded upon dissection, that it is a rare occurrence. Thickened.

A hernial sac, when small, does not adhere to the parts amongst which it is placed, but can then be readily drawn into the cavity of the abdomen, which I have several times done in the dead subject, and have then seen the sac lying loosely within the cavity of the belly, at the orifice through which it had descended. This however can only happen whilst the hernia is small, and in the most recent state; for, if it has been of long standing, or has descended far, it has always contracted very firm adhesions to the surrounding parts, from which dissection alone can separate it. At first the adhesions are few and weak, but they gradually become strong, and uniformly spread over the surface of the sac. Adhesion.

The opening by which the sac communicates with the abdomen is generally its smallest part, and is called its mouth; but when it has passed a short way from the abdomen, and has quitted the tendons which surround its mouth, it enters parts more easily distensible than tendons, and then dilates into a bag of a pyriform shape. Shape.

As the hernial sac generally passes through openings which are designed for the passage of blood-vessels, its exact situation with respect to these vessels should be most carefully attended to. Nor is this all, for in the two most important herniæ, the inguinal and femoral, an artery passes near the orifice of the sac, the course of which it is of the utmost importance for the surgeon to observe, as an ignorance of it must often expose the life of the patient to imminent risk in the operation for hernia. Vessels connected with it.

One of the coverings of the hernial sac is generally a tendinous fascia, and often more than one; a circumstance which should be always kept in mind, to prevent great embarrassment during the operation. Coverings.

Several hernial sacs are sometimes found in the same subject, at different parts, an instance of which will be afterwards given, that occasioned a difficulty in determining which was to be the subject of operation. Sometimes more than one hernia exists in the same situation. I have a preparation of two hernial sacs at each groin, with another in an incipient state on the left side; and the subject of one of the plates to this volume, represents two herniæ on one side and one on the other. When this is the case, they seldom are all at the same time in a state of protrusion, and the second sac is often formed after the cure of the first disease, two examples of which will be hereafter related. Several sacs.

A hernial sac will sometimes be burst by a blow. When this happens, its contents escape out of the sac, and diffuse themselves under the contiguous skin, so that the viscera require to be returned into the sac before they can pass from the sac into the abdomen. I attended a case of inguinal hernia under these circumstances, with Mr. Brickenden, a surgeon in Southwark: the viscera had escaped under the skin of the scrotum, through a hole in the fore part of the sac, and were obliged to be returned into the sac before the reduction of the hernia could be effected. Burst.

The protruded parts in this disease are not always however contained in a sac; for, when hernia arises from a mal-formation of the muscles allowing of unnatural apertures in them, these holes are not always covered by peritoneum, the elongation of which membrane produces the hernial sac. This was the case in a hernia through the diaphragm that I met with some years ago, in which the colon, the viscus that had protruded into the chest, was lying upon the lungs without any peritoneal covering. It is not every hernia of the diaphragm, however, No sac.

that is thus destitute of a sac, for I have known an instance of that disease in which the viscera were included in a process of peritoneum. The hernia congenita has no peritoneal covering distinct from the tunica vaginalis testis, excepting in a very uncommon variety of the disease. The hernia cystica is described as being equally destitute of this membranous coat.

Dr. Marshall has a preparation of umbilical hernia in which no sac appears, but the protruded parts lie in direct contact with the skin. This variety is very rare; but the possibility of such an occurrence should be known, as in performing the operation for hernia extreme care should, on this account, be taken to avoid wounding any of the protruded viscera.

CHAPTER II.

Of the Anatomy of the Parts concerned with Inguinal Hernia.

FIVE pairs of muscles with their tendons form the principal covering of the abdomen. These are, on each side, the obliquus externus, the obliquus internus, the transversalis, the rectus, and the pyramidalis. It is only the three first of these, however, that are concerned in the production and course of inguinal hernia.

External oblique muscle. The external oblique muscle arises on either side from the eight lower ribs, passes obliquely downwards with an easy slope towards the front of the abdomen, and terminates in a broad tendon that covers the anterior part of the belly; at the middle of the fore part of which it unites with the tendon of the corresponding muscle coming from the opposite side, forming by this union a straight white line, extending from the ensiform cartilage to the pubis, and called the linea alba. The tendon of this muscle is also fixed into the pubis, partly on the same side from which it originates, and partly on the opposite side: it is also inserted into the spine of the ilium.

From the ilium to the pubis a tendinous border is stretched, which will be more particularly described hereafter, formed by a doubling-in of the lower edge of the tendon of the external oblique muscle, under which pass the femoral vessels and nerves, and the iliacus internus and psoas muscles. It has been called the ligament of Fallopius, or Pourpart's ligament, or lately, the crural arch. Lines may be also observed in the tendon which covers the fore part of the abdomen, one on each side of a semilunar figure extending from the cartilage of the seventh rib to the symphysis pubis, and called the linea semilunaris; and others called the lineæ transversales, which pass from the linea semilunaris to the linea alba.

Abdominal Ring. In the lower part of the broad tendon of the external oblique muscle, a little above and to the outer side of the symphysis pubis, is a hole called the abdominal ring, which is formed for the passage of the spermatic cord in the male, and the round ligaments of the uterus in the female. The mode in which these openings are formed is the following: the tendon of the external oblique muscle, as it proceeds towards the pubis, splits into two columns, leaving a space between them for the passage of the spermatic cord: the lowest of the two columns, after being doubled under the spermatic cord, is inserted into a small process of the pubis, which may be felt in the living subject, and may be called its spinous process, and from thence onward to the crest of the pubis to the extent of an inch, as will be distinctly seen in Plate I; the upper tendinous column is inserted into the symphysis pubis, and extends across the cartilage to the bone of the pubis on the opposite side.

These columns are united together, an inch from the pubis, by a small process of tendon which proceeds from the anterior and superior spinous process of the ilium, and from the crural arch, crossing the upper and outer part of the ring so as firmly to bind the columns to each other; and also by a few semicircular tendinous fibres, which pass from the edge of one column to the other. The direction of the fibres of this tendinous process from the spine of the ilium is at right angles with those of the external oblique muscle. See Plate I.

Direction. The direction of the abdominal rings is obliquely upwards and outwards, in a line from the pubis to the spinous process of the ilium. Though called a ring, it is not a true circle, for, the diameter in length, which is the direction from the pubis to the transverse column, is about one inch; but the breadth, from one column of tendon to the other, is only half an inch. The center of this aperture is one inch and a quarter from the symphysis pubis. A fascia which originates from the tendon of the external oblique muscle, pusses over each ring, and uniting with the spermatic cord, accompanies it in its descent into the scrotum, to which, as well as to the spermatic sord, it closely adheres.

Surgeons have very generally believed that the aperture was continued into the abdomen immediately behind the ring. This however is not the case, for all direct passage of the spermatic cord into this cavity is shut out by tendons and a fascia, which are probably intended as a guard against protrusions of the contents of the belly. The tendons that close the opening are those of the internal oblique and the transversalis muscles. *No opening behind it.*

The Internal Oblique muscle arises from the spine of the ilium, from Poupart's ligament, and from the three inferior vertebræ of the loins: it is inserted into the six inferior ribs, into the ensiform cartilage, and the linea alba. The lower edge of this muscle arises from the outer half of Poupart's ligament, passes over the spermatic cord, and gives off a tendon, which runs behind the upper part of the ring, and is inserted into the lower part of the linea alba and into the symphysis pubis. If the finger be passed through the ring this tendon may be felt immediately above it and towards its inner side. *Internal oblique.*

The Transversalis muscle arises from the seven inferior ribs, from the lowest vertebra of the back, and from the four superior of the loins. It is inserted into the greater part of the linea alba. The lower edge of this muscle arises also from the crural arch, crosses the spermatic cord, and sends off a thin tendon which joins with that of the internal oblique and passes behind the abdominal ring, and is inserted tendinous into the body of the pubis; and I have seen it send out a semi-circular slip into a fascia, which will be presently noticed. Therefore if the finger be thrust into the abdominal ring, the tendon of the transversalis opposes a resistance to its direct passage into the abdomen, which can only be overcome by a violence capable of tearing the tendon. *Transversalis.*

The foregoing description will shew that there is no natural aperture into the abdomen immediately behind the ring; and therefore the opening must be sought for elsewhere. It will be found one inch and a half above and to the outside of the ring, in a line passing from the ring to the spine of the ilium, the direction of which is obliquely upwards and outwards. The line is the course of the spermatic cord, and the opening which allows its exit immediately from the abdomen is formed in a fascia, to understand the nature of which, Poupart's ligament and its fasciæ must be more particularly described.

Poupart's ligament, or the crural arch, is connected to the spine of the ilium, whence it passes down in a vaulted form over the femoral vessels, and terminates on the inner side of those vessels in a semicircular sweep, from which extends a triangular portion connected with the spinous process of the pubis, and extending from it to the upper part of the symphysis pubis. Its insertion is best seen, as well as the parts hereafter described, by dissecting them as in Plate I. If there had been no other defence to the lower part of the abdomen than that afforded by this arch, few persons would escape herniæ; but this part is fortified by other means. *Poupart's ligament or the crural arch.*

Three different fasciæ are connected with Poupart's ligament, two of which pass upwards and one downwards; and in addition to these a thin tendinous expansion covers the abdominal muscles and their tendons, and quits them at the lower part of the abdomen, passing upon Poupart's ligament to be lost in the adeps and the absorbent glands of the groin, and upon the spermatic cord below the abdominal ring. *Fasciæ.*

The fascia which passes from Poupart's ligament downwards, is the fascia lata of the thigh, which, being continued from the crural arch and from the pubis, gives a strong covering to the muscles of the thigh. The two fasciæ which pass upwards are, first, one which is given off by the crural arch from the ilium to the place at which the femoral vessels pass out from the abdomen, and which adheres to the iliacus internus muscle and to the crest of the ilium. This is united to the crural arch at a white line, which is readily seen when the peritoneum is stripped from the inner part of the abdominal muscles; it is the great means of strengthening the lower part of the abdomen under the arch. This will be seen in Plate II. It has been described by Gimbernat in his work on femoral hernia, and will be more particularly mentioned in a future part of this work. Secondly, a thinner fascia is sent upward from the crural arch immediately behind the abdominal muscles, to which it gives a lining similar to that tendinous expansion which covers them on the fore part. This is the fascia which leaves an opening from the abdomen for the spermatic cord in the male, and for the round ligament of the uterus in the female. It is continued from Poupart's ligament, and passes upwards to the inner side of the transversalis muscle and its tendon, to which it is united by a cellular membrane; and it is extended from thence on the inner side of the same muscle to the upper part of the abdomen, but becomes thinner as it ascends. Above the middle of Poupart's ligament it passes on each side of the spermatic cord, leaving a hole for its passage. The lower part of this hole has a thin tendinous margin; its upper part is shut by the internal oblique and transversalis muscle. From the edge of this fascia a thinner is sent off, which unites itself to the spermatic cord. A part of the same fascia descends under the middle of Poupart's ligament, and becomes united to the femoral artery and vein, and a part of it is fixed into the pubis. (See Plate II.)

The best mode of discovering this passage is to pass the finger into the abdominal ring, and by carrying it obliquely upwards and outwards in the course of the spermatic cord, towards the abdomen, the border of the fascia will be distinctly felt. To expose it to view, the abdominal ring and the tendon of the external oblique muscle should be first dissected, then, by making an opening midway between the ring and the spinous process of the ilium, and raising the lower edge of the internal oblique and transverse muscles, the situation of this aperture will be most distinctly seen. (See Plate I.)

The strength of the fascia differs in different subjects. In some subjects it appears only as condensed cellular membrane, but in all cases of inguinal herniæ it becomes of considerable strength and thickness, especially on its inner edge; and if it had not existed the bowels would, in the erect posture, be always capable of passing under the edge of the transversalis muscle, so that without it no person could be free from inguinal hernia. The inner edge of the passage which this fascia forms, and which is strengthened by the situation of the epigastric artery, is distant about an inch and a half from the abdominal ring, the outer edge is two inches and a half from the ilium, and the diameter of the orifice for the spermatic cord is half an inch. These measurements, however, must of course vary according to age and stature, but the relative distances will always be the same; the inner margin of the opening being invariably half way between the spinous process of the ilium and the symphisis pubis.

Spermatic cord. Through the opening, which I have just described, and through the abdominal ring of the external oblique muscle, the spermatic cord passes down to the testis. The cord is composed of arteries, veins, nerves, absorbent vessels, an excretory duct called the vas deferens, a membranous sheath, and the cremaster mucle. As soon as it quits the abdomen midway between the spine of the ilium and the symphisis pubis, it turns suddenly inwards and downwards, passing in its course to the ring along the edge of the transversalis and internal oblique muscles, before the epigastric artery, and in a groove formed by the doubling of the tendon of the external oblique muscle. On its emerging from the ring, the cord takes an almost perpendicular direction into the scrotum.

Artery. The spermatic artery, on each side, is derived from the fore part of the aorta in the middle of the abdomen a little below the superior mesenteric arteries. It passes to the lower part of the abdomen, opposite the middle of Poupart's ligament, into the upper opening which I have before described. As it here forms a part of the spermatic cord, its course to the testis is the same.

Vein. The spermatic vein, on each side, arising from the testis, passes along with the cord into the abdomen. Hence it accompanies the spermatic artery to the middle of the abdomen, where they separate; the right vein terminating in the inferior cava opposite the kidney, and the left uniting with the left emulgent vein. (See Plate IV.)

Vas deferens. The vas deferens on each side arises from the posterior part of the testicle, to which it is the excretory duct; and, with the cord, passes into the abdomen; here it quits the spermatic artery and vein, sinks into the cavity of the pelvis, and runs behind the bladder to open into the urethra.

Tunica Vaginalis. These three vessels together with their appropriate absorbents and nerves, receive a double covering of peritoneum from the part at which they quit the abdomen, which closely unites them together. This covering is called the Tunica Vaginalis of the Spermatic Cord. Just above the testis the two layers of the tunic recede from each other, so as to form a bag for the purpose of covering this organ, and this is named the Tunica Vaginalis Testis.

Besides the spermatic arteries, the cord contains two other arteries, one arising from the internal iliac branch and accompanying the vas deferens; and the other a ramification given off from the epigastric artery midway between the pubis and ilium, the latter however is sometimes wanting.

Cremaster. The cremaster muscle is added to the cord between the upper and lower rings. It arises under the external oblique muscle, from the edges of the internal oblique and the transversalis, descends into the scrotum upon the vessels which I have described, covering the tunica vaginalis of the cord, and is finally attached to the tunica vaginalis testis.

It appears therefore that the portion of the spermatic cord contained between the testis and the abdominal ring is composed of several vessels, covered, first with a double peritoneal coat, formed by the tunica vaginalis, next with the cremaster muscle, and, over all, with a fascia given off by the external oblique muscle. The portion of cord above the ring, included between it and the upper aperture, is equally covered by the peritoneal coat and the cremaster muscle; but instead of the fascia given off by the external oblique, it is covered by the tendon itself of this muscle. Higher up, within the cavity of the abdomen, the only covering to the spermatic vessels is derived from the peritoneum.

The course of the spermatic cord from the upper opening to the ring is very oblique, verging downwards towards the middle of the upper part of the thigh, after which it suddenly takes a more perpendicular direction towards the testicle. _{Course of the cord.}

This first obliquity in the direction of the cord appears to be intended to prevent the ready protrusion of the abdominal viscera, for had the cord emerged from the abdomen immediately behind the abdominal ring, scarcely any person who was in the habit of much bodily exertion would be free from hernia. As it is, the protrusion of the viscera is opposed, by the obliquity of the passage, and especially as this contrivance causes the tendons behind the ring, when pressed upon by the abdominal viscera, to shut up the oblique aperture in the manner of a valve, which acts with a force proportional to the pressure. _{Use of its obliquity.}

The epigastric artery is situated so near to the spermatic cord, and is so much concerned in the operation for hernia, that a most accurate knowledge of its course is absolutely requisite. This vessel arises from the iliac artery behind Poupart's ligament, (See Plate II.) and passes upwards and inwards close to the under and inner side of the spermatic cord, between it and the symphysis pubis. Here it sends off a branch which runs upon the spermatic cord. For one inch and three quarters of its course it lies posterior to all the abdominal muscles, between them and the peritoneum, after which it enters before a tendon which is placed behind the rectus muscle. It then passes upwards on the middle and posterior part of the rectus muscle to the top of the abdomen, where it anastomoses with the internal mammary artery. In its course this artery sends lateral branches to the abdominal muscles. The spot at which the epigastric artery is concerned with hernia is at the beginning of its course, close to the inner and under side of the spermatic cord, where the latter issues from the abdomen through the upper opening which has been before described. Here the epigastric artery is generally three inches from the symphysis pubis, and the same distance from the spine of the ilium. _{Epigastric artery.}

CHAPTER III.

Of the Inguinal Hernia.

First appearance. THIS disease makes its first appearance in the form of a small tumour, situated about an inch and a half to the outer side of the abdominal ring, in a line extending from the pubis to the anterior superior spinous process of the ilium.

Direction. If its progress is uninterrupted, it proceeds gradually obliquely downwards and inwards in the direction of the spermatic cord as far as the abdominal ring.

Unsuspected. As long as it remains above the ring its existence is often not suspected by the patient, because it requires a careful examination to detect it; but to a surgeon acquainted with the natural feel and appearance of the parts it is sufficiently obvious. The length of the swelling above the ring will be found the same as the part of the spermatic cord included between the upper opening and the abdominal ring; that is, about an inch and a half in the adult subject.

Descent into the scrotum. The tumour next descends through the abdominal ring into the scrotum, (here taking the name of scrotal hernia), and being now less confined than before, it forms a distinct swelling, sufficient to awake the patient's attention, who now, generally for the first time, is led to require surgical assistance. As the growth of the tumour, when in the scrotum, is little restrained by external pressure, it increases to an almost unlimited, and

Size. sometimes enormous size. One of the largest of these swellings which I have ever seen was in a man who was sent to me to Guy's Hospital by Mr. White, surgeon at Lambeth. It reached to the patient's knees, its length was then twenty-two inches, and its circumference thirty-two. Another measurement taken by Mr. White when it had been for some hours strangulated, gave thirty-four inches for the circumference, and twenty-two for the length.

Dissection. When an inguinal hernia is dissected, immediately under the skin of the scrotum is found a fascia of greater

Fascia. or less thickness according to the duration and size of the tumour. This fascia is given off by the tendon of the external oblique muscle above the abdominal ring. In general it appears little more than a condensed cellular membrane, but I have seen it in old herniæ as dense as the fascia that covers the muscles on the outer part of the thigh.

Cremaster. Under this fascia is the cremaster muscle, which forms another covering to the hernial sac; for this muscle, in passing down through the abdominal ring, is united both to the fascia and to the sac, separable from both however by an easy dissection. This muscle becomes much more extended and thicker in hernia, than in the natural state.

Sac. When the fascia and the cremaster muscle are removed, the proper hernial sac becomes exposed to view. This is thinner than the two former coverings, but somewhat thicker than the peritoneum from which it is immediately derived. Many writers have represented the sac as much denser than it really is, mistaking the two above-mentioned coverings for the sac itself, (See Plate III.)

Spermatic cord. Behind the hernial sac lie the spermatic cord on the upper part, and the testicle on the lower; so that the sac is situated between the cord and the cremaster muscle, anterior to the former and posterior to the latter. The direction of the hernia above the abdominal ring is obliquely upwards and outwards towards the spine of

Situation of the sac above the ring. the ilium, the same as that of the spermatic cord. Above the ring, the hernial sac is covered by the tendon of the external oblique muscle; the spermatic cord is still behind it, and further backwards are the tendons of the internal oblique and transversalis muscles and the fascia before mentioned. At the upper aperture in the fascia the sac penetrates the abdomen along with the spermatic cord. This part is called its mouth, and is generally, though not always, its narrowest dimension. Between the mouth of the sac and the symphysis pubis passes the epigastric artery. This vessel runs in some degree under the sac and along its inner side. There is no vessel of importance above the mouth of the sac, nor externally, that is, between it and the spinous process of the ilium, (See Plates III. and IV.)

The relative situation of hernia with the abdominal openings above described, applies only whilst it remains of small size; for when hernia has existed a considerable length of time, and has carried with it a large portion of the abdominal viscera, the constant pressure dilates the parts in each direction, extending the opening through which it passes from the abdomen, both towards the spine of the ilium, and especially towards the symphysis pubis. Hence it is that in old and large herniæ the orifice of the sac into the abdomen is brought to be almost in contact with, and opposite to, the abdominal ring.

This difference will be distinctly seen in Plate IV, in which a hernia on each side is represented: in the right, a small hernia, where the mouth of the sac is at the greatest distance from the abdominal ring; in the left a large hernia, the mouth of which approaches very closely to the ring. This change by gradual enlargement, however, makes no alteration in the relative position of the epigastric artery, except in giving it a greater curve; for its course is still on the inner side of the mouth of the sac. *Gradual enlargement of its mouth.*

It has been stated that the hernial sac in its descent is anterior to the spermatic cord. This is its most frequent situation, but varieties occur in this respect which the surgeon should keep in mind during the operation. Thus the cord is sometimes found separated, and the hernial sac protruded between its vessels. This circumstance is represented in Plate V, taken from a preparation in my possession. The vas deferens is seen passing on one side of the sac, and the spermatic vessels on the other. In another case, which I shall afterwards describe, I met with the spermatic artery and vein passing before the sac and the vas deferens behind it. It has been stated, but this I cannot give from my own observation, that the whole of the cord is sometimes anterior to the sac. *Varieties in situation.*

The inguinal hernia is very generally pyriform, small towards the ring, and enlarging as it descends. It occurs much more frequently on the right than the left side. *Form of the hernia.*

The symptoms and circumstances whereby this disease may be distinguished from other tumours with which it is liable to be confounded, are the following: *Distinguishing symptoms.*

First, When the patient is desired to cough, the tumour becomes immediately distended, owing to the pressure of the abdominal muscles forcing down into the sac more of the viscera or their contents.

Secondly, When the patient can state from his remembrance, that on the first appearance of the tumour in the groin, it had used to return into the abdomen when he was in a horizontal posture, and to reappear on standing erect; though circumstances may have long prevented this symptom from continuing.

Thirdly, When the progress of the tumour has been from the groin gradually downwards to the scrotum.

Fourthly, When the tumour contains intestine it is elastic and uniform to the touch; and on being pushed up into the abdomen, it returns with a *guggling* noise. But when omentum is contained, the tumour is less equal on its surface, receives an impression from the fingers, is heavier than in the former case, and does not make the same noise when returned into the abdomen. Most commonly, however, both intestine and omentum are the contents of the hernia, a circumstance which impairs the accuracy of any very nice distinctions by the touch; though still on pushing back the contents of the tumour, the presence of intestine, which returns the first, will often be indicated by the guggling noise, whilst the more solid omentum may be felt going up after it.

Lastly, The functions of the viscera are somewhat interrupted. Eructations, sickness, constipation, colicky pains, and distention of the abdomen occur; and pain is produced by violent exertions, coughing, or sneezing. These are the symptoms that generally give the patient some suspicion of the nature of the complaint.

However there are several diseases of the groin and scrotum with which hernia is liable to be confounded; so that there are few surgeons who have seen much of hernia who have not frequently witnessed mistakes, made even by medical practitioners, which have led to the application of trusses in diseases where they not only are useless, but even productive of much injury. The reputation of the surgeon, and the safety of his patient, require of him a very accurate attention to this point. *Diseases with which it is liable to be confounded.*

A hydrocele of the tunica vaginalis testis resembles hernia in its form, but may be distinguished from it by the following marks. *Hydrocele.*

The hydrocele begins to form at the lower part of the scrotum, and gradually extends towards the ring. It also involves the spermatic cord and testis, so as to render them with difficulty distinguished by the touch; whilst in hernia they may, in general, be felt with ease behind the tumour. Hydrocele gives a fluctuating feel

F

when struck with the fingers, does not become dilated when the patient coughs, and appears considerably transparent when a lighted candle is held by its side.

I have seen cases of hydrocele, however, in which there was unusual difficulty in deciding upon the nature of the complaint. When it becomes so large as to extend upwards through the abdominal ring to the abdomen, the form of the tumour is precisely the same as that of hernia, and it even dilates when the patient coughs, owing to the sudden pressure upon that part of it which lies above the ring. The transparency, the fluctuating feel, and the observed progress of the swelling from below upwards are then the only distinguishing marks.

A tumour sometimes appears in the scrotum which descends in the erect posture, returns when the body is recumbent, distends upon coughing, fluctuates, and is transparent. This disease is a collection of water which runs backwards and forwards from the cavity of the abdomen within the tunica vaginalis, owing to the opening of this membranous sheath never having been closed. When this disease is complicated with ascites it becomes distended to an enormous size. It is readily distinguished from hernia by its transparency, which may always be observed.

Cyst upon the cord. Water sometimes collects in a cyst upon the spermatic cord, forming a hydrocele of the cord. When it is placed entirely below the ring, its want of connexion with the abdomen readily distinguishes it from hernia; but when it passes within the ring to the abdomen some difficulty occurs in understanding its nature. If from its situation the transparency cannot be examined, and if the fluctuation is not very distinct, a surgeon should be very cautious in operating on such a tumour.

The following case occurred to me. I was desired to see a boy, a patient of Mr. Clarke, surgeon in the Borough, who had a tumour which extended from the upper part of the scrotum through the abdominal ring along the cord to the abdomen. The lad's father was anxious for the removal of the disease, but on examination it did not project sufficiently to enable me to judge whether there was either fluctuation or transparency. However as it interfered with the boy's usual occupation, I resolved to cut down upon it with extreme caution. When I had reached by incision the surface of the cyst, I found the spermatic vessels running upon it, and was obliged to open the cyst by its side to avoid these vessels. The cyst contained a portion of the small intestine, every where adhering to its inner surface, which had prevented the return of the bowel into the abdomen. The vas deferens could be discerned behind the sac, so that this was a hernia, the sac of which had insinuated itself between the spermatic blood vessels and the vas deferens.

Enlarged testis. Nothing but great want of attention can cause a hernia to be confounded with an enlargement of the testis. This latter is sufficiently distinguishable by the form of the organ, which is retained under morbid enlargement, by its weight, by the pain with which it is generally accompanied, and by that peculiar and intolerable sensation always produced by pressure upon this part.

Hematocele. Hematocele, or a collection of blood in the tunica vaginalis testis, as it generally arises from a blow, is of the same form with hernia, and liable to be confounded with it. But the firmness of hematocele, the redness of the skin with which it is accompanied, its refusing to dilate under coughing, and a freedom from swelling of the spermatic cord at the abdominal ring, which is generally the case, will usually afford the means of distinction from hernia.

Varicocele. But of all the diseases of the scrotum, which are ever mistaken for hernia, none is so much so as the Varicocele or enlargement of the spermatic veins. Often have I known persons (even the children of medical men) to wear trusses for a supposed hernia, which they complained did not fit, gave them pain, and could not prevent the descent of the tumour, when it was found that the disease was this enlargement of the spermatic veins.

Varicocele has indeed many of the marks of hernia. When large, it dilates upon coughing, but not otherwise; it appears in the erect position and retires when the body is recumbent; and it is first observed near the ring. The only sure method of distinction with which I am acquainted is this: place the patient in the horizontal posture, and empty the swelling by pressure upon the scrotum, then putting the fingers firmly upon the upper part of the abdominal ring, desire the patient to rise: if it is a hernia, the tumour cannot reappear as long as the pressure is continued at the ring; but if a varicocele, the swelling returns with increased size owing to the return of blood into the abdomen being prevented by the pressure.

Some judgment may also be formed by the feel of the tumour, for that of varicocele is always ropy as if a bundle of cords were contained within the scrotum.

There are however some cases of a complicated nature which demand much judgment and accurate discrimination. For instance, hernia is sometimes complicated with hydrocele of the tunica vaginalis; and sometimes the sac contains omentum, adhering to its upper part, and a collection of water below. If the adhesion of the omentum is complete, there is no danger of attempting the cure of the hydrocele by injection; however, if the case clearly appears to be of this kind before operation, it is best to use the method of incision.

Sometimes the case is still more complicated. A man of the name of Freeman, now a patient in Guy's Hospital, has a diseased testis and hydrocele on each side, the latter of which is open to the abdomen; together with a large hernia on the left side and a smaller one on the right.

Complicated cases.

CHAPTER IV.

Of the Causes of Hernia.

All the causes of hernia usually alledged may be resolved into two kinds: those which diminish the resistance of the abdominal muscles, and those which increase the pressure of the viscera.

The principal predisposing cause of this disease is weakness, in whatever way produced; for weakness occasions relaxation, which allows of the dilatation of the orifice through which the spermatic vessels naturally pass, and consequently opens a passage for the protrusion of the abdominal viscera. The same cause also operates in elongating the attachments of the viscera, rendering them thereby more extensively mobile, and consequently more easily liable to be displaced from their natural situation.

If a person debilitated by fever returns to a habit of violent exertion before his strength is fully re-established, a swelling of the groin will often occur, which proves to be a hernia.

Old age also, from the general relaxation which it produces, is very frequently accompanied with this disease, so much, that I have been surprised to find but few old men entirely exempt from it. Since I have had this publication in view I have neglected no opportunity of procuring specimens of this disease, and on inspecting the bodies of old people I have scarcely ever been disappointed in finding either inguinal or femoral hernia. The subjects which I have examined, however, have principally been old persons who have been obliged to labour for their subsistence after their strength became unequal to great exertions.

Those who work hard, and live more on fluid than solid food, are also very subject to hernia; whence its frequency among the poor of this town, who work to the utmost of their strength, and subsist very much upon liquids.

Heat of climate and seasons, warmth of cloathing during the day, and warm covering at night, must also be reckoned as predisposing causes of this disease. Herniæ, though frequent in England, are much less common here than in the south of Europe, or in Africa. A gentleman thus writes from Malta, " This is the place where " hernia should be studied; for, from the extreme relaxing heat of the climate, assisted by the constant exertions " which the inhabitants are obliged to make in passing their rocky paths, few persons escape the disease, and " it is often of an enormous size."

In Egypt too we have the testimony of medical men who attended the late expedition, that herniæ are extremely common there, and often of an unwieldy bulk. Of this, Sir Robert Wilson mentions the following instance. " I saw a man who had a belly hanging down from his navel to his ancles, a blue skin contained his " bowels, but which seemed so thin, as to be liable every moment to burst. The weight was enormous, and " the size appeared much larger than an ox's paunch. The unfortunate wretch was otherwise in good health, " and crawled about gaining his bread by begging."

There are also other causes which diminish the resistance of the muscles and their tendons. Thus a person naturally fat, who has become suddenly lean, is in consequence generally the subject of hernia; for, the fat which had loaded the spermatic cord, and had extended the apertures to and from the abdomen, being suddenly absorbed, room is left for the viscera to supply its place. In some respect it appears to depend on hereditary conformation. I have frequently been consulted by fathers, themselves wearing trusses, for more than one of their sons afflicted with the same complaint. In such cases as these, I have found by attentive examination the abdominal ring very imperfectly formed; so that instead of the ring extending an inch and a half in length, it could be traced nearly half way to the ilium. Hence it would seem, that in these persons the tendon which shuts in the superior margin of the ring, either does not exist at all, or is at least very imperfect; for whoever is in the habit of dissecting the abdominal ring will often find it varying both in extent and in the firmness with which it is closed, being in some subjects carefully shut by the transverse tendon from the ilium, and in others this tendon is very small, or even entirely wanting.

In such persons the slightest cause is sufficient to produce hernia, on account of the diminished resistance to protrusion of the intestine at the aperture of the abdomen through which such protrusion generally passes.

Hernia is often suddenly produced by blows. A gentleman consulted me concerning a tumour which had appeared in his groin after he had been thrown from his horse in hunting. He fell upon the post of a gate which struck against his groin, and he immediately felt great pain, and found a swelling in the part, which proved to be a hernia. Blows.

A young gentleman from America, who had a hernia, told me that it appeared immediately after having received a kick from his schoolmaster.

Neither of these, however, was common inguinal hernia, but a variety that will be hereafter described, produced, I believe, by a laceration of the tendon of the internal oblique and transversalis muscles.

Violent actions of the abdominal muscles, by the pressure which they exert upon the viscera, become frequent causes of hernia. It is in this way that coughing produces this disease. Few persons who have long been asthmatical are free from it, and those who play upon wind instruments are more subject to it than others. Coughing.

But of all the causes of hernia the most frequent is lifting heavy weights, an action which strongly exerts the abdominal muscles at the time that the body is bent. In this position the lower part of the abdomen is not contracted to the same degree as the upper, the viscera are forced downwards by inspiration, and compressed by the abdominal muscles above, whilst the openings of the groin are relaxed by the posture of the body. I am informed that few persons are more subject to hernia than the men who work in our dockyards: the great weights which they are in the habit of lifting, and the stooping positions in which they often work, will, I think, sufficiently account for this circumstance. Lifting weights.

Persons who suffer under habitual costiveness, are not only subject to hernia, but have the symptoms of strangulation often brought on whilst at stool, owing to the strong pressure made on the abdominal muscles during the difficult expulsion of fæces. Hence the practical caution of persons subject to hernia to avoid every cause of constipation. Costiveness.

Strictures in the urethra appear often to produce this disease, for the difficulty in passing urine must necessarily occasion strong action of the abdominal muscles. In the body of a man who had a stone in the urethra, which I opened with Mr. Weston, Surgeon in Shoreditch, we found several hernial sacs. Difficulties in voiding the urine.

There are causes of this disease that principally affect the viscera, and in which the abdominal muscles may be said to be nearly passive. Thus the viscera become too large for the cavity of the belly in an extreme degree of obesity, which loads the omentum and mesentery with fat, and they are compelled to protrude through any opening that presents itself. If the fatness comes on very rapidly, it seldom fails to produce this disease, as the abdominal muscles cannot immediately accommodate themselves to the enlargement of the belly. Obesity.

The same effect is produced by constant external pressure which tends to diminish the cavity of the abdomen, the size of its contents remaining the same. It is thus that hernia is brought on by wearing the breeches very tight about the waist, which pinch up the belly, and do not leave sufficient room for the variations that occur in the size of the viscera after taking food, or from exertions of different kinds. External pressure.

The enlargement of the uterus in pregnancy sometimes occasions hernia, but less frequently the inguinal, than the other species. Distention of the stomach operates in a similar manner. A frequent and forcible pressure or shaking of the viscera downwards, as happens in riding in rough carriages, is a common cause of this complaint. In the town of Yarmouth, where I formerly lived, I knew many persons among my friends who had this disease brought on by riding in the small carts peculiar to this town, and which from being constructed without springs were rough and uneasy, and shook the rider in a very severe manner. Coachmen who are much upon the box, and persons who ride rough-going horses, are for the same reason liable to this complaint. The cavalry are much more subject to it than the infantry, and I have known children in which it has been produced by frequent riding in company with older persons, and constantly going a pace uneasy to them. Pregnancy.
Rough Horses or Carriages.

Jumping operates in the same way, often suddenly. I have known many persons, after much of this exercise, complain of a pain in the groin, which was soon followed by hernia. In these, and every other cause of the complaint, an upright posture of the body strongly contributes to its formation by keeping up the pressure of the viscera on the lower part of the abdomen. Jumping.

CHAPTER V.

Of the reducible Inguinal Hernia, and Use of Trusses.

Reducible.

HERNIÆ are found in the three following conditions: reducible; irreducible; and strangulated.

The reducible is that state in which the protruded parts may be returned into the cavity of the abdomen. This generally happens in the night during sleep, and the tumour returns in the morning on changing to the erect posture. Sometimes the reduction of the tumour is attended with difficulty, and requires the assistance of pressure. A person under these circumstances lives in a constant state of danger. Any accidental fall, violent effort, or slight inattention to the state of the bowels, may produce a strangulation of the prolapsed intestine, the consequence of which will be fatal, unless early and well-directed skill be employed.

To prevent this accident a constant pressure should be applied at the part where the hernia opens into the abdomen, to shut the mouth of the sac, and thus oppose an effectual resistance to the protrusion of its contents.

Truss.

For this purpose bandages of different kinds, and elastic trusses, have been invented, but the only instrument that can be safely relied on is a truss of steel; all other bandages affording only a false security, more dangerous even than a total omission of this kind of support, since they encourage the patient to take violent exercise without apprehension of the probable consequences. An elastic steel truss, if properly made and well applied, ensures the security of the patient during any degree of moderate exercise, and is no hindrance to any of the common occupations of life.

Its construction.

A steel truss is composed of a pad made of a supporting piece of iron, and stuffed so as to take a conical form, the apex of which immediately compresses the abdomen at the part whence the hernia threatens to descend.

The pad is rivetted upon a long flat piece of steel, tempered to a great degree of elasticity, and curved to the shape of the lower part of the body, which it embraces like a belt. The length of this steel should be sufficient to pass from the hernia round the region of the groin to about an inch beyond the spine behind, forming somewhat more than a semicircle, but compressed. Both the pad and truss are quilted with leather. A strap of leather proceeds from the hinder end of the truss, which passes round the body, completing the circular belt by fastening upon the pad.

An under strap is added to the truss, which passes down between the patient's thighs behind, and is brought round in front, to the opposite side of the truss, to prevent its slipping when applied. However if the pelvis is well formed, that is, standing outwards, or the abdomen is large, this under strap is not necessary, and is generally discontinued, but when the pelvis inclines towards the abdomen, the truss will slip from its proper position, unless retained by this strap.

Many surgeons, and almost every surgeon's instrument-maker, have thought proper to vary the form of the truss, and to prescribe different rules for the duration and force of the pressure, but almost all have agreed in determining that the pressure should be made upon the abdominal ring.

Its application.

This is precisely the circumstance, however, in which they are all defective; and indeed it is the frequent failure of the purpose for which they are designed, when made according to this principle, that has led to such a variety in the mode of their construction. The object in applying a truss is to close the mouth of the hernial sac, and destroy its communication with the abdomen; and this object can never be perfectly fulfilled by any truss which is applied in the usual manner upon the abdominal ring, and extending from it upon the os pubis. In this case the cure must be incomplete, because a considerable portion of the hernial sac remains uncompressed towards the abdomen, which portion is that situated between the abdominal

Sac imperfectly closed.

ring and the opening of the sac into the cavity of the belly. In Plate 5th will be seen a hernial sac closed opposite to the abdominal ring, but still open to the abdomen above and outwards. In the same plate, is another sac imperfectly closed from the same cause. This sac has several partitions in it dividing it into cells, the formation of which is to be explained in the following manner: The patient first applies his truss to the abdominal ring, which, after being worn for a time, shuts or contracts the sac at this part, and the patient thinking himself cured, leaves off the bandage. The sac, however, is still open higher up towards the abdomen, though closed at the ring, the hernia again protrudes, and the truss is resumed, but being still applied upon the ring, only a partial cure is a second time produced, and the cause of the disease remains as before. Nor is this all the mischief that attends this practice, for the pressure of the spermatic cord by the truss against the os pubis, frequently occasions great pain, to relieve which the patient is constantly shifting its situation, and destroying its effect, and often the testes themselves become wasted by the interruption of the passage of the blood along the spermatic vessels. Septa in the sac.

The proper method of completely obliterating the mouth of the hernial sac is to apply the truss, not upon the abdominal ring, but upon the part at which the spermatic cord, and with it the hernia, first quit the abdomen; for in this way only can a descent of the hernia be prevented entirely, and a cure by pressure, if practicable, can be performed.

The effect of wearing a truss at this part is to bring the sides of the mouth of the sac together, to prevent its being opened by the insinuation of the viscera, and after, gradually contracting it, to cause an adhesion between its sides, and at last, if the pressure is continued long enough, to obliterate the sac, and prevent the hazard of a future descent in the same cavity. Effect of the truss.

In Plate 6th is shewn the mode of applying the truss so as to ensure the most favourable effect, the pressure being here exerted just opposite to the aperture into the abdomen. Therefore, when a hernia has been returned by the surgeon into the abdomen, he should lay his fingers obliquely above and without the ring, and direct his patient to cough; and the furthest part from the ring towards the spine of the ilium, where the hernial sac is felt to protrude, is the point which should be noted for the application of the pad of the truss, and the instrument made accordingly. Measurement is taken for making the truss by laying one end of a piece of string upon this spot, and carrying the other round the pelvis, midway between the trochanter major and spine of the ilium, till it meets the fixed point at first determined, and completes the circle. This is the proper length for the truss. In the above manner I have been in the habit of measuring persons for trusses, excepting when the hips have projected unusually, when it is advisable to substitute for the string a piece of iron wire, which, by retaining the precise outline of the patient's hip, serves as a necessary direction for the instrument-maker to copy. Mode of measuring for the truss.

It will be found that the pad of the truss must be applied proportionally nearer to the abdominal ring in large than in small hernias. Where the protrusion is small, the pad may be fixed midway between the symphysis pubis and the spine of the ilium; but as the dimensions of the hernia increase, the mouth of the sac moves gradually nearer the abdominal ring, and the artificial pressure must, in some degree, be regulated accordingly; always remembering, however, that the truss should never be brought upon the pubis, as a pressure on the outer and upper part of the ring will still be sufficient to keep the viscera within the abdomen. Different application in large hernia.

It happens not unfrequently that hernia appears on both sides of the body. When this takes place a double truss, or one with two pads and springs must be worn, made of materials similar to the single truss. To make them sit easy, and fit properly, they should buckle behind, and be made longer or shorter at pleasure. This is done by constructing them in such a manner that one spring will readily slide upon the other. The principle of application, and the degree of pressure required, are to be regulated as the single trusses. Double truss.

As it is often an object of importance for the patient to use the bath whilst wearing a truss, I have directed the spring to be covered with oil-skin to prevent its wetting, for the patient should on no account remove it at the time he is making such a considerable exertion as that of swimming.

A truss when first applied produces some uncomfortable feelings for about a week, after which they wear off, unless the force of pressure is unnecessarily great, in which case the spring must be weakened. On the contrary, if the hernia ever comes down whilst the truss is duly applied, a stronger spring must be provided. The best made truss will chafe at first, however well put on, but this inconvenience of a few days is a good deal prevented by interposing a piece of linen between the pad and the skin, which generally puts a stop to the uneasy chafing. Truss occasions uneasiness at first.

It is usual for the patient to enquire how long his truss must be worn. This is difficult to be determined. I have known a hernia completely cured by wearing a truss only nine months, and instances are not at all uncommon, of the truss being left off at the end of a year without any relapse of the complaint. But I would at all events advise it to be worn at least two years even by young persons, in whom alone the complaint is curable by this method. As to elderly persons, they must continue to wear it for the remainder of life, for in Time it should be worn.

Worn at night.

them there is no probability of much change taking place in the mouth of the sac. I have never known them long omit its use without experiencing some relapse: during growth, parts will readily accommodate to pressure, extending or diminishing according to circumstances, but in adults, and in the old, this process is much more tardy. The truss should be worn even during the night lest any unexpected occasion should call the patient from bed unprepared for the sudden change of posture; for if the hernia descends a single time during the wearing of the truss, the cure must be considered as recommencing from that moment.

Another sac forms.

There is one circumstance which will always render a prudent surgeon guarded in promising a complete cure of hernia from wearing a truss: it is that although the original sac may be completely shut at its mouth by adhesion or perfect contraction, it is possible that another sac may be formed contiguous to the first. An instance of this may be seen in Plate 5th. In this case two hernial sacs are found side by side, one open and capable of containing the bowels when protruded, the other contracted so much as not to admit of a goose's quill. In the latter therefore the disease was cured, but remained in the former. A similar instance of a second descent is seen in Plate 9th, and another example of the same kind will be mentioned hereafter.

Hydrocele of the sac.

When a hernia has been cured by adhesion, as the peritoneum which forms the sac is a secreting membrane, an accumulation of water sometimes collects in it, forming a species of hydrocele, an instance of which is represented in Plate 5th. The treatment of this disease should be similar to that of hydrocele from other causes.

During the application of a truss it is proper that every part of the protruded contents should be carefully returned, so that no compression be made on them; and if the patient should find that any part has again descended, he should place himself in a recumbent posture, take off the truss, push back the hernia with his hand, and again apply the truss. A person obliged to use a truss who allows of the descent of a portion of the hernia whilst this instrument is worn, is in greater danger of strangulation of the part than if he wore no truss at all. For, when unprotected by this bandage, he always feels his danger, and is ready to guard against it, but a bad truss gives the idea of security without ensuring its reality.

CHAPTER VI.

Of the irreducible Hernia.

When a hernia is incapable of being returned into the abdomen by outward pressure, it is termed irreducible. Irreducible.
The following are the causes to bring the disease into this state. Causes.

First, When the protruded parts are suffered to remain long down they increase so much in size as to be incapable of reduction.

Secondly, When membranous bands form across the sac, and thus entangle its contents, preventing their free motion.

Thirdly, When the protruded parts become closely united by an adhesion to the sides of the sac, sufficiently firm to render them immoveable.

In whichever of these ways a hernia becomes irreducible, the patient is thereby made subject to many inconveniencies and dangers. The principal danger is of strangulation of the protruded parts; however this is Dangers. certainly less in the irreducible hernia, than in one that descends only occasionally; for in the former, the sac is already nearly full, and cannot readily admit of any great increase of its contents. But the patient is liable to danger from other causes, as will be seen by the following case.

A man was brought into St. Thomas's Hospital who had fallen from a ladder, and his scrotum, in which was a large hernia, struck upon the edge of a piece of wood. After complaining of violent pain and tension in his abdomen, in four hours he died. On examining his body after death, a portion of the ilium which had formed a part of the hernia, was found ruptured.

Mr. Norris, surgeon in the Old Jewry, also shewed me a preparation of hernia and ruptured intestine, which he had taken from a man of whom he gave me the following account.

" Whilst running, and suddenly turning the corner of a street, he struck violently against a post. The
" middle of the abdomen was the part that received the shock, from the effects of which he soon appeared
" to have recovered, but on proceeding a little way he felt great pain in the belly, and became very
" faint, which obliged him to sit down on the steps of a door. In about ten minutes he was just enough
" recovered to be able to crawl to his home, which was about two hundred yards off. I saw him on the following
" morning. There was not the slightest appearance of injury on the part that had received the stroke, but on
" the course of the spermatic process on the left side extending into the abdomen, there was a fulness and
" enlargement equal to a moderate sized hernia. He vomited frequently, his pulse was quick and extremely
" feeble, his countenance was pale, and expressive of the greatest anxiety, and he complained of acute pain all
" over his belly. The abdomen, however, was quite soft, and the contents of the tumour were easily returned
" into its cavity, but quickly came down again when the pressure was removed. These symptoms continued
" with the most torturing pain till the evening, when he expired. Having obtained leave to open the body,
" Dr. Yelloly and myself met the day after his death for that purpose. The tumour was now larger than before,
" discoloured, and contained air, discoverable to the touch. The contents of the tumour were found, on opening
" it, to be air, blood, and water. On examining the abdomen a similar fluid, to the quantity of a quart, was
" found effused. An irregular aperture was perceived in the ilium, which readily admitted my finger, and
" through which every thing that had descended into the stomach found a ready passage into the cavity of the
" belly. No other injury of any kind to any of the contents of the abdomen could be detected."

Another danger incurred by irreducible hernia is that of ulceration. This may happen when any pointed body is swallowed, and follows the course of the food down the intestinal canal into the hernial sac; when arrived in this place, it has been known to make its way out by ulceration, leaving a passage for the fæces.

A boy, aged thirteen, was admitted into St. Thomas's Hospital for an irreducible scrotal hernia, from which a quantity of fœculent matter was constantly discharging through a small hole in the scrotum. He remembered having accidentally swallowed a pin, and five weeks afterwards his hernia began to swell, and to become very painful. A poultice was applied, and an abscess formed, which soon after burst, and on looking at the orifice by which the matter had discharged, the point of a pin appeared projecting from it, which was easily extracted. A fistulous opening of the intestine remained, for which he was admitted into the hospital. Attempts were made to unite it by paring off the edges of the wound and encouraging adhesion, but without success.

Enormous size.

An irreducible hernia sometimes becomes of a most enormous size when it has remained entirely unconfined, and it then produces various other inconveniencies, of which the case of Mr. Gibbon, the celebrated historian, will furnish a striking example.

Mr. Gibbon had been for thirty years subject to a scrotal hernia on the left side, of which he made no complaint, and to which he applied no remedy to prevent its increase. But in the summer of 1793, finding it grow suddenly uneasy he became alarmed, and consulted Sir Walter Farquhar and Mr. Cline. The tumour was then of uncommon size, reaching to his knees, and very large at its connexion with the abdomen. As some water was perceptible at the lower part of the tumour, it was tapped in the month of November 1793, and a large quantity of water was drawn off. In a fortnight after it was again tapped, and three quarts of water were evacuated without any very sensible diminution of the swelling. Six weeks afterwards, the skin over the tumour having inflamed, and shewn a disposition to ulcerate, the tapping was again repeated, Jan. 13, 1794, when six quarts of water were discharged. Two evenings afterwards he began to complain of a pain in his stomach and soreness in the abdomen, and in the tumour on pressure. He passed the night restlessly, but the next morning when he rose he seemed in better health and spirits than usual. Soon after he became insensible, and expired about eleven o'clock.

Mr. Cline asked me to accompany him to inspect the body. We found the abdomen nearly emptied of all the moveable viscera, no omentum remaining within its cavity, and of the intestines only the duodenum and cœcum. Even the pylorus was drawn down so low as to lie upon the orifice of the hernial sac, into which all the omentum, and all the intestines, except those I have just mentioned, had descended. They were all uncommonly loaded with fat, and slightly inflamed. The hernial sac extended nearly as low as the knee, its orifice was so large as to admit my hand within it. Below the sac appeared a separate bag large enough to hold several quarts of water, which, by its containing the testicle, proved to be the tunica vaginalis testis.

Consequences such as these result from a neglect of proper bandages in hernia. A tumour of such magnitude as that above described, requires to be concealed by a particular dress. The penis is deeply sunken into it, so that the urine can only be carried off by trickling over the surface of the scrotum, which must keep it constantly excoriated.

Scrotum diseased.

Besides these inconveniences, a very large hernia produces a disease of the scrotum itself; an abscess is formed, which is kept fistulous by the constant distension of parts, and can hardly ever be healed without confining the patient to his bed.

Cure by fasting.

When the contents of hernia have become so large and incumbered with fat as to render the disease at that time irreducible, it has been recommended previous to any attempt at reduction, to make the patient undergo a course of extraordinary fasting, accompanied with cathartic medicines, and every means used to keep up a free perspiration. It is scarcely to be doubted that such a plan would, after a considerable time, be attended with ultimate success; but I have never met with any one who would submit to so severe a regimen, to free himself from a disease, which only gives a present inconvenience, and does not alarm the patient for the future event.

Laced bag truss.

A more easy and equally effectual remedy is to apply a bag truss to support the scrotum, and made to lace before. In this way a considerable pressure is steadily preserved upon the parts, which occasions a gradual absorption of the adipose matter of the protruded hernia; and thus after some days confinement, the tumour becomes very much diminished, and at last may be returned.

Cold.

In some cases the application of ice also occasionally procures the return of the hernia which appeared irreducible.

I was asked by a physician to examine a hernia which had come down about a fortnight before, and had ever since resisted all attempts at reduction, without being painful. I found it was an omental hernia, and I ordered ice to be kept upon the tumour for a considerable time. In twenty-four hours it was so much diminished, as to encourage a perseverance in the plan, and in four days the hernia was entirely removed.

Mr. G. a surgeon in the East India service, called on me to shew me an omental hernia on the right side, which, though not painful, gave him some anxiety, as it could not be returned, and he was apprehensive of its becoming strangulated at some future time: I ordered him to bed, and put him on the same plan as in the former case, which produced a very gradual diminution of the tumour, and at the end of five days its entire removal. It appeared to me, in both these cases, that the good effects attending the use of the ice, was owing to a consequent contraction of the scrotum, which thus performed the office of a strong and permanent compression on the tumour.

Hernia sometimes becomes irreducible, as I have before stated, from the formation of membranous bands across the sac, which entangle the protruded parts. They are seen in Plate 5th, but in the preparation the viscera, are in part removed to afford a good view of these bands. Irreducible from membranous bands.

They appear to be produced in the following manner: during the reducible state of the hernia inflammation takes place both in the contained parts, and in the inner surface of the sac, but by using proper means, the protruded parts are reduced, and the sides of the sac collapse and adhere together. However, while the adhesions are still in a glutinous state, a fresh descent takes place from the abdomen, and the hernial contents again disunite the surfaces of the sac every where, except at the points of union of these inflamed parts, the cementing lymph of which, instead of bursting asunder, elongates with the fresh pressure, and forms these membranous bands which are seen passing from one side of the sac to the other. Between these the intestine and omentum get entangled, a circumstance which adds so much to the difficulty of reduction, as to make it, in general, considered as impracticable; but unless the hernial contents themselves adhere, there appears no reason why the means already pointed out may not here also prove successful. After all there is scarcely a possibility of detecting by the feel this variety of the disease in the living subject.

They also become irreducible, though rarely, from a contraction in the sac, which I have seen take place in its middle so as to produce an hour-glass appearance, and a portion of omentum has been confined below and above the contracted part. Contraction of the sac.

Herniæ are irreducible from adhesion having taken place between the contents of the tumour and the sides of the sac, they are sometimes universal, but more commonly partial; they exist most frequently at the lower part of the sac, but sometimes at its mouth only, and must remain unreturned for the rest of life, unless it be expedient or necessary to undertake an operation. The cases in which such an operation may be proper and necessary will be mentioned in a future place. All that can be done in an irreducible intestinal rupture is, to apply a bag truss of the size of the tumour, which, by affording a constant pressure, will check the increase of the disease. But if the hernia be omental only, its increase and the subsequent descent of the intestine may safely be prevented by a spring truss. There is so much difficulty, however, in these instances in the living subject, in determining the precise nature of the hernia, and deciding whether or not some small convolution of intestine may be descended, that the spring truss should only be fixed after the most careful examination, the spring itself weak, and it should be entirely thrown aside if it produces any pain or interrupts the functions of the bowels. From adhesion.

In old irreducible hernia the omentum often becomes diseased. I have seen it affected with schirrus, that is, not the schirrus which terminates in cancer, but forming a large and very firm tumour. A specimen of this form of the disease is preserved at the Museum of St. Thomas's Hospital. Hydatids have been known to be produced in it; but I have never seen an instance of it. Schirrous omentum.

When suppuration occurs, it produces an external abscess. An instance of this happened last year in a woman, who had an abscess in the omentum which had arisen from an old irreducible omental hernia.

CHAPTER VII.

Of the strangulated Hernia.

Symptoms.

This form of the disease consists, not only of an irreducible state of the intestine and omentum, but of such a compression of the blood-vessels as to excite inflammation, and totally to interrupt the passage of the fæces through the strangulated portion. Its symptoms are, considerable pain in the tumour, and a sensation as if a cord were tied tight around the upper part of the abdomen, or sometimes only round the navel. To these succeed frequent eructations and vomiting; first, of the contents of the stomach, and presently, as an antiperistaltic motion is established through the intestine, bilious matter is brought up. Indeed, when the strangulation has happened in the colon, I am certain that I have seen portions of feculent matter discharged by vomiting, a circumstance which is accounted for, when it is considered that the valve at the end of the ilium is often imperfect, and especially that an antiperistaltic motion will reverse the operation of this valve, as well as of the rest of the intestinal canal. I have seen this symptom so often, that I can entertain no doubt on the subject.

An obstinate constipation attends the vomiting, so that no stools can be obtained, except from the portion of intestine below the strangulation, by means of glysters. The pulse is quick, and at the beginning of the complaint, hard. If effectual relief be not obtained, the tumour becomes red and painful, and when handled, the mark of each finger is left in a white hollow impression, the same as occurs on pressure of a dropsical limb. This indicates an effusion of fluid into the cellular membrane covering the hernial sac, produced by the continuance of the inflammation. The abdomen now becomes slightly tense and sore upon pressure, the vomiting very frequent, and the whole body is bedewed with sweat. The constipation remains obstinate, and instead of eructation, hiccough comes on, whilst the countenance sinks and shews great anxiety, and the pulse now becomes extremely small and thready, so as to lead those unaccustomed to the disease to think the patient dying. These symptoms, however, are subject to exacerbations; they are for a time very violent and described by the patient as spasmodic, after which the patient becomes comparatively easy, so that the surgeon is flattered with hopes that the means he has employed have been successful, till the symptoms again return with more than their former severity.

After having suffered most intolerable pain throughout the first stage of the complaint, the patient becomes suddenly easy, and expresses great satisfaction at this change. The tumour, which still continues, generally assumes a purple or leaden colour, and gives a crackling feel, owing to air being contained in the cellular membrane. The abdomen becomes more tense, the hiccough more violent, a cold sweat covers the body, and the pulse, though now fuller and softer than before, if attended to for a little time is found to be intermittent, but still the patient remains perfectly sensible, full of hopes, and generally continues so till death, which now speedily puts an end to the complaint. So remarkably strong is this delusive feeling of amendment, that I have known a patient at this extremity insist upon rising, and expire in the very act; and another who sat up in bed, called for something to drink, and died as he was putting it to his lips.

Dissection.

If the tumour be examined after death, a quantity of clear serum will first be found under the skin. The hernial sac contains a portion of bloody serum of a coffee colour. The intestine is of a chocolate brown, with here and there a black spot, which easily breaks down on being touched with the finger. A coat of coagulable lymph, of the same colour as the intestine, may be peeled from its surface, and adhesions of no great strength are found to extend from the intestine to the sac. At the particular part where the intestine is strangulated by the constricting membrane, it is either ulcerated through, or readily pulls asunder under slight pressure. If the inflammation has been very extensive there is a quantity of air in the surrounding cellular membrane.

Inflammation different to most others.

The inflammation which takes place in strangulated hernia is different from almost every other species: in most cases it is produced by an unusual quantity of blood sent by the arteries of the part which become enlarged; but still the blood returns freely to the heart, and the colour of the inflamed part is that of arterial blood: whilst in hernia, the inflammation is caused by a stop being put to the return of the blood through the veins, which produces a great accumulation of this fluid, and a change of its colour from the arterial to the venous hue.

This will be seen in Plate VI. Fig. 2. which exhibits the true colour of strangulated intestine, as taken from the body; and this ought to be perfectly understood, that it may not be mistaken for mortification, which last shews itself in separate black spots dispersed over the inflamed bowel.

On dissection the cavity of the abdomen is found inflamed, red lines are to be traced in the course of the intestines, and at these parts they are slightly glued together by effused coagulable lymph. No general effusion takes place within the belly, but the tension of this cavity seems to arise principally from a great secretion of air within the intestinal canal. *Appearance of the abdomen.*

In strangulated omental hernia the symptoms are much less violent than in the intestinal species. The vomiting is not so frequent, the pain in the tumour but inconsiderable, the tension not so great over the abdomen, and the constipation is by no means so complete; for stools can, in general, be procured through the whole duration of the disease, both by glysters and by cathartics. The hiccoughs are less violent and less constant; and the pulse, though small and frequent, is not so remarkably small and thready as in the intestinal hernia. Likewise the patient survives the fatal event a much longer time, sometimes as many as fourteen days. In this species, inflammation occasionally takes place on the skin, though more rarely than in intestinal hernia; and when an extensive slough is thrown off, it is attended with much less constitutional irritation. *Omental hernia.*

On examination after death from strangulated omental hernia, the omentum is found scarcely changed from its natural appearance, its colour is a little, and but little, darker than usual. I have found it in some cases, even during the operation, extremely offensive to the smell. There is scarcely any fluid in the sac. Though the cavity of the abdomen is inflamed, and the intestines slightly adhering to each other, they never appear to have suffered so much as by intestinal hernia.

On examining the seat of the strangulation in inguinal hernia, it will sometimes be found at the abdominal ring, which from its unyielding nature has operated like a tight cord upon the protruded omentum or intestine, when more of these abdominal viscera have passed down, than the aperture would readily admit or allow to return. This is the principal point of strangulation in old and large herniæ, but in other cases it is more commonly seated above the ring, at the place where the spermatic cord first quits the abdomen. The strangulating pressure is here made by the transversalis muscle and its tendon, which pass over the hernial sac in a semicircular direction, and by the fascia arising from Poupart's ligament, the semicircular border of which passes under the sac, and which has been mentioned in the anatomical description of these parts. In Plate XI. Fig. 4. is represented a preparation of a hernia thus strangulated by pressure above the ring. Hereby may be explained the opinion which some surgeons have entertained of the *spasmodic* nature of the stricture, a state which it was difficult to account for when the seat of strangulation was supposed to be confined to the ring, as this tendinous aperture possesses no muscular action, and therefore cannot assume the state of spasm. But when the strangulation is above the ring, a portion of intestine protrudes under the edge of the internal oblique and transversalis muscles, compressing them, which in their turn being excited to contraction by the irritation of this pressure, react upon the intestine with a force sufficient to produce a strangulation, accompanied with spasmodic symptoms. So if the surgeon, during the operation for hernia, examines accurately into the seat of the strangulation, he will find that, except in large herniæ, cutting through the ring is insufficient to release the protruded parts; but he must proceed with his knife further up towards the spinous process of the ilium, before he can return the swelling. For the truth of this assertion I would appeal to those surgeons best acquainted with the structure of the parts, who have performed this operation the most frequently, and with the greatest attention. *Seat of strangulation. At the ring. At the aperture to the abdomen. Spasmodic stricture.*

On account of this frequent insufficiency of dividing the abdominal ring, some surgeons have supposed the stricture to be occasioned by a preternatural thickening of the sac at its mouth. But though this sometimes happens, I find from dissection that it is an extremely rare occurrence; and even where it exists, a very inconsiderable degree of pressure is sufficient to return the hernial contents, by mere dilatation of the sac with the finger, without cutting it through, provided the surrounding parts have been properly divided. *Mouth of the sac thickened.*

Moreover though the abdominal ring be dilated with freedom, the hernia will in many cases still retain its colour of strangulation, and remain as irreducible as before; but if the sac be traced up with the knife about an inch and a half, midway between the ilium and the pubis, the stricture will there be found; and when this is divided the intestine recovers its colour, and can be readily returned.

Strangulated hernia is almost always fatal unless the tumour is reduced, but now and then an instance will occur of the parts sloughing off, and a fistulous opening remaining for life at the wound, through which the fæces *Hernia sloughs.*

are evacuated. This dreadful termination of the disease leaves the patient constantly offensive, incapable of considerable exertion, and renders life itself rather a loathsome burden than a prolonged enjoyment.

Medical men liable to be deceived by the patient.

Whenever any medical attendant is called to a person suffering under the symptoms which I have described above, he should carefully inquire whether his patient has had no tumour coming down in the day, and returning when in the recumbent posture at night, placed in the groin or any other known seat of hernia; and he should not be content with mere inquiries, as persons are sometimes unconscious of this disease, and sometimes unwilling to acknowledge it, but he should himself carefully examine the abdomen with his hand, to discover, if possible, any tumour to which these symptoms may be attributed.

Strangulation from one convolution.

Though the cause of strangulation is the descent of an additional portion of intestine and omentum into the hernial sac, it might be thought that the mere protrusion of a greater length of a single fold of intestine would not increase the stricture at the narrow ring of compression; but the chief reason that it does so is, that a proportionally larger quantity of mesentery descends along with the bowel, and thus increases the pressure made by the stricture upon the blood vessels of the hernial contents.

Causes of strangulation.

The same causes that produce herniæ render them strangulated, such as, sudden distension of the abdominal viscera, exertion of the abdominal muscles, particularly in positions which compress the bowels on the upper part of the abdomen, and leave the lower part relaxed, and the apertures unguarded, violent exertions in expelling the fæces, raising a heavy weight from the ground when the body is stooping, straining to reach a great height, coughing, sneezing, and the like. Eating flatulent vegetable food is peculiarly apt to induce strangulation. This latter cause operates by distending the intestinal canal, causing it to occupy more space than before in the abdomen, and consequently pushing out part of the viscera into the hernial sac.

Small and recent hernia most readily strangulated.

A small hernia is much more easily strangulated than a large one, the pressure upon the contents being more violent; and a hernia which appears suddenly is more liable to this accident than one of long standing which has been in the habit of constantly passing up and down.

CHAPTER VIII.

Of the Treatment of strangulated Hernia.

As all the symptoms that have been described in the preceding chapter originate from the compressed state of the protruded parts, it must be the surgeon's object to return them as soon as possible into the cavity of the abdomen; and he is only wasting time by any attempts to alleviate the violence of the symptoms independent of this principal object. Object to return the parts.

The return of the part is first to be attempted by what is called the Taxis. This is done by making pressure with the hands upon the tumour, and at the same time placing the patient in that posture which gives as much room as possible in the abdomen, and relaxes its muscles and apertures. Taxis.

The best position for this purpose is supine, with the body moderately incurvated. This is effected by laying the patient upon his back, and putting one pillow under the pelvis and another under the shoulders, which will cause the loins to sink down between them. Both the thighs should also be elevated to a right angle with the patient's body, and the knees should be brought so close together as only to admit of the surgeon's arm between them: this last is a most essential point, since it relaxes the fascia of the thigh, and consequently the aperture through which the hernia first quits the abdomen, which, as we have before described, is ultimately connected with this fascia. The patient should also be desired to void his urine, and then to keep himself as quiet as possible. Position of the patient.

The surgeon then places himself by the patient's right side, and, embracing the tumour with his right hand, he presses it towards the abdominal ring so as to keep it from receding: then applying the finger and thumb of his left hand upon the neck of the tumour at the part where it enters the abdomen, he gently presses it from side to side, thus endeavouring to get a small portion of it within the abdomen. If any part can be forced up, the rest generally follows without difficulty. Of the surgeon.

The pressure should be maintained from a quarter to half an hour. I have known it succeed after a trial of twenty minutes, and it should not therefore be hastily abandoned. The degree of force should be but moderate, as the chief dependance should be placed on continuance rather than violence of pressure, the latter being sometimes known to produce a laceration of the protruded parts. Of this the following case is an instance. Pressure. Degree of.

A woman of the name of Chilton, a patient in Guy's Hospital, had an irreducible hernia, for the reduction of which a very considerable force was improperly used, when it suddenly gave way, but the tumour did not entirely disappear. In a week afterwards the part became very red and painful, a poultice was applied, when it broke, and a large quantity of bile, or rather of the contents of the small intestines, was discharged. This continued for several days, and afterwards gradually diminished, and the wound healed up entirely. Probably an adhesion had taken place between the ruptured intestine and the mouth of the sac, so as to prevent the effusion of bile from the bowel into the cavity of the abdomen, which would have produced fatal consequences.

The longer the hernial tumour has been strangulated, the more dangerous is it to use any considerable pressure for its reduction, as the parts have then a much less power of resistance than in their natural state. The force of the pressure should be directed towards the anterior and superior spinous process of the ilium, in the course which the tumour takes obliquely upwards, and not towards the abdomen immediately behind the abdominal ring.

If the attempts at reduction in the posture which I have described do not prove successful, it has been recommended to sling the patient by his knees, with his head hanging downwards, over the shoulders of an assistant. This position, however, does not provide for that relaxation of the abdominal muscles which is so desirable, and it is altogether painful to the patient, and renders it difficult for the surgeon to apply proper pressure upon the tumour. From frequent experience of it by my own trials, and by witnessing those of others, I can affirm that I have never found it answer, where the other method, fairly and fully performed, has previously failed. Slinging the patient.

The intestinal hernia will be found more easy of reduction than the omental. The former goes up suddenly with a guggling noise; the latter returns gradually, excepting the last remaining portion, which does indeed Intestinal most easy of reduction.

rapidly slip up from beneath the fingers, but unaccompanied with any noise. If from want of elasticity in the hernia the surgeon is clear that it is merely omental, the force used for reduction may be much greater than it would be safe to employ for the intestinal species.

If a fair trial of the plan which I have just mentioned should not prove successful, other means should be resorted to. One of them is the drawing of blood, the object of which is, first, by the general languor which it occasions to produce a relaxation of the strictured part, and next, to prevent the local inflammation from running so high as to occasion mortification, which would render the case fatal though the protruded parts were afterwards returned.

Bleeding.

The quantity of blood to be drawn should be from fourteen to twenty ounces, according to the strength of the patient's constitution. So much should be taken away as to bring on a degree of faintness, in which state of general relaxation the attempts at reduction should be repeated.

A surgeon unaccustomed to the small thready pulse of a person suffering under strangulated hernia, feels apprehensive of taking away blood, conceiving the patient's strength to be fast sinking. But this fear is groundless, as the pulse becomes larger after this evacuation.

Warm bath.

If this fail of success the patient is usually put into the warm bath, and indeed I generally employ the warm bath immediately after the bleeding, before the second attempt at reduction by the taxis. The first heat of the bath should be about one hundred degrees, and it should be gradually raised till the patient faints, or feels disposed to do so, which mostly takes place in fifteen or twenty minutes. The attempt at reduction is then to be repeated.

However, although bleeding and the warm bath appear likely to produce a state of body highly favourable for reduction, I must confess that I have seldom been gratified by seeing a hernia reduced by them, though the fairest trial of them had been made.

Still the patient scarcely ever fails to express feeling much less pain after the bleeding and the warm bath than before, at the same time that it too often happens that no advantage is gained in the essential point of reduction.

The two remedies on which, as far as my observation goes, the firmest reliance is to be placed, are, the tobacco glyster, and the application of cold; and if these fail I should be little inclined to await the trial of any other remedy.

Tobacco glyster.

Tobacco has been used in hernia both in form of smoke and as a liquid glyster. To use the smoke with any effect requires a complicated apparatus, and consequently is often very badly managed; it is besides uncertain in its effects, and hence its use has long been discontinued in the Hospitals of the Borough, and in the private practice of their surgeons.

Mode of administering.

The tobacco glyster, which is by far the most convenient, is made by infusing a dram of tobacco in twelve ounces of boiling water for ten minutes, after which it is fit for use. But as the effect of this potent remedy varies very much in different constitutions, and perhaps according to the quality of the tobacco, it is best to inject only half the quantity at first, and the remainder half an hour afterwards, if the first portion has not proved sufficient. To those who have commonly heard of two drams being thrown up at a time without bad consequences, this may appear an useless precaution; but, instructed by personal observation, I can venture to assert that whoever practises this often, will meet with effects which will lead him to repent his rashness.

I once saw a man with whom the tobacco glyster had been used in the quantity of two drams, without a reduction of the tumour, who about half an hour afterwards was put upon a table to have the operation for hernia performed; when his pulse was found so low, his countenance so depressed, and his body covered with cold sweats, that he was ordered back to bed, and on carrying him thither he expired.

A girl who laboured under strangulated hernia, and who was sent to Guy's Hospital by Mr. Turnbull, surgeon, had a single dram of the tobacco in infusion injected. It produced most violent pain of the abdomen, with vomiting, in which was thrown up a matter, which smelt strongly of tobacco, and she died in thirty-five minutes after the glyster had been administered, and most evidently from its effects.

These are my reasons for advising the above cautious manner of using this remedy, but at the same time it should be observed, that there are some persons on whom even the quantity of two drams produces little effect.

Its action.

When the tobacco acts in the manner to be desired, it produces extreme languor, a weak and quick pulse, a cold sweat, and such universal relaxation, that the patient has not power to exert any of the voluntary muscles of the body. In this state the hernia will often return into the abdomen with a very slight pressure, though it had previously resisted a considerable degree of force. I have felt a hernia, which had been previously tense, under the operation of a tobacco glyster, become perfectly soft and relaxed, which state was produced not by any partial return of its contents, as no pressure had been used, but simply by the temporary removal of the force of circulation from the protruded intestine.

The other powerful method of assisting the reduction of hernia is the application of cold. To produce it, brandy and vinegar, vinegar and sal ammoniac, or simply dashing cold water upon the naked abdomen and tumour, have all been employed. The most simple and effectual, however, where it can be procured, is to apply ice. For this purpose it should be broken in small pieces and put into a bladder as about to half fill it, which being tied up and wiped dry is to be laid upon the hernia to cover the inflamed and swollen parts. Its effect is almost immediately to diminish pain, to contract the skin over the tumour, and by the pressure thus produced to compel the return of the protruded parts. Another great advantage of this remedy is, that it arrests for a length of time the progress of the symptoms, so that it may be continued for several hours upon the part without incurring the risk of losing too much time. If after a trial of about four hours the symptoms become mitigated, and the tumour lessens, this remedy may be persevered in some time longer, but if they continue with unabated violence, and the tumour resists every attempt at reduction, no further trial of the ice should be made. *Cold.*

The degree of cold may be increased to any extent, even beyond what can be safely employed, by the mixture of salt with the ice.

It is improper to apply the ice to the part, wrapped up between folds of cloth, as is often done, as the melted portion constantly keeps the patient's bed wet and uncomfortable, and besides, if long continued, it produces the effect of being frost-bitten, and the part sloughs off. An instance of this kind occurred to Mr. Sharp and Mr. Cline, in a case which they attended in February 1780. They directed ice to be applied to a strangulated hernia, which being continued for thirty-six hours, occasioned the integuments to become frozen about four inches in circumference. The part was white and hard, but when the ice was removed it thawed, becoming again red and warm, and soon after the hernia was reduced. The integuments which had been frozen continued red and inflamed for ten days, when they became livid, and sloughed as far as they had been frozen, but the ulcer afterwards healed without difficulty. *Mode of application.*

As ice cannot be procured in many situations, some substitute for it must be had. The most convenient is a mixture of sal ammoniac and nitre, first finely powdered, and mixed in equal proportions. On sixteen ounces of water put into the bladder, ten ounces of the mixed salt is to be thrown, and the bladder then tied up and laid upon the tumour. The degree of cold produced by this mixture is lower in the hottest weather than the freezing point of water, and if the water be previously cooled the cold will be greater. *Substitutes for ice.*

Nitrated ammonia and water in equal parts produce a still greater intensity of cold, but as this salt is not used in medicine, it is not easily procurable. Vinegar and sal ammoniac, and vinegar with spirit of wine, generate too slight a degree of cold to be much depended on for this purpose.

In addition to the means hitherto described, it is proper to give opium to allay the violence of the vomiting. After copious bleeding opium is of particular service and much assists the subsequent attempt at reduction. *Opium.*

With respect to cathartics, the most drastic kind were formerly employed, but they have so repeatedly been found not only ineffectual in this complaint, but positively injurious, that their use is now entirely laid aside, excepting when the symptoms are very slight. If the strangulation has produced vomiting, purgatives only increase it, for the stomach is so irritable that the medicine is rejected as soon as swallowed, and hence cannot have a purgative effect, whatever be the state of strangulation in the intestine; and if the hernia be omental, little advantage could be derived from purgatives. *Cathartics.*

Where the symptoms are but slight, aperient medicines may be given, if there is either no vomiting or only at distant intervals. In such cases I have known opium, joined with calomel and cathartic extract, produce stools and relieve the patient.

In slight cases fomentations and poultices may be applied to the part with advantage, but still, even in the less urgent cases, I think them much inferior to the application of cold. In one case in which the tumour was tense, and the scrotum much inflamed, I found the application of leeches, and the subsequent application of fomentations, occasion a return of the protruded parts. *Fomentations and poultices.*

CHAPTER IX.

Circumstances to be considered previous to the Operation.

<small>Operation necessary.</small>
IF all the methods above described have failed of success, it becomes necessary, to preserve the life of the patient, to perform an operation to liberate the protruded parts from their confinement.

<small>Operation little dangerous.</small>
The operation, if well performed, in an otherwise healthy person, is attended with little if any danger, and it is therefore natural to enquire why it has so frequently been followed with the death of the patient. The great reason of want of success in this operation is its being performed too late; so that the protruded contents have proceeded to a state of gangrene, or so nearly approaching to the gangrenous condition, that the long-inflamed parts are unable to recover their natural functions; or else that the inflammation has extended to the viscera in the cavity of the abdomen, continuing the consequences of the disease after the stricture which caused it has been removed.

<small>Much time lost.</small>
It cannot be too much lamented or condemned that so much time is commonly lost before the operation is performed. To reduce the hernia, trial after trial is made, the same means are often repeated, the tumour by being often compressed becomes excessively tender, so that the mere cessation of the efforts at reduction gives a comparative ease, which flatters the patient and his medical attendant that a part of the tumour has gone up; hopes are still entertained that an operation may be avoided, till the rapid progress of the symptoms of danger points out the fatal error of delay, and when the operation is performed, too clearly demonstrates the impossibility of success.

<small>Criterion of time.</small>
It would be a fortunate thing if surgeons were possessed of any criterion which, by shewing the exact state of the protruded parts, would enable them to judge of the latest time to which the operation could be safely delayed. Hiccough has been named as the deciding symptom of the presence of mortification, but this is now known not to be accurate, since the operation has several times been performed in the Hospitals of the Borough after this symptom has occurred, when parts have been found free from mortification, and the patients have recovered. On the other hand, I dissected a woman who died of strangulated hernia, in which a portion of the ilium was mortified, who had not shewn the slightest hiccough during the progress of the disease.

<small>Performed before tension of the belly.</small>
In every case to which I have been called, I have been anxious to perform the operation before the occurrence of soreness of the belly under pressure. Soon after the symptoms of strangulation appear, the abdomen becomes tense, owing to the flatulent distention of the intestines, but still the patient does not immediately complain of soreness upon pressure; but when, in addition to the tension, pressure on the abdomen gives much pain, it is a proof that the inflammation has extended into that cavity. In this state there is peritoneal inflammation to contend with, which, unfortunately, the operation itself, though the only method of removing the stricture, is calculated to increase; so that on opening into the cavity of the abdomen this inflammation spreads through its cavity and destroys the patient.

Therefore as soon as bleeding, the warm bath, the tobacco glyster, and topical cold, have been fairly tried, and have proved unsuccessful, if the abdomen is becoming affected, the operation should be no longer delayed; and indeed if the warm bath cannot be conveniently and quickly procured, it is better to omit it altogether, than to endanger the patient's life by further delay.

<small>Patient's consent quickly gained.</small>
It will be said that it is difficult to obtain the patient's consent to an early operation. But this I have never found, where the precise state of the case was fairly represented. The almost certain fatal consequence of delay, and the inconsiderable degree of pain which is inflicted here, compared with many other operations, seldom fail to gain the patient's consent of submitting to the only remaining method of relief from his sufferings and his dangerous situation.

This soreness, upon pressing the abdomen, is a much better criterion than the time which has elapsed since the occurrence of the first symptoms of strangulation, for there is the utmost variety in the time that elapses between these symptoms and a fatal termination. There is a drawing of a large intestinal and omental hernia in the Museum at St. Thomas's Hospital, which Mr. Else used to state in his lectures proved fatal in eight hours from the first appearance of strangulation; under these circumstances death is not occasioned by mortification, but by the constitutional irritation which the inflammation of so large a surface occasions. On the other hand, I have known the operation successfully performed at the end of eight days after the accession of the symptoms of strangulation, although death generally happens on the sixth or seventh day from the commencement of the symptoms.

Some judgment may be formed from the pulse, and from the patient's general appearance: if the pulse be so small as to be scarcely perceptible, and the countenance anxious and sunken, no time is to be lost; but even under these circumstances, and with hiccough superadded, I have known the operation succeed. *Pulse a criterion.*

Indeed there is scarcely any period of the symptoms which should forbid the operation; for even if mortification has actually begun, the operation may be the means of saving life by promoting the ready separation of the gangrenous parts. *Operation at any time.*

Though a large hernia, when completely strangulated, is more rapidly fatal than a small one; the latter, being commonly the most severely compressed by the stricture, demands the operation more frequently than the larger hernia. *Operation required most frequently for small herniæ.*

An omental hernia, though much more difficult to reduce than an intestinal, is not so dangerous; being slower in its progress, and producing much less violent symptoms, so that the operation may be delayed to a later period with every prospect of saving life. *Omental least dangerous.*

When the omentum and the intestine have descended, the disease takes a middle course in the violence and duration of its symptoms, and the intestine generally suffers less from the strangulation, than when unaccompanied with omentum.

When more than one irreducible hernia exists in the same person, it is sometimes difficult to determine which it is that requires the operation. This will be illustrated by the following curious case which occurred during the last spring at Guy's Hospital. *Several herniæ.*

A woman was admitted with three herniæ, two in the groin, and one at the navel. The umbilical hernia, and that of the left groin, were irreducible; that of the right groin felt extremely sore upon pressure. A doubt arose which was the hernia that required the operation; but as the symptoms of strangulation were not extremely urgent, though the woman was very low, it was agreed to wait till the next day for a consultation. During the night, however, she died, and upon inspecting the body, the tumour in the right groin was found to be an enlarged and inflamed absorbent gland lying over an empty hernial sac. In the left groin was a portion of inflamed intestine, and at the navel was an irreducible omental hernia which had suppurated, and contained about a table spoonful of matter. This woman complained chiefly of pain in the right groin, and if the operation had been performed, this would have been the tumour laid open. This case also furnished another observation; though this woman had several herniæ, yet the operation, on whichever it had been performed, would have given no relief; as she died, not of strangulated hernia, but of peritoneal and omental inflammation. When the abdomen was opened the intestines were found adhering to each other, with matter interposed in some places; and a considerable quantity of pus had been effused into that part of the omentum which was contained in the cavity of the abdomen. In this case, therefore, the abdomen was first affected, and the inflammation, after having extended through it, was continued to the protruded parts. Soreness of the abdomen, therefore, which in strangulated hernia is a late symptom, must here have been one of the earliest. *Case.* *Disease began in the abdomen.*

As a recent hernia is more difficult of reduction than one which has been long accustomed to descend, it therefore more frequently requires the operation. The latter is situated amidst parts relaxed by repeated dilatation, the recent is surrounded by parts which have great powers of resistance, and are already in a state of contraction. *Recent hernia most difficult to reduce.*

The herniæ of the very young and the very old require the operation less frequently than those of the middle period of life, when the fibres are firmer, and the muscular strength more robust: in the tenderness of youth, and the relaxation of age, a reduction of the hernia by the taxis is almost always practicable; and it is principally in old persons that much time elapses before the strangulation produces fatal effects, the period of their sufferings having been known to be protracted sometimes to twenty days. *Most difficult in the adult.*

CHAPTER X.

Of the Operation of Inguinal Hernia.

<small>Object of the operation.</small> The object of the operation, is to liberate the protruded parts from their confinement, and to return them into the cavity of the abdomen, if they are found upon examination to be in a state likely to recover from the effects of the strangulation.

<small>Position of the patient.</small> For this operation the patient is to be placed upon a table about three feet six inches in height, his body lying in a horizontal posture, excepting that the shoulders should be a little raised, his legs as high as the knees hanging down over the edge of the table, and the thighs a little bent in order to relax the abdominal muscles. The bladder should be emptied, and the diseased side must be shaved.

<small>Incision.</small> The surgeon then, standing between the patient's thighs, grasps the tumour with his left hand, and with a common scalpel in the other, makes an incision through the whole length of the tumour, unless it is very large; beginning opposite to the upper part of the abdominal ring, at the middle of the sac, and extending it to the bottom of the tumour in the same direction.

<small>Bleeding.</small> This incision, by which the skin and cellular membrane over the sac are cut, also divides the external pudendal artery, which always crosses the sac near the abdominal ring, and sometimes affords rather a free hemorrhage. This circumstance however is in no degree alarming to a surgeon who expects it, as the bleeding may be stopped by the vessel being compressed by an assistant, or if the artery is larger than usual, owing to the scrotum being long distended by the disease, the blood may be stopped by a ligature. This artery may be seen in Plate VI. It arises from the femoral artery just below Poupart's ligament, and passes to the skin of the penis and scrotum, crossing the spermatic cord near the abdominal ring.

<small>Fascia exposed.</small> This incision which divides the skin and cellular membrane exposes the fascia which passes off from the external oblique muscle, and which forms the first and thickest covering of the sac. The middle of this fascia is next cut through, and a director introduced beneath it, is carried upward to within an inch of the abdominal ring, and the fascia is divided upon it; and again by turning the director downwards, a similar division of the fascia is made to the bottom of the tumour.

<small>Cremaster muscle.</small> This opening through the fascia exposes the second covering of the hernial sac, viz. the cremaster muscle; which must be also divided both upwards and downwards with the assistance of the director, precisely in the same manner as the fascia.

<small>Sac.</small> When these coverings are cut through, the sac itself becomes perfectly exposed. It should be remarked that to those not accurately acquainted with the anatomy of the part, the division of these layers causes great embarrassment and delay; for the operator expecting to see the sac itself as soon as he has divided the common integuments, cuts the fascia with extreme caution, fibre after fibre, from fear of injuring the intestine beneath, mistaking this thickened covering and the cremaster muscle for the hernial sac.

<small>Fluctuation.</small> When the sac is completely exposed, if the hernia is intestinal, and the intestine does not adhere to the sac, a sense of fluctuation may be generally perceived at its anterior and inferior part, when the tumour is grasped, and the fluid which it contains is pressed forward.

<small>Sac opened.</small> The surgeon is next to pinch up some of the cellular membrane which closely adheres to the anterior and inferior part of the sac, by means of a pair of dissecting forceps, and when the sac is thus raised, and separated from the intestine, he is to place the edge of the knife horizontally, and to cut a small hole just sufficiently large to admit the blunt end of a probe or that of a director, upon which the sac is to be further divided, being cut upwards to within an inch of the abdominal ring, and downwards to the bottom of the sac. The reason that the anterior and inferior part of the sac is selected for the first incision into it is, that the intestine seldom descends so low, and if it does, the fluid which it contains is generally found interposed between the intestine and that part of the sac. The sac should not be divided higher than to an inch below the abdominal ring, as its division near the abdomen makes it more difficult to close the wound, and exposes the patient to greater danger of peritoneal inflammation.

As soon as the sac is opened, a quantity of fluid escapes; its colour, if the strangulation has not been long continued, is that of serum, but if the intestine has been for a long time compressed, it becomes of a coffee colour, and sometimes offensive to the smell. Its quantity, if there is no adhesion of the intestine to the sac, is proportioned to the quantity of intestine strangulated, for if adhesion exists, little, if any, is found, so that the surgeon who depends upon meeting with it, would wound the intestine in the operation. In the omental hernia also there is seldom any fluid in the sac, and if any, a comparatively small quantity; for this fluid seems to be principally a secretion from the surface of the intestine. *Fluid escapes. Its quantity.*

When the sac is opened, the contents of the hernia appear; and if both the intestine and omentum have descended, the latter is the first that presents, and generally covers, and sometimes entirely envelopes the intestine. The omentum retains much of its usual appearance, its colour being only a shade darker than natural; but the intestine is covered with a coat of coagulable lymph, and appears red if it has not been long strangulated, but of a chocolate brown colour if the stricture has been very tight, or the strangulation long continued. The veins upon it are turgid with blood, and I have seen the lacteals upon the jejunum and ilium distended with air. *Contents of the sac. Omentum. Intestine.*

The next part of the operation is the division of the stricture, and the surgeon carries his finger into the hernial sac to examine accurately into its situation, which he will find in one or other of the three following parts. *Situation of the stricture.*

First, at the abdominal ring.

Secondly, above the ring from one inch and an half to two inches, and inclining outwards toward the spinous process of the ilium.

Thirdly, in the mouth of the hernial sac.

If the stricture is owing to the pressure of the columns of the tendon which form the abdominal ring, it is then to be divided in the following manner. The surgeon passes his finger into the sac as far as the stricture, and then conveys a probe pointed bistory on the fore part of the sac, and insinuating it within the ring, cuts through it in a direction upwards opposite to the middle of the sac, and to an extent proportioned to the size of the tumour. The dilatation of the ring should not be larger than is sufficient to return the protruded parts; but it should allow them to pass without committing any violence by the pressure exerted in effecting their return. In general, if the finger can be readily admitted into the abdomen, by the side of the protruded parts, the dilatation is sufficiently free. *Division of the abdominal ring.*

It is best to divide the stricture by passing the knife between the ring and the sac, as a larger portion of peritoneum is thus left uncut, and the cavity of the abdomen is afterwards more easily closed. The direction given to the knife in dilating the stricture has been usually upwards and outwards towards the spine of the ilium, but I prefer doing it directly upwards, for the two following reasons.

First, as the higher aperture must only be dilated directly upwards, it is better that the surgeon should have one general rule for the use of the probe-pointed bistory, applicable to every case of inguinal hernia, than to be perplexed in the operation by a variety of directions, which only partially apply to one or other seat of the stricture; and secondly, the division of the tendon in this direction weakens the abdomen less than upwards and outwards, because as the cord passes towards the abdomen in that direction, and the hernial sac is parallel with the cord, a dilatation in that course takes off the resistance which the tendon would otherwise make to any future descent. When the ring is divided directly upwards, the upper column of tendon which forms it is cut, when it is dilated upwards and outwards, the transverse fibres uniting the columns, are divided. The dilatation upwards is equally safe with the other, for if this were not the case, no subordinate advantage ought to interfere with the most important one of security. *Reasons for preferring the division upwards.*

A frequent situation of the stricture, however, is not at the abdominal ring, but at the place at which the sac opens into the abdomen, that is an inch and an half or two inches above, and to the outer side of the ring; and it is there occasioned by the pressure of the tendon of the transversalis which passes over it, and by the resistance of the border of fascia which passes under it. *Stricture above the ring.*

If the stricture is at this orifice it is to be divided as follows.

The surgeon passes his finger up the sac, and through the abdominal ring, until he meets with the stricture; he then introduces the probe-pointed bistory with its flat side towards the finger, but anterior to the sac, and between it and the abdominal ring, his finger being still a director to the knife. Thus he carries the knife along the forepart of the sac until he insinuates it under the stricture formed by the lower edge of the transversalis *Mode of dividing it.*

and internal oblique muscles, and then turning the edge of the knife forwards, by a gentle motion of its handle he divides the stricture sufficiently to allow the finger to slip into the abdomen: the knife is then to be withdrawn with its flat side towards the finger as it was introduced, to prevent any unnecessary injury of the parts.

Upwards. The direction in which this orifice is divided is straight upwards opposite the middle of the mouth of the sac, as in this way the epigastric artery can scarcely be cut, whatever be its relative situation with respect to the sac. The truth of this is evinced by examining Plates III, IV, VII, VIII, and IX, of this work, and the mode of performing the operation is shewn in Plate XI.

Advantage. An advantage is derived from dilating the stricture without cutting the sac itself, for there is no danger of injuring the intestine with the naked edge of the knife, which I have twice known to happen when the stricture was divided from within the sac; in one case the patient died from the contents of the intestine escaping into the cavity of the abdomen, in the other the intestine was obliged to be retained in the sac to allow of the escape of the fæces by the external wound. An additional advantage is derived from this mode of dilatation, viz. that if by any mistake of the operator the epigastric artery is cut, as the peritoneum is undivided, the flow of blood would be immediately perceived, and then the vessel might be secured; whereas if the sac is included in the incision, the artery would bleed into the abdomen, and the consequences might be fatal, without the cause being known but by dissection.

Case. In the following case, the stricture existed both at the abdominal ring, and at the aperture two inches and an half above it, and it is here introduced to illustrate the foregoing observations.

David Sugmund, aged sixty years, was admitted into Guy's Hospital, under the care of Mr. Lucas, on Sunday the 25th of December 1803, for a large strangulated scrotal hernia on the right side. The disease had existed for twenty years, but it had become strangulated only twenty-four hours preceding his admission, in consequence of a hard day of labour. As the disease resisted every attempt to reduce it, the operation was determined on, and was performed on Monday the 26th at one o'clock.

On opening the sac no other contents were found than the cæcum and its appendix, little altered in colour, but covered with a coat of lymph on its anterior surface, and firmly adhering to the sac at its posterior and upper part. When the finger was passed into the sac a stricture was found at the abdominal ring, which being freely divided, attempts were made to return the intestine. Trial after trial was made, considerable pressure was exerted, but without effect. When the finger was passed further up the sac, another stricture was found there, situated two inches above the ring, which prevented the finger from being passed into the abdomen. This stricture was formed by the edge of the transversalis above, and by the semicircular border of the fascia below, both of which could be distinctly felt. A probe-pointed bistory was passed under the edge of the transversalis muscle, between it and the hernial sac, and the edge of the former was divided, when the finger readily passed into the abdomen, and the intestine, by slight pressure only, was immediately returned. The dilatation of the transversalis was made directly upwards, with considerable freedom, to give as much room as possible, as the intestine was much thickened and enlarged by frequent descent.

Stricture of the mouth of the sac. The third seat of the stricture is the hernial sac itself, from its becoming thickened or contracted; but I have already said it is not so frequent an occurrence as has been imagined; for the pressure of the surrounding parts above the ring has been often mistaken for it. It is, however, undoubtedly true, that it does sometimes occur, as the instance proves which I have already stated, of septa forming in the sac, as will be seen in Plate V, Fig. 3, a preparation in the Museum at St. Thomas's Hospital. It is also proved by another drawing in the same Plate, from Fig. 4. From the seat of the contraction in the sac in the latter instance, it would seem that it had been induced by the pressure of a truss at the abdominal ring. I lately also dissected a subject in which the peritoneum, at the mouth of the sac was considerably thickened, and had pressed upon a portion of the intestine, which it included so as to occasion its strangulation.

A membranous band crossing the mouth of a hernial sac, might produce strangulation, by its pressure upon the intestine.

Mode of dividing it. If the stricture is placed within the sac, it will be known by the dilatation of the transversalis being insufficient to liberate the intestine, and when this is found to be the case, it is necessary to proceed in the following manner. The finger being carried within the sac up to the stricture, a probe-pointed bistory like that in Plate XI, is placed with its side upon it, and is carried into the stricture; the cutting edge being then turned towards the stricture, it is to be divided by a gentle motion of the knife's handle forwards and upwards, opposite to the middle of the anterior part of the sac.

It is necessary to be very careful in using the knife within the sac to avoid injuring the intestine, which is otherwise liable to be cut. The bistory should be sharp only on a small part of its edge, as in that which is shewn in Plate XI. *Knife.*

It is stated, but I have never seen it, that the omentum is sometimes the cause of the stricture, by enveloping the intestine, and becoming thickened around it. Such an occurrence is possible, and ought to be looked for, and if found the stricture will be easily divided. *Omentum sometimes the cause of the stricture.*

When the stricture has been completely removed, the protruded intestine is to be attentively examined, to observe whether the brown colour which it assumes under strangulation, lessens or disappears; as this is a proof of the return of circulation in the part. The veins on its surface may be also emptied by pressure, and their sudden filling noted, and the intestine should be pulled down a little to make these observations on the part which has immediately been compressed by the stricture. If the intestine appears to have a free circulation, the surgeon should directly, but gradually, return it, thrusting up about an inch at a time, and securing each part with his fingers until the whole is returned into the abdomen. All violence and improper haste should be carefully guarded against, for the intestine is tender, and will easily tear at the strictured part. The portion of intestine shewn discoloured by strangulation in Plate VI, was taken from a woman, in whom under this operation, but a slight degree of pressure had been used to return it; and though it had been strangulated only forty-four hours, it gave way, and the contents were extravasated into the cavity of the abdomen. I shall also have occasion to mention another instance of a similar kind. *Intestine examined.* *Mode of returning it.*

In returning the intestine after the operation, it is proper to put the patient in the same position as when the attempt at reduction is made without the use of the knife; that is, to elevate the thigh on the diseased side, and to relax, as much as possible, the aperture into the abdomen.

If the intestine is connected with the sac by adhesion, an extraordinary degree of caution is required on opening the sac, as it contains little or no interposed fluid. If the bands which form the adhesion are long enough to allow of the intestine being drawn a little from the sac, they may be completely separated by dissection; but if they are so short that the intestine and sac are agglutinated together, it becomes necessary to cut off portions of the sac, and to return them, still adhering to the bowel, into the cavity of the abdomen. Sometimes the adhesion exists only at the orifice of the sac, all the lower part being perfectly free; a circumstance which requires great caution in the operation to ensure the entire return of the protruded intestine, as otherwise the operation will fail of its object. *Adhesions.*

On Feb. the 26th, 1799, a person was taken into St. Thomas's Hospital, for a strangulated inguinal hernia; the attempts made to reduce it were unsuccessful, and the operation was performed on the day of his admission. The omentum was very much thickened, and a large portion of it was removed. The intestine was found very difficult to reduce, from an adhesion between it and the mouth of the hernial sac; but it was at length apparently returned into the cavity of the abdomen. Two stools were procured by glysters on the 27th, but from that time till the 9th of March, on which day he died, he had no stool. On examination of the body, the ilium, which was the intestine that had been strangulated, was found in the mouth of the hernial sac, and doubled back within it; the small intestine above this portion was inflamed and greatly distended, and the jejunum was in a state of mortification. The large intestines were empty and much contracted. These adhesions therefore, by preventing the complete return of the intestine, occasioned the death of the patient. *Adhesions of the intestine to the mouth of the sac.*

It is an operation of extreme difficulty and delicacy to divide these adhesions at the mouth of the hernial sac. It requires that the sac should be dilated to its mouth, and that the tendon of the external oblique should be slit up to the part at which the hernia descends from the abdomen. Great danger of wounding the intestine, even when the parts are thus completely exposed, attends the division of the adhesions. *Difficulty of removing them.*

It sometimes happens that the convolution of intestine in the hernial sac has its sides glued together by recent adhesions. When this happens, it is right to separate them before the intestine is returned, because the stools do not readily find their way through an intestine which is thus doubled. A man who was operated upon in Guy's Hospital, and had the intestine returned in this adhering state into the cavity of the abdomen, had no stool after the operation; and upon examining his body, no other cause for his death was found, than that the portion of intestine had not entirely recovered its natural colour, and that one portion of it was placed parallel to *Folds of intestine adhering.*

R

the other, confined in that situation by adhesion. The fæces had accumulated above this part, having found no passage through it.

<small>Appendices epiploïcæ removed.</small>
If the colon has protruded, and the person be corpulent, the fatty appendages of this intestine are found more diseased than the intestine itself, so that it becomes necessary to remove them. A lady, a patient of Mr. Pidcock's of Watford, had a large hernia, which became strangulated, and required the operation. When I opened the sac, I found that it contained the colon. This intestine was much discoloured, but the appendices epiploïcæ were still more so, and did not recover their natural hue when the stricture was removed; I therefore cut off all those appendages from the surface of the colon, and returned the bowel. No hemorrhage ensued, and the lady recovered, contrary to my expectations, as besides extraordinary obesity, she actually laboured under ascites, and a large quantity of water was discharged during the operation.

<small>Omentum returned.</small>
When the intestine has been returned, the omentum is to be examined with attention, and if it is in a healthy state, and not of very considerable bulk, it should be returned into the cavity of the abdomen by as slight a pressure as possible. But if it is very bulky, a part of it should be removed; which may be done by the knife with great freedom, and if properly managed, without any danger. I have myself removed it in several instances

<small>Removed.</small>
without the patient seeming to suffer any subsequent inconvenience. The surgeon raising the omentum, whilst an assistant grasps it higher up to prevent its return into the abdomen, cuts it off near the mouth of the sac. Some small arteries always bleed, which are to be secured by a fine ligature; and when the hemorrhage is stopped, the omentum is to be returned into the abdomen, with its divided surface applied to the mouth of the sac, from which the ligatures are suspended, and it thus forms a plug that shuts up its cavity.

<small>Tied.</small>
The practice of applying a ligature round the whole of the protruded omentum, to make it slough away, though it has had its advocates, is now very generally laid aside. Indeed it appears extraordinary that it should ever have prevailed. The very object of the operation for hernia, is to take off from the omentum the stricture derived from the pressure of a surrounding tendon, which acts as a cord upon the part; and no sooner is this removed, than the surgeon applies a ligature, which produces a more perfect constriction than that which had previously existed. A man, twenty years of age, was admitted into St. Thomas's Hospital in the year 1790, for a strangulated omental hernia. Upon performing the operation, the quantity of omentum was found to be so large, that there was no possibility of its being returned, and for the purpose of its removal a ligature was applied around it. He experienced no relief from the operation, and died on the seventh day from that on which it had been performed. I have, however, several times known the omentum tied, and the patient still recover; but it appeared to me that its living powers had been already destroyed by the pressure of the stricture; and if the part is mortified, a ligature cannot excite constitutional irritation, or produce any dangerous consequences, but, on the other hand, its application is attended with no utility, as the omentum would have sloughed if the thread had not been used.

<small>Mortified.</small>
If mortification has taken place in the omentum, it is to be removed by excision at the sound part, in the manner I have already described. Even if there is only suspicion, and not positive certainty, of the omentum being mortified, it should be cut away; as the removal is, so far as I have seen, unattended with danger; and its return into the abdomen, if mortified, or even approaching to that state, attended with the utmost hazard, and generally proves fatal. One exception, however, to this opinion, I have seen. A man underwent the operation

<small>Omentum sloughing.</small>
for hernia in Guy's Hospital, and the sac was found to contain both omentum and intestine, which as they appeared not mortified, although considerably changed, were returned into the abdomen. On the sixth day after the operation the man appeared to be dying, his pulse was extremely feeble, and he complained of severe pain in the abdomen. The ligatures upon the scrotum were cut away, fomentations and poultices were applied to the wound, and on the following day a small portion of omentum protruded in a gangrenous state. More of it continued to come down, in this state, from time to time, during seven days, after which the whole portion which had been originally contained in the hernial sac, appeared in the wound, and gradually sloughed off. The wound then healed, and the patient recovered. This favourable termination could only have happened in a case in which the mouth of the hernial sac was wide, and where the omentum was lying in the abdomen just opposite to its orifice.

<small>Adhesion of the omentum.</small>
If the omentum adheres to the sac, the adhesions may be cut through with considerable freedom, and the bleeding vessels being secured, the omentum should then be returned into the cavity of the abdomen.

<small>Scirrhous omentum.</small>
It is sometimes necessary to cut away the omentum on account of its being in a scirrhous state. A case of this kind occurred in a man who was operated upon for a hernia congenita; and the omentum being thus diseased, formed a large and hard tumour, which is preserved in the Anatomical Museum at St. Thomas's Hospital.

CHAPTER XI.

Mortification of the Intestine.

THE symptoms by which this state of the intestine is known are, that the tumour which was tense and elastic becomes soft and doughy, and air can be felt crackling in the cellular membrane; that its colour which was at first of a florid red becomes purple. The hiccough and tension of the abdomen still continue, but the vomiting is less frequent. The pulse is intermittent, but fuller and softer than during the inflammatory state; the eyes are glassy. The hernia now sometimes returns into the cavity of the abdomen without assistance, and the patient survives but a few hours, but sometimes the skin over the tumour sloughs, the intestine gives way and the fæces being discharged at the opening, the symptoms of strangulation soon after cease. When this happens the intestine contracts adhesions to the hernial sac. The portion which has been mortified sloughs away and an artificial anus becomes established, through which generally during the remaining part of the patient's miserable existence the fæces are constantly discharged. However, it sometimes happens when the intestine has sloughed that a reunion takes place of its extremities, the external wound gradually heals, the artificial anus is closed, and the fæces resume their natural course. My friend, Mr. John Cooper, surgeon, of Wotton Under Edge, Gloucestershire, gives me permission to insert here the following curious fact which proves the truth of the foregoing statement.

Mary Perkins, aged sixty, a poor woman, who resides at Kingswood, desired Mr. Cooper to see her on account of a crural hernia. She appeared to be sinking fast, and the hernia was in a state of mortification; she had fallen down stairs a fortnight before, and soon after discovered a tumour in her groin which gave excruciating pain, produced vomiting and constipation, which had continued from that period to the time at which he saw her. As mortification had already begun, it was thought that there was little chance of saving her life; no other direction was given but that her strength should be supported by every means which were in her power to procure. In a few days the mortified parts began to slough, and the whole of the fæces passed through the artificial anus for three months, during which time several inches of one of the small intestines was discharged at the wound. At the expiration of three months a small portion of the fæces began to take their natural course, and the quantity gradually lessened, until at the period of six months from the commencement of the symptoms, the fæces passed entirely by the rectum, and the wound became perfectly healed. A few days after the mortification had begun in the groin, a tumour formed near the ilium, on the same side, which proceeded to mortification, and an inch of intestine was discharged; the wound continued open for a month, and then healed. She took large quantities of bark and cordials during her confinement, and is now as well as she has been for many years.

The degree of danger which attends an artificial anus depends upon the vicinity of the sphacelated intestine to the stomach, for if the opening is in the jejunum, so little space is left for the absorption of the chyle that the patient dies from inanition.

A man aged fifty years was admitted into Guy's Hospital for an umbilical hernia, the surface of which was red and very painful to the touch. He did not vomit, but no stools could be procured. The tumour was ordered to be fomented and poulticed. Its surface became black, and the skin having sloughed, exposed a portion of gangrenous intestine, which also separated. During the period of sphacelation the man's pulse was feeble, his countenance generally flushed, and he seemed to be sinking under the disease; but when the intestine had sloughed his strength seemed to recover, and great hopes were entertained that he would ultimately do well. However when he began to take food in any considerable quantity, a part of what he ate was observed in half an hour to be discharged at the artificial anus. What he drank came away in less than ten minutes, and although he ate and drank a sufficient quantity to support a healthy person, yet he wasted rapidly, and died in three weeks after the tumour first began to slough.

Upon examination of the abdomen, there was no effusion into the cavity, nor did the intestines appear inflamed. The jejunum being traced downwards was found proceeding through the umbilicus, and there it opened into the hernial sac, the aperture being situated in the lower part of this intestine.

s

When the artificial anus is in the ilium, it is attended with less danger than in the jejunum. I have already mentioned one instance of recovery, and shall have occasion to give another in the course of this chapter. If it is situated in the large intestines patients scarcely appear to suffer in their general health, for I have seen several instances of this disease in the colon, all of them in women, and from umbilical or ventral hernia; and they seemed to possess the same bodily health with others, some of them being afterwards extremely corpulent.

Treatment of artificial anus. With respect to the treatment which is required in these cases of sloughing hernia, I believe that very little more can be done than to quicken the process of separation by fomentation and poultice, and to support the strength by cordial medicines and bark; and that any attempt made to lead the fæces into their natural course, prior to the sloughing being completed, will only irritate the parts, prevent the regular progress of separation, and endanger the destruction of the patient. When the artificial anus is completely established, all that can be done is to lessen as much as possible the offensive state of the patient, by confining the fæces until it is convenient to discharge them. For this purpose a square cushion, covered with oil silk, is to be placed over the artificial anus, and a steel truss, which exerts but a slight degree of pressure, being placed upon it confines the fæces so as to lessen the offensive smell, and allows the patient to seek a convenient situation for an evacuation. This plan answers extremely well if the fæculent matter has some consistence, but if the aperture is in the ilium the contents of this intestine are with difficulty confined.

Inversion prevented. When the mortified parts have sloughed, if any part of the fæces pass by the natural aperture, it is proper to guard against the inversion of the intestine at the artificial anus, as the consequence of that inversion is to establish the false passage, and prevent all hopes of the patient having a cure performed. The following case of inguinal hernia will illustrate this position. A patient of Mr. Cowell's, in St. Thomas's Hospital, who had long had an irreducible omental hernia on the right side, had a second protrusion forming a distinct tumour on the outer side of the old hernia. This last became strangulated, and the operation was performed, when the protruded intestine was found mortified and was therefore left in the hernial sac.

Case. For three weeks after the operation, the fæces were discharged in part from the wound, and in part by the anus, but most by the latter. In a month after the operation the intestine began to protrude at the wound, and became inverted, and from that time the fæces ceased to take their natural course by the rectum. This man lived eleven years discharging his fæces by the protruded intestine at the groin. He died in the year 1778, and when his body was examined it was discovered that a part of the colon, opposite the entrance of the ilium, and the ilium itself had sloughed away, but the adhesions of the intestines to the orifice of the wound, and to each other, had prevented any of the fæces escaping into the cavity of the abdomen, and whilst the ilium was preserved from protrusion, the fæces escaped in part from it into the colon, and were discharged by the rectum, and in part passed out at the artificial anus; but when a protrusion of the ilium happened, its communication with the colon was stopped, and the fæces were then all discharged at the wound. To prevent this occurrence in future it is proper, during the progress of the healing of the wound, to support the intestine and prevent its inversion, for this circumstance will otherwise establish an artificial anus in every case in which a lateral opening of the intestine exists.

Operation. In performing the operation for strangulated hernia, if the intestine is mortified, the appearance which it assumes is that of a dark purple, or leaden coloured spot, or spots, which readily break down under the impression of the finger. The other part of the intestine is of a chocolate brown colour, which has been often mistaken for mortification, but its colour and its firmness prove that it has not advanced to that state. Every part of the surface of the intestine is covered by a layer of coagulable lymph of a brown colour.

Mortified intestine. As the intestine cannot when mortified be returned into the cavity of the abdomen, the surgeon is to consider in what manner he is to proceed to save the patient from that most miserable state of existence, which is produced by an artificial anus. In forming his judgment upon this subject he will be directed by the state in which the part is found.

Treatment of small opening. If a small hole only has been produced, the intestine should be returned into the abdomen, excepting that portion of its cylinder in which the hole exists. A needle and ligature should be passed through the mysentery at right angles with the intestine, to prevent its including the branches of the mysenteric artery which supply that part of the intestine, and then through the mouth of the hernial sac; and tying the thread, the intestine becomes confined to the mouth of the sac, and the fæces pass readily from the opening by the wound, but will in part take their course by the rectum. As granulations arise, and the wound becomes closed, the opening in the intestine is gradually shut, and an artificial anus is effectually prevented.

Mr. Turner, a very excellent surgeon at Yarmouth, in Norfolk, was called to a man near Lowestoff, who had long laboured under an inguinal hernia, which was then strangulated. The operation being proposed and consented to, a large part of the omentum, and a small portion of intestine were found in the hernial sac. A part of the omentum was removed, and a ligature passed through the remainder, and loosely tied, and both the intestine and the remaining portion of the omentum were placed at the mouth of the hernial sac, probably from a suspicion of what afterwards happened being likely to occur. The edges of the wound being brought together, the symptoms of strangulation soon ceased, and he had regular stools for nine days; but upon the tenth, fæces were discharged at the wound, though a part still passed by their natural channel. The fæces continued to pass for eleven weeks, in part by one channel and in part by the other; when the wound healed, and the natural course of the fæces was restored. Under these circumstances, that portion of the cylinder of the intestine which had been lost, was most probably reproduced by the adhesion of the inner side of the sac to the intestine. *Case.*

When the whole cylinder of the intestine is mortified, it is necessary to proceed very differently. Then the mortified part of the intestine should be cut away, and the ends are to be brought in contact and confined by means of four ligatures. *Whole cylinder mortified.*

As far as a judgment can be formed from experiments made upon animals, it will be seen that this operation is in them both safe and effectual; for I have made the experiment of dividing the intestine and afterwards sewing its extremities together, and was pleased to find it succeed. That I might have an opportunity of showing the united intestine, during my lecture on wounds of the intestine I requested Mr. Phillips, then a pupil at the Hospitals, now a surgeon in Southwark, to make the experiment for that purpose. *Experiments.*

EXPERIMENT I.

The abdomen of a dog being opened, one of the small intestines was divided; a cylinder of isinglass was then introduced into the bowel, and three sutures were made upon it: one at the part at which it joins with the mesentery, and the other two on each side of the intestine. In three days the animal had regular stools. On the sixteenth day he was killed, and the united portion of the intestine was shown to the students.

EXPERIMENT II.

It appeared in the foregoing experiment that the animal derived no advantage from the cylinder of isinglass, as it became shut by the contraction of the intestine. I therefore divided the intestine of another dog, and sewed it with three threads, without including the isinglass. On the second day the dog took food, on the third appeared playful, on the fifth I pulled the ligatures away; after which he suffered nothing from the experiment. I have not yet had an engraving made of the portion of the intestine, but it shall be included in the second part of this work.

In both these experiments the intestine was returned into the abdomen, where it rested against the wound in the parietes; and the ligatures were left hanging externally. But my friend Mr. Thomson, lecturer in surgery at Edinburgh, made these experiments in a different manner, and their result is so curious as to deserve attention.

EXPERIMENT I.

Assisted by his friends Drs. Farre and Jones, he divided the intestine of a dog. The cut edges were sewn together, first by an interrupted suture going round the cylinder of the intestine, and then four other stitches were introduced at nearly equal distances from each other. The ligatures being cut close to the intestine he returned it into the abdomen, and sewed the external incision. No swelling or tension succeeded. The dog was killed on the tenth day. On opening the abdomen he found a portion of intestine, thickened and more vascular than usual, adhering to the parietes at the site of the external wound; on slitting this up he could see distinctly on the inside, but not on the out, the place at which the intestine had been divided. Three of the ligatures had disappeared, but the place of their former attachment could be distinctly seen on the inner and thickened surface of the wound. Two of the threads still remained adhering to the side of the wound. *Mr. Thomson's experiments.*

pleased to find that the ligatures had passed from the outer to the inner side of the intestine, and that they had been discharged by stool, he determined to repeat the experiment, and to give a longer time to learn the result of it more completely.

EXPERIMENT II.

In a full grown dog the first experiment was repeated, five stitches only being put in the intestine. The dog was killed at the end of six weeks.

On opening the abdomen he could see no distinct mark of division in the intestinal canal; but upon cutting out a piece and inverting it, he found two stitches still adhering to its inner side. He could also perceive, as in the former case, but less distinctly, the marks made by the stitches which had disappeared.

It appears then, by these experiments, that in the animals which were the subject of them, not only the intestine may be returned into the cavity of the abdomen, but the ligatures which are applied upon it; and that no apprehension need be entertained of these ligatures being separated into the cavity to produce the inflammatory effects of extraneous bodies.

Treatment of the divided intestine.

However, as the protruded parts in hernia are so much inflamed as to endanger a speedy separation of the ligatures; and, as it appears by the first experiments which I have related, that the animal did not suffer from the ligature hanging from the abdomen; I should still prefer performing the operation of uniting the divided intestine, in such a manner as to give an opportunity of extracting the ligatures, if any inconveniences arose from their application.

The practice, therefore, which ought to be followed in an intestine divided by mortification, is to cut off its mortified extremities, and then to pass four stitches through them, one at the mesentery, and the three others at equal distances round the intestine. Then returning it to the mouth of the hernial sac, which should be opened higher up than usual, it must be there firmly confined by a ligature being passed through the mesentery, in the manner already directed. If stools pass the ligatures, and the patient goes on well, the ligatures may remain untill they are thrown off by ulceration; but if there are no stools, and the patient suffers from a distended abdomen, three of the stitches should be cut away, leaving that which attaches the intestine to the hernial sac, as well as that which joins its edges at the mesentery. The fæces can then readily escape at the external wound; and as granulations arise, and the wound heals, the mouths of the divided intestine will become united, so that the fæces will take their natural course, as they did in the case which I have related, where many inches of the intestine sloughed.

The necessity of having the ligatures within reach, so as to enable the surgeon to remove them if they do not answer the purpose of restoring the natural course of the fæces, is evinced by the result of the following case, which was sent me by my friend Dr. Cheston of Glocester, whose superior talents and extensive information are too well known to require any panegyric from me. This case also points out a curious fact respecting the absorbent power of the intestine.

CASE.

Dr. Cheston's case.

In the month of July, 1794, I was called to a young man twenty-two years of age, who had, for six days, laboured under a strangulated hernia of the right groin; the symptoms of which had been for five days so mild, that they had not excited sufficient alarm at his danger.

In the state in which I then found him, of constant sickness, tight belly, extreme soreness of the tumour, without any evacuation per anum for the above mentioned period, I could not but consider him in the most imminent danger, and therefore urged the necessity of an operation, without any further delay.

Mr. Nayler, one of the surgeons of our County Hospital, was then sent for to perform it, and proceeding with that caution which an experienced and dexterous operator ever does on such occasions, he divided the sac, which he found without any fluid whatever, closely embracing a considerable portion of the ilium, which, with the sac, was in a gangrenous state.

On endeavouring to separate, in the most tender manner, the gut from its adhesions, it unfortunately burst, and its contents immediately escaped. Perceiving, however, the intended separation, and having at last effected it so as to draw out the whole of the diseased part, with a sufficient portion of the mesentery, near four inches of the intestine were found so completely destroyed as to require removal; which, with that of the gangrenous portion of the sac, was accordingly done, under such further intentions as circumstances must warrant, most likely to serve the patient in this most deplorable situation.

The first thought which occurred, was the truly pitiable state to which the patient would be reduced in the event of his recovery, by having an artificial anus. Desiring therefore, if possible, to avoid such a composition for existence, we agreed to bring the gut together by the usual recommendation of gastroraphy. This being effected, and to guard against any ill consequences on the failure of the intention, from a retraction of the intestine into the cavity of the abdomen, two stitches were passed through the mesentery on each side of the divided intestine, and secured to the parietes of the wound. In this manner the operation was finished, and the patient being properly dressed was removed to his bed, when an emollient glyster was thrown up, and cloths moistened with spirits applied over the abdomen. He was ordered an opiate, and directed to take food sparingly of the lightest kind.

As the patient lived fifteen miles from Gloucester, he was left under the immediate care of his attending surgeon, an able and experienced practitioner, to act as circumstances might require; at the same time it was proposed, that Mr. Nayler should visit him again on the morrow evening.

On his arrival he found the young man by no means benefited by the operation. No evacuations had passed by stool, his belly was rather more distended, he was equally sick as before, and now and then teased with hiccough. In this alarming state Mr. Nayler thought it necessary to remove the dressing for the inspection of the part, when observing the wound to bear a very unhealthy aspect, he thought it necessary to remove the stitches on the intestine, bringing its open extremities just without the edges of the wound, to allow of an easy discharge of air or fæces contained in the superior part of the canal *.

In the course of the night, when he appeared almost expiring, a sudden and violent discharge of air and fæces burst forth from the wound in immense quantity, to his immediate relief. His pulse rose, a comfortable warmth succeeded, his stomach became settled, and his hiccough left him; in short, every prospect brightened, and from that day each symptom became more promising.

On the tenth day the parts looked so well and healthy, that Mr. Nayler, hoping there was still a possibility of diverting this most loathsome evacuation from the groin into its natural channel by another attempt to procure an union of the divided portion, once more brought the extremities together by suture. Unfortunately this likewise failed in the extent proposed, most of the stitches giving way to the continual pressure to which they were exposed.

One advantage, however, and that eventually a material one, was thereby gained, an union being effected at the sides of the intestine, so that the sections there consolidated formed an appearance very similar to that of a double-barrelled gun. Notwithstanding this partial union of the intestines the fæces still continued to pass wholly through the wound, till the patient accidentally having made a slight pressure upon the part, he soon afterwards felt a sort of natural inclination for a stool, which, encouraging by the usual efforts, he passed off to his great joy.

It instantly occurred to him, that probably a similar pressure, by compress and bandage, might assist him in future, so as to gain the power of a natural discharge.

This expedient most fortunately answered, and I received the greatest pleasure by the information from Mr. Nayler that he had a daily discharge of fæces and wind per anum, and that he was now become so expert in the application of his bandage, that he could prevent any escape of fæces by the wound, however liquid they might be.

As it now became desirable to assist him with some better and more manageable contrivance, he was accordingly supplied with a truss, whose pad fully made the desired pressure, and completely answered the purpose.

From the time of the operation the wound underwent very considerable changes. At first, from the patient's being quiet in bed making little or no exertion of the abdominal muscles, it remained on a level with the surface of the integuments; but when he began to give his body more motion, the wound sunk inwards,

* Qr. Might it not be proper, upon any such occasion, to allow some time for the escape of any accumulation above the divided part?

or became deeper, and the extremities of the intestine returned likewise; so that they appeared at the bottom of a sulcus, forming near half a cylinder of a full inch in diameter.

He was now enabled to move about as usual, to take greater liberties in his exercises and amusements, to walk about his grounds, or get on his horse, without any restraint or inconvenience whatever. In this state having a call to London, I wished him to meet me there, as well to shew his case to Mr. Cline and Dr. Babington, as that he might derive any assistance from their well-known abilities. The result, however, of this meeting, was their surprise at his extraordinary and unfortunate state, and an acknowledgement that they knew no plan more promising than that he was then following.

At this time the appearances of the part were singularly curious. The upper portion of the intestine, in its action of protruding its contents, shewed that approximation of its internal surface which may have been frequently observed in the expulsion from the rectum of a horse of the last remaining fæces; but which was, in this instance, thrown forward with such a degree of projectile force as to clear the edge of the upper portion of intestine, whilst the inferior mouth was in that kind of relaxation or diastole as to form a temporary cavity for its reception and absorption; when immediately closing again, nothing more was seen of what it had received; so regularly and promptly did these divided parts continue to act, and most probably perform their functions, according to their original powers and peristaltic motion.

The above process was, however, only to be seen when the supply from the upper portion of the gut was rather scanty; for when (which was frequently to be observed) an increased quantity of fæces was brought forward which the inferior portion could not receive, some, consequently, overflowed; but the manner in which it went on under cover, proved the assistance it received either from pressure, or the formation of an artificial canal.

M. Ramdohr's proposal.

Under a complete division of the intestine it has been recommended by M. Ramdohr to put the upper extremity of the intestine within the lower, and to confine it there by ligature; but besides the difficulty of knowing in a hernia which is the upper and which the lower part of the intestine, I find, by experiments on living animals, that it is impracticable. Some years ago I divided the intestine of a dog, with a view of trying to introduce the one intestine within the other; but I had no sooner made the division than the intestine inverted, and became so bulbous at each extremity, that I found it impossible to pass one within the other; and that this also takes place in the human subject, is proved by a preparation of wounded intestine, in the Museum at St. Thomas's Hospital, taken from a man who had been kicked by a horse. The jejunum was ruptured, and it appears inverted.

Large lateral opening.

If the intestine has a large opening in its side, occupying one half of its cylinder, it is, if left to nature, sure to produce an artificial anus. Sufficient of the intestine is not then remaining to conduct the fæces in their proper channel. The wound heals so as to form an orifice sufficiently large to permit the escape of that portion of the fæces which the intestine cannot convey, and if it heals further than to that point, abscesses frequently form, which when they burst, discharge with the matter a considerable quantity of fæces.

Case.

This is evinced by the case of a Mrs. S—, in Duke-street, Smithfield, whom I have frequently attended on account of a hernia of the ventral kind, from which a portion of intestine has sloughed. The wound has since several times healed; but at the interval of a month, and sometimes of six weeks, an abscess forms, and produces a discharge of purulent and fæculent matter for four or five days, when the wound again closes; and in this way she has been teased for many years.

If the wound in the integuments is small, and the intestine has more than half its cylinder, it would be naturally supposed easy to unite it, and cases of success are related; but in the instances in which I have known it attempted, it has not been attended with success. In a former part of this work, I mentioned an instance of a boy who had an artificial anus in the scrotum, produced by swallowing a pin, which made its way from the hernia through the scrotum. In this lad the edges of the wound were pared and brought together by suture, but still they did not show any disposition to unite, and no advantage was derived from the operation.

Cases.

I also attended a lady who had an umbilical hernia, which had sloughed and left a small fistulous orifice, which Mr. Cruickshank endeavoured to unite, by passing stitches through the wound after paring its edges; but this attempt brought on, in four days, such symptoms of pain and tension of the abdomen, with constipation of the bowels, that he withdrew the threads, and a very large quantity of fæculent matter issued, by the discharge of which she became immediately relieved.

As it appears, therefore, that there is little probability of relief to the patient when this state is once established, the surgeon should attempt, by all the means in his power, to prevent its occurrence.

The means which will occur to the mind as being most likely to effect this object, will probably be to make an uninterrupted suture upon the opening in the intestine; but this treatment would leave the intestine with only half its cylinder, the fæces will not pass, they will either soon burst the stitches from the wound, or it will become necessary for the surgeon to cut them to unload the intestine, and prevent the death of his patient. *Treatment of.*

There is a curious difference in the facility with which a longitudinal and transverse wound of the intestine unite. It has been already shown, that the transverse heal readily; but with respect to the longitudinal, they have a contrary tendency. Mr. Thompson, whose name I have already mentioned, made the following experiments, the result of which will be found extremely curious.

EXPERIMENT I.

Exposing the intestine of a dog, he made an incision into it of an inch and an half in length, in a line opposite to, and parallel with the mesentery. The cut edges were brought together by four stitches, which were cut away close to the knots by which they were tied, and the intestine was returned into the belly. *Mr. Thompson's experiments.*

The dog became uneasy in the evening, and continued so the next day. The belly became tense, and he shewed an aversion to food; and in less than forty-eight hours he died.

Upon opening the abdomen strong marks of peritoneal inflammation were apparent, and a quantity of fluid was found consisting in part of exudation from the inflamed surface, and in part of the contents of the intestinal canal. The edges of the wound were torn open. One of the stitches had disappeared, but the three others remained, each adhering to one side of the wound.

EXPERIMENT II.

He repeated the foregoing experiment, and, to prevent the escape of the fæces, sewed up the interstices between the interrupted stitches with a fine thread. This dog, like the former, soon became uneasy and restless, the belly became tense, and he died in less than forty-eight hours from the experiment. The appearances, upon opening the abdomen, were the same as in the former experiment. The circular marginal fibres of the intestine had torn open the wound, and had detached the continued as well as the interrupted stitches.

This experiment, although it produces a greater degree of constitutional irritation than sewing the intestine after a complete division of it, does not always destroy the animal, as the following experiment proves.

EXPERIMENT.

Saturday, January 14, I made a longitudinal incision of one inch and an half into the small intestine of a dog, and then having sewed the edges of the wound together with great care by an uninterrupted suture, I cut off the ligature close to the intestine, and returned it into the abdomen. In twenty-four hours after this experiment the animal was so ill as to make his recovery doubtful; but in forty-eight hours he was much better, and able to take food. From that time he recovered quickly, running about the house and taking whatever was offered to him. On the seventh day I killed him, and found, upon examining the abdomen, the intestines glued together so as to prevent my seeing the ligature upon the outer side of the intestine; but upon cutting them open, I found the thread loosely adhering to the edges of the wound, but the knot which I had made upon the outside was hanging on the inner side of the bowel. The intestine was uninflamed upon its internal surface, and the lacteals were loaded with chyle. Although this animal did not die from the experiment, it was certainly in greater danger, and suffered more, than in that in which the intestine was divided, and it requires much greater care to perfectly close the longitudinal wound than is necessary in the transverse.

Treatment.   These experiments greatly assist in elucidating the treatment of the mortified intestine in hernia. Instead of endeavouring to maintain a diminished canal by sewing the intestine longitudinally, the surgeon should not only cut out the mortified part, but all the remaining part of the cylinder of the intestine, and then approximating the extremities of the intestine, he should endeavour to unite it in the manner in which a transverse division of the intestine is treated, by making four sutures upon it, and confining it by means of the mesentery to the mouth of the hernial sac.

CHAPTER XII.

Of the Treatment after the Return of the protruded Parts.

When the operator has returned the protruded contents of the hernial sac, he should clear it of any blood which it may contain, and bring the edges of the wound together, confining them by two sutures. The needle and ligature should only be passed through the integuments, and great care should be taken to avoid penetrating the sac, which might occasion a dangerous extension of the inflammation. A piece of lint should then be laid on the wound, with a compress of linen over it, and these pressed pretty firmly down upon the groin by the T bandage, so as to close the orifice of the hernial sac. *Dressings.*

The patient is then to be carried to bed in an horizontal posture, and whilst this is doing, the surgeon should support the wounded part with the palm of his hand, to prevent the intestine from again falling down.

It is usual, immediately after the operation, when the patient is laid on his bed, to give him a dose of opium, with a view of procuring him sleep after his sufferings. But when a person has been for many hours in violent pain, with constant vomiting and perpetual watchfulness, a sudden removal of his sufferings will generally be followed in a few minutes by profound sleep, without the use of opium; and this medicine becomes, in this case, not only useless, but positively detrimental, as it occasions a torpor of the bowels, and prevents their ready evacuation. The patient, if left to himself, will have natural stools in two or three hours after being put to bed, unless the parts have suffered a very high degree of inflammation; but this will always happen much later after opium has been given; and its use is therefore to be avoided, if possible, since the patient is never completely relieved till the bowels are unloaded. *Opium.*

If several hours elapse without an evacuation, a purgative glyster should be given, composed of Magnesia Vitriolata, Infusum Sennæ, and a large quantity of liquid, as warm as the patient can bear it. If this does not succeed, they may be followed by the Oleum Ricini; but no purgatives should be used, till it appears probable that stools cannot be procured without them. Spirituous fomentations to the abdomen will assist the natural action of the bowels. *Purges.*

It sometimes happens that the vomiting continues for some time after the operation, notwithstanding the patient has had stools. This arises from an extreme irritability of the stomach which still remains, and under these circumstances opium becomes absolutely necessary to remove it. *Vomiting.*

In like manner opium sometimes is required to remove a troublesome cough which comes on after the operation; it both prevents the patient from taking rest, and endangers a return of the protrusion by the sudden pressure on the abdominal contents. *Cough.*

The patient must be particularly enjoined on no account to move from the horizontal posture during cure, particularly whilst having stools, otherwise the intestine will be very liable again to descend. Of this the following case is an instance. A gentleman, who had just undergone the operation, having had no injunction as to posture, was found by his surgeon on the evening of the same day sitting upon the night-chair, and straining violently. On examining the hernia, it was found that the intestine had not only forced its way again into the sac, but had passed between the ligatures so as to project through its interstices beyond the external wound. It was again returned, and the patient did well. *Horizontal posture preserved.*

The wound should be dressed on the third day, and every day afterwards. If much inflammation comes on, or the hernia is large, the scrotum must be supported by a small cushion, and fomentations and poultices applied.

The ligatures should be drawn away on the fifth day, unless a high degree of inflammation renders it necessary to remove them earlier. After this the cure proceeds as in a common wound, only the patient should be kept in bed till it is complete. *Sutures withdrawn.*

If the operation has not been too long postponed, the patient's recovery is generally regularly progressive; but if much time has elapsed, various dangerous syptoms arise.

First. The intestine sometimes does not recover its function, the vomiting and constipation continue, and the patient falls a victim to the disease.

Secondly. If inflammation continues in the peritoneum, and the abdomen remains tense and sore although stools can be procured, the disease proceeds until the patient dies; and upon examination the intestines are found glued together and greatly distended with flatus. This state must be prevented by bleeding, fomentation, leeches to the abdomen, and purges.

Thirdly. A violent purging sometimes succeeds, and continues for many days, which exhausts the patient's strength so as to prevent his recovery. Under these circumstances, small and repeated doses of opium, with glysters of starch and opium, and feeding the patient with isinglass and milk, is the practice I have known to answer best in stopping this disease.

Fourthly. In a very irritable person tetanus will sometimes occur when every other circumstance appears favourable. This happened in a case of Mr. Spry's, Surgeon, in Aldersgate-street. He operated upon a man of the name of Ashby, aged fifty years, who had a hernia which became strangulated on the twenty-third of December, 1803, and which resisted every attempt to reduce it, made by himself and by Dr. Yelloly. On the twenty-fifth the operation was performed in the most satisfactory manner. By the eighth day after the operation the wound was healed, excepting at one small spot; but upon the morning of that day he complained of stiffness and soreness about the neck, with a difficulty in swallowing, and the jaw became soon completely locked. Opium and the cold bath were tried with some slight temporary abatement of the symptoms, but without any permanent advantage, and the man soon fell a victim to the disease.

Hernia returns.

When the patient has recovered from the operation, he is still, as before, exposed to a descent of the hernia; and more indeed than at first, as the division by the knife must have enlarged the aperture into the abdomen. I have now under my care in Guy's Hospital, a man who, twenty years ago, was the subject of operation for strangulated hernia, and he has now again this complaint on the same side. A truss must therefore be always applied after the cure, before the patient can be allowed to walk about and return to his usual occupation. A man who lived opposite the gates of St. Thomas's Hospital, had the operation of strangulated hernia performed on him many years ago, and on his cure the surgeon warned him of the necessity of wearing a truss to prevent future danger. But having neglected this caution, two years afterwards he was again seized with symptoms of strangulation, and anxious to avoid the operation, he tried every means to reduce the hernia without effect, and at last he only sent for a surgeon when his approaching death made it useless to perform the operation. On opening his body, I found the hernia strangulated in the former sac.

Truss necessary.

Hence it becomes absolutely necessary that the surgeon should see his patient fitted with a proper truss, to prevent him from future danger.

It is also proper that the patient should be confined to his bed until the wound is healed, that the adhesions which form in the sac may acquire considerable firmness before he exposes himself to the danger of a future descent; and he should not quit the horizontal posture without a truss, which must have a compress of linen under it, to prevent its injuring the recently healed wound.

Sac removed.

As, therefore, the operation itself only removes the present disease, and does not effect a radical cure, some surgical writers, to accomplish this end, have proposed the cutting away, or tying, the hernial sac during the operation, or returning it into the cavity of the abdomen. To ascertain the effect of cutting away the sac, I took the following opportunity in a favourable case that occurred: A woman of the name of Bispham, a patient of Mr. Holt's, of Tottenham, had for many years a femoral hernia, which, in the summer of 1801, became very painful, without, however, interrupting the regular course of her bowels, and confined her to her bed on account of the extreme pain she felt upon attempting to put her leg to the ground. Having remained several days in this state, incapable of using any exertion for her maintenance, Mr. Holt requested me to see her. I made several fruitless attempts to reduce the hernia, and a week afterwards, as the pain and inability to move still continued, I advised the operation, which Mr. Holt performed. When he had opened the sac a minute portion of intestine was found just at the mouth of the sac, adhering to it firmly, and inflamed, but not gangrenous. It was so small a portion of the circumference of the intestine that the fæces were able to pass it, and therefore no constipation was produced by this partial strangulation; but it became painfully compressed at every attempt to extend the thigh, which was the cause of the inability to move. Mr. H. with great care separated the adhesions, and returned the intestine into the cavity of the abdomen. As the hernial sac was large, and had been considerably detached from the surrounding parts during the operation, I thought it would be a very favourable opportunity of trying what would be the effect of removing it, and requested Mr. Holt to permit me to do it. I dissected away the whole of the sac, which was easily done; then passed stiches through its mouth so as to bring the edges into perfect contact. The ligatures were drawn out of the external wound, which was treated in the usual way. On the sixth day the ligatures came away, and the wound was healed on the tenth. A month afterwards I saw the woman, and was surprized to find that another hernia had formed on the same spot, which was already as large as that for which the operation had been performed. She came to request a truss, finding that on every attempt at exertion she felt a powerful forcing-down in the tumour, which was also rapidly increasing in size. I saw her again two years afterwards, at which time, immediately on removing the truss, which had been worn ever since the operation, the hernia freely descended.

It appears, therefore, that the removal of the sac will not prevent a return of the disease; and, indeed, when it is recollected that the aperture from the abdomen continues of the same size after, as before the operation, and that the peritoneum will still remain the only obstacle to the descent of the intestine, it does not appear probable that this highly extensible membrane should succeed in preventing a return of the same hernia, the first formation of which it was unable to resist. *Does not succeed.*

The plan of making a ligature round the mouth of the hernial sac has been also recommended, and in some instances adopted; but it is liable to so many objections, particularly in the inguinal hernia, that it is never likely to come into general practice. The sole intention of this operation is gradually to cut away the sac, but I have just shown that this would be insufficient to produce a cure, could it even be done with perfect safety to the patient. But it cannot even be securely done, for, *Tying the sac.*

First, the spermatic cord is often divided by the sac, so that one part of it passes behind, and the other before, or on the side of the sac. When this happens, it would be extremely difficult, if not impossible, to conduct the operation in such a manner as to avoid injuring parts which should never be touched.

Secondly, this operation is founded on mistaken ideas of the hernial sac; for a ligature applied as proposed, at the abdominal ring, if it cut through the sac, must leave a hernia above it, with a sac still open as before; and the ligature cannot be employed to the part of the sac lying above the ring without splitting up the tendon of the external oblique muscle, which would take off so much of the natural support of the parts as almost certainly to allow of a future descent.

Thirdly, the danger of the operation is besides a principal objection. A ligature applied around a part of the peritoneum must inflame it, and as this membrane is continued without interruption along the sac into the cavity of the abdomen, the inflammation will follow the same course, and expose the patient's life to hazard. Extended surfaces very rapidly propagate inflammation, as we see in the skin under erysipelas, or in the veins and absorbent vessels when inflamed; but if the surface is broken by adhesion, the inflammation extends only to the adhering part, and there stops. Thus, when a ligature is applied round the spermatic cord in the operation of removing the testicle, the inflammation thereby excited does not extend into the abdomen, because the tunica vaginalis of the cord is closed by adhesions. In animals where that is not the case, the disease takes a more extensive range, as will be seen in the following example:—A surgeon, who thought he could castrate a horse much better than a farrier, who employs red-hot irons to burn off the spermatic cord and seer the vessels, persuaded a friend of his to allow him to castrate a fine young horse. He cut down upon the cord, made a ligature around it which stopped the bleeding, and proceeded to remove the testicle, as it is done in the human subject. However, in four days the animal died; and on opening the body it was found that the inflammation produced by the ligature had extended along the tunica vaginalis (which in the horse is open to the abdomen) into the cavity of the belly, so that the animal died of peritoneal inflammation. Petit has noticed the danger incurred by tying the hernial sac; in one case the pain was so great after this operation, that he was obliged to cut away the ligature to check the inflammation which was spreading into the abdomen; in another case where this practice was pursued, symptoms of strangulation came on, and the patient died. On inspecting the body the peritoneum was found inflamed, both where it lines the abdomen and where it covers the intestines.

<small>Returning the sac.</small>

With respect to returning the sac into the abdomen, that is in a large hernia often impracticable, and the only use attending it, will be in those cases in which adhesions have, to a great extent, taken place between the intestine and the hernial sac, where it will be more easy to return the intestine and sac with it, than to remove the adhesions; but of this I shall treat farther in the Chapter on Small Herniæ.

CHAPTER XIII.

Of very large Hernia.

WHEN an inguinal hernia is very large, and especially when, at the same time, there is reason to believe that the parts which it contains adhere to the inner side of the hernial sac, a different operation is required to that which has just been described as applicable to common circumstances; and for the following reasons: Require a different treatment.

First, in very large old hernia, the cavity of the abdomen is so much diminished by the habitual loss of the protruded intestine and omentum, that it becomes scarcely able to receive them again; and, if a reduction is attempted, the force necessary to effect it endangers the bursting of the intestine.

This happened in a case that occurred at St. Thomas's Hospital, an engraving of which is seen in Plate X. fig. 3. The hernia was very large, and the diminished size of the abdomen made it necessary to use great efforts in the reduction, during which the intestine burst, and the man died five days afterwards.

Secondly, a large surface of the intestine is exposed and handled for so long a time as to produce, even if it does not give way, the risk of an inflammation, which will probably be attended with fatal consequences.

Thirdly, even if by great pains the intestine be returned, it is scarcely possible to keep it in the now over-distended abdomen, so that the slightest cough or effort of any kind is sufficient to bring it again down into the sac, and thus to induce a high and dangerous inflammation.

Lastly, when great adhesion occurs, so much time is necessarily required in performing the operation to separate the united surfaces, that fears may be justly entertained of the patient not surviving the operation. It has been recommended, under these circumstances, to dissect the sac from the surrounding parts, and to return it into the cavity of the abdomen after the stricture has been removed; but although this operation is practicable in small hernia, it becomes extremely dangerous in one that is large, connected as it is with the spermatic cord, and sometimes splitting the vessels which compose it.

Hence, in these cases, I would advise only the division of the abdominal ring; or, if the stricture is higher up, of the lower edge of the transversalis muscle; but not the opening of the hernial sac, unless the stricture is situated in the sac itself. Division of the stricture only.

The following case will shew the advantage of this practice in this variety of the disease. Charles Beegey, aged fifty-four years, was admitted into St. Thomas's Hospital, on Friday, the 4th of February 1803, for a strangulated hernia. He had been subject to the disease from his earliest years, and it had been produced by a bruise on the pummel of a saddle. It had always been in a great degree reducible, but not entirely so; for whenever he had emptied the sac as much as he could, something might still be perceived to remain within it. On Monday, January 31st, it became painful whilst he was at work, and could not be in any degree reduced; and almost at the same moment he was seized with the sensation of colic, and with vomiting. Case.

Tuesday, February 1st, all the symptoms were increased; he had had a small stool, but not more than could well be supposed to come from the large intestines below the stricture; which was the more probable, as it afforded him no relief. On Wednesday, Thursday, and Friday, the symptoms continued to increase, and he was then admitted into the Hospital. Mr. Birch, whose patient he was, being absent, I was requested to see him.

The tumour was of an enormous size, reaching halfway to the knees; it was hard, and painful on pressure. The abdomen was hard and tense, though but little painful. He was sick, and occasionally vomited, and had had no stool since Tuesday. Many attempts were made to reduce the hernia, but without success; and his situation was such, as to leave no hopes of preserving his life but by an operation; but even this alternative appeared desperate, on considering his age, the size of the swelling, and the adhesion which its contents had contracted. To these discouraging circumstances was added the presence of an habitual cough, which would render it almost impossible to keep the parts in the abdomen when returned. I therefore resolved, before opening the sac, to ascertain whether it were practicable to perform the operation of cutting the ring and the parts above it, and returning the reducible portion without exposing it.

With this view I made an incision, three inches in length, immediately over the abdominal ring, exposing it with the knife, as well as the fascia which it sends off. I then made a hole in the fascia large enough to introduce a director, which I thrust up behind the abdominal ring, between it and the hernial sac; and passing a curved probe-pointed bistory upon it I divided the ring. I then introduced my finger, and feeling some resistance from the transversalis, I carried the bistory upon the director up to it, and divided this also. I was immediately gratified with finding that a slight pressure was now sufficient to return into the cavity of the abdomen all the protruded part, which did not adhere, and it went up with a guggling noise as soon as my hand was laid upon the tumour. The man was soon relieved of his pain, and the edges of the wound being brought together, he was put to bed.

On visiting him about sixteen hours after the operation, I felt happy at having performed it in the manner above described, as I found him free from every symptom of strangulation, and scarcely suffering from the wound; but what convinced me of the propriety of the practice which I had pursued, was to find that whenever he coughed, the tumour again increased largely in size, and, though easily reducible, the intestine again descended at the next fit of coughing, nor could any endurable degree of pressure on the wound keep it supported. Although under these circumstances this descent was of no importance, yet if the sac had been opened the continual irritation kept upon its exposed contents, must probably have been followed with fatal consequences. As it was, he had no bad symptom; in a week he could bear the application of a laced truss, like that which I have described to be used for large irreducible hernia, and in three weeks the wound was perfectly healed.

Case.

The following unsuccessful case, in which an opposite practice was pursued, will equally illustrate the advantage of the plan above recommended. I was desired by Mr. Johnson, Surgeon, of Swan-street, Minories, to see a patient of his, a lady sixty-eight years of age, who had long suffered under an irreducible ventral hernia of enormous size, which was now strangulated. As various unsuccessful attempts had been made to return the parts, the operation was proposed, to which the patient consented. When the sac was opened, the omentum and intestine were found adhering both to it and to each other, so as to make a return of the protruded parts absolutely impracticable; and the sac itself was too large to allow of its being separated from the surrounding integuments and returned into the abdomen. I therefore had to regret that I had opened the sac. All that could be done was to dilate the stricture, and to bring the integuments closely together, confining them by sutures, so as to close the hernial sac. The symptoms of vomiting and pain in the abdomen immediately ceased, and she had a passage through the bowels. However, on the succeeding day inflammation took place in the integuments and hernial sac, the abdomen became very tender, and in thirty-seven hours after the operation she died.

If I had, in this case, performed the operation without dividing the sac, merely by dilating the stricture, the patient's life would probably have been saved.

Dr. Monro, of Edinburgh, to whom it would be ingratitude not to acknowledge the obligation I feel for the instructions conveyed in his lectures, has strongly urged the propriety of dilating the abdominal ring without opening the sac, in hernia in general; and I feel convinced that this operation will be gradually introduced into general practice when it has been fairly tried, and found, if performed early, to be free from danger, and attended with no unusual difficulty.

Objections.

It has been objected to this practice, that if there is a probability of the intestine being mortified, it does not afford the means of ascertaining it, or of relief, if this state of the bowel exists. This objection is certainly well founded, when, from the duration of the disease, there is reason to suspect this event to have happened; but still the operation in which the sac is not opened may be employed with safety, in those cases where the surgeon is convinced, from his general experience, that if a reduction by the tobacco glyster, or any simple means, could be brought about, the parts would resume their healthy functions.

It is also objected, that this operation would not apply to those cases in which the stricture is at the mouth of the sac occasioned by a thickening of the sac itself. But to this I would answer, that this is not so frequent an occurrence as has been imagined, the stricture above the ring on the outer part of the sac having been frequently mistaken for it, as I have explained in a former part of this work. But even if the stricture has arisen from a thickening of the sac, a division of the parts on the outside of the sac would expose the patient to no danger, and would even be a necessary step to take in the dilatation of the part where the stricture existed.

Lastly, against the objection that, in case of adhesion of the contents of the sac, this operation would leave the patient with an irreducible hernia, I would contend that this very adhesion ought to be a strong inducement not to open the sac, on account of the great additional risk to life which such a proceeding would produce.

CHAPTER XIV.

Of small Inguinal Hernia.

Hernia between the ring and abdomen.
HERNIÆ sometimes become strangulated when they are so small as to protrude no lower than within the space lying between the abdominal ring and the upper aperture at which the spermatic cord first quits the abdomen. An example of a hernia in this state will be seen in Plate III, V, and VI.

Its covering.
This hernia is covered with the tendon of the external oblique muscle: the spermatic cord, and the epigastric artery lie behind it; Poupart's ligament below it; and the internal oblique, and transverse muscles, extend above it in a semicircular direction. In short it is the two first inches of inguinal hernia.

Difficult to detect.
An attentive examination is requisite in the living subject to detect it, as it does not exhibit that detached circumscribed tumour which is produced by the hernia after it has passed the ring, but appears merely as a fulness above the ring and Poupart's ligament. When strangulated it is very sore on pressure, and coughing produces much pain. Before strangulation comes on the patient is sensible of a weakness at the part under every exertion.

Very frequent.
This tumour occurs much more commonly than is usually supposed, for I have frequently found it in the dissection of bodies of persons who have never been suspected of labouring under the disease, nor have ever worn a truss. When strangulated these cases more commonly fall under the care of the physician than the surgeon; for, as the patient himself is often not conscious of having a tumour at the groin, the symptoms of strangulation are ascribed to inflammation of the bowels, and the patient dies, as is supposed, of iliac passion.

Case.
A man was admitted into St. Thomas's Hospital with symptoms of strangulated hernia, which for five days had been treated as a case of simple inflammation of the bowels, without a suspicion of the true cause having been excited.

On examination, a fulness could be perceived above Poupart's ligament, and when this was compressed, a small tumour, like the end of the little finger, appeared at the abdominal ring, which again receded to its former place, on withdrawing the pressure. Pain was felt at the same time, and on coughing much uneasiness was produced at that spot.

As five days had elapsed between the first accession of the symptoms, and his admission into the Hospital, the performance of an operation afforded but little prospect of success; for, besides vomiting, he had a hiccough for forty hours, his belly was sore on pressure, and his pulse so small as scarcely to be distinguishable. However, as it was the only possible chance for recovery, the operation was undertaken. On cutting down to the tumour, it was found to be produced by a hernial sac an inch and a half long, and when this was opened, about half the circumference of one of the small intestines was found to be contained within it, together with a quantity of sanious serum. The stricture which existed an inch and a half above the abdominal ring was then divided. The intestine was discoloured, but the point of the knife having accidentally touched one of its superficial veins, blood issued from it freely, proving that the bowel was in a fit state to be returned; which was accordingly done as soon as the bleeding ceased. The patient had stools in twelve hours, and, although he afterwards suffered from a severe purging, he ultimately recovered.

Operation for it.
In this variety of hernia the operation should be performed in the following manner. The incision is to be begun over the tumour, half way between the symphisis pubis and the spinous process of the ilium, and extended downwards parallel to Poupart's ligament, as low as the abdominal ring. This incision, which only divides the integuments, exposes the tendon of the external oblique muscle, which being next cut through in the same direction, without cutting the abdominal ring, the hernial sac comes in view, extending from the abdominal ring to the opening at which the spermatic cord quits the abdomen. The sac is then to be opened in the manner described in a former chapter, and the intestine examined. A probe-pointed bistory being then introduced behind the stricture which is formed by the tendon of the transversalis, this is to be divided in an

upward direction. In this case, however, it is of little consequence whether the stricture be divided straight upwards, or outwards and upwards, towards the ilium; as the epigastric artery, to avoid which the straight-upward direction has been recommended in a former chapter, is in this variety of hernia on the inner side of the hernial sac. But for the same reason a direction of the incision inwards or towards the pubis, must always be carefully avoided; and to prevent any doubt at the time of the operation, the incision upward at the middle of the mouth of the sac will be the most proper.

After this operation, as this part of the abdominal parietes is weakened by the division of the tendon, a truss must be put on as soon as possible.

It has been proposed to return into the abdomen the hernial sac, without opening it. For this purpose the stricture is first to be divided, the intestine and omentum returned from it if possible, and the sac is then to be pushed into the cavity of the abdomen.

In a very small hernia this operation is practicable, because the sac has then contracted no strong adhesion to the surrounding parts, and it can be also readily done in the female; but if the hernia is comparatively large, it cannot be effected without much dissection, which in inguinal hernia in the male could not be always safely performed, on account of the frequent varieties in the course of the spermatic cord, the vessels of which in large herniæ are always more or less turned from their usual course. *Sac returned.*

As there would be often much difficulty in executing this part of the operation, it will be best to push back the contents only, without attempting to return the sac, as the patient is equally liable to a future protrusion, although the sac is returned, as the following case will prove.

Mr. Weld, jun. Surgeon at Romford, was called on May the twenty-fourth last, to a woman of the name of Moore, in that place, who laboured under symptoms of strangulated hernia, proceeding from a tumour of this description at the abdominal ring. All attempts to reduce the hernia having failed of success, the operation was performed of cutting down upon the tumour, separating it from its adhesions, and dividing the stricture which was at the abdominal ring. The sac and its contents were then returned into the cavity of the abdomen, as there was no reason to suspect the existence of mortification. The wound healed in the space of a fortnight, and the woman recovered. *Case.*

This operation was so far completely successful, and does Mr. Weld great credit; but he has since written to inform me, that the hernia has reappeared, as the woman would not wear a truss upon a part, which was still tender from the operation. However she experiences no inconvenience from it, as it can be now readily returned into the cavity of the abdomen. As it appears, therefore, that the return of the sac into the abdomen will not be attended with a radical cure, if there is any danger from the size of the tumour, or from the position of the spermatic vessels, it is an attempt which should not be made unless the intestine adheres, and it ought never to be done under any circumstances, unless the sac is first either emptied of its contents, or the stricture is clearly divided, as there is danger of the symptoms of strangulation continuing, if the mouth of the sac is contracted and it remains undilated. *Objections.*

I shall conclude this chapter with an account of a highly interesting case, which has been sent to me by my friend Mr. Thomas Blizard, under whose care the patient was. The disease was a small hernia, which descended behind the spermatic cord, and the person also laboured under a hydrocele of the tunica vaginalis testis. The following is Mr. Blizard's account of the case. *Hernia behind the spermatic cord.*

CASE.

A man was admitted into the London Hospital, who had been troubled with a bubonocele of the right side upwards of six years, during which period he had almost constantly worn a truss. About two years ago a swelling took place in the testis of the same side, which he describes to have been similar to a swelling he now has on the left side, which is a hydrocele. That swelling in a few months gradually disappeared, and left the testis wasted and drawn up towards the groin. This is the man's account.

When first called to him I found a small bubonocele of the right side, and could distinctly feel the testis of the same side, but very small, lying at the bottom of the hernia, having an inclination forwards. The means employed for reduction having failed, at the expiration of about twenty hours from the descent I performed the operation. Having dissected down to a membrane, which I considered to be the hernial sac, I punctured it at the upper part, and then laid it open its whole length. It extended within the ring, which, to obtain room for examination, I dilated. Upon further enquiry I found the hernia was seated more deeply, and that the membrane which I had laid open was the tunica vaginalis testis, extended by the hydrocele, which had entirely disappeared. I then, of course, dissected through this tunica vaginalis at the posterior part, and laid open the hernial sac, which contained a small portion of intestine, nearly black from strangulation. Having already dilated the ring, I could pass my finger some way above it, by which I discovered the obstacle to reduction to be a contraction at the mouth of the sac. By the assistance of a director I removed the stricture, and returned the intestine. The man is doing well. In this case the hernia must have been seated behind the cord.

CHAPTER XV.

Of the Inguinal Hernia on the inner Side of the Epigastric Artery.

An inguinal hernia very generally takes the course of the spermatic cord, and it is therefore situated on the outer side of the epigastric artery, at the orifice where it first quits the abdomen. But sometimes the hernial sac protrudes nearer to the pubis than usual, descending from the abdomen immediately behind the abdominal ring; and then the hernia is situated on the inner side of the epigastric artery.

This variety of hernia has now very often fallen under observation, and has been, for more than twenty-five years, described in the lectures delivered at St. Thomas's and Guy's Hospitals.

Mr. Cline, on May the 6th, 1777, in opening a Chelsea Pensioner, with Mr. Adair Hawkins, found a hernia on the right side, the mouth of which was situated an inch and a half on the inner side of the epigastric artery; and I have in my possession four other preparations of this species, which, with one that I destroyed in ascertaining the exact course of the disease, make six instances of this variety of inguinal hernia occurring within my knowledge; besides the cases which remain to be described in this chapter. *Cases.*

There is, besides these, a preparation of this kind in the Museum at St. Thomas's Hospital, made by Mr. Baynham, now Surgeon in America, more than twenty years ago. In Plate VII. it will be seen that the hernia on the right side was of this species, the epigastric artery being on its outer side; whereas that on the left is situated in the common way with regard to this artery.

Plate VII, VIII, IX, and X, show an external and internal view of this disease, and its situation with respect to the tendons of the abdominal muscles and the epigastric artery.

The abdominal ring is closed towards the abdomen by the tendons of the internal oblique and transversalis muscles. The lower parts of these tendons are inserted into the pubis, and connected with the fascia which passes upwards from the external oblique muscle at Poupart's ligament. If this tendon is unnaturally weak, or if from mal-formation it does not exist at all, or from violence has been broken, a protrusion of the viscera may then take place immediately behind the ring. I have only seen it produced by the first and last of these causes; that is, by weakness, and by rupture of the tendon of the latter: the following is an instance. *Abdominal ring closed by a tendon of the internal oblique and transverse muscles*

A gentleman applied to me who had been thrown from his horse, and had received a blow upon the groin which gave him great pain at the time, and produced a fulness at the part, which proved afterwards to be a hernia of this description, which could only have been thus suddenly produced by a rupture of the tendon of the transversalis.

Below the abdominal ring the appearance of this tumour differs from that of common bubonocele in being situated nearer the penis; and the spermatic cord passes on its outer side instead of its posterior part, particularly at and above the abdominal ring. (See Plates VII. VIII. and IX.) *Appearance of the tumour.*

Above the abdominal ring the sac passes directly upwards, so that no part of it takes the usual oblique direction towards the anterior superior process of the ilium, but rather the contrary direction inwards towards the navel. Examined by accurate dissection its course is as follows:—The sac first protrudes between the fibres of the tendons of the transversalis, nearly an inch directly above the ring. It then passes under the lower edge of the tendon of the internal oblique muscle. The epigastric artery runs upon the outer side of the hernial sac. The spermatic cord has no connexion with it above the ring. The hernia then emerges from the abdominal ring, the spermatic cord being on its outer side, and it is covered with the fascia given off by the tendon of the external oblique, but not by the cremaster muscle. (See Plate VII. and VIII. which contain a view of this hernia.) *Dissection of it.*

I have never seen it acquire the same size as the common inguinal hernia often does, but I have met with it somewhat larger than that which is shown in Plate VII. An increase of bulk, however, does not render it more dangerous. In the greater number of cases I have found it accompanied by diseases of the urethra. One of the specimens in my possession contains six herniæ of this kind; it was taken from a patient of Mr. Weston's, Surgeon in Shoreditch, who had long laboured under a difficulty in discharging his urine, and his health was too much broken, as well as his urethra too irritable, to admit of the common means of cure. On inspecting his body I found several strictures in the urethra, a stone impacted behind one of them, and six herniæ, three on each side, all of which were of the species above described. (See Plate X.)

I shall mention the treatment of this hernia, as of the others, in its three different states.

Reducible. When reducible, the truss should be longer than that required for common hernia, because the hole through which the sac emerges from the abdomen is one inch and a half further inwards towards the pubis; so that the pad of the truss must reach round as far as the abdominal ring itself, but still is not to rest upon the pubis. In other respects the form of the truss does not require to be changed.

If irreducible, the same means must be employed as in the common species of inguinal hernia.

Strangulated. When strangulated, the attempt at reduction should be directed differently to the usual mode. The tumour is, as before, to be grasped with one hand, but the fingers of the other are to be placed at the abdominal ring to *knead* the hernia at that part, directing the pressure upwards and inwards, instead of upwards and outwards, to return the tumour into the abdomen.

Case. A man was admitted last summer into Guy's Hospital, who had a hernia of this kind strangulated. He came in on account of other complaints, but on complaining to Mr. Stocker, Apothecary to the Hospital, that he was frequently sick, so as to vomit, Mr. S. examined him, and found a hernia on the right side of the scrotum. I was desired to see him, and found that the tumour extended no higher than the abdominal ring, where it was lost; the spermatic cord passed upon the outer side of the hernia, which last took a direction *Mode of reduction.* towards the region of the pubis, instead of being inclined towards the spinous process of the ilium. I desired him to draw up his thighs at right angles with his body, and to place his knees together, and then, by grasping the tumour with my right hand, and pressing it at its mouth upwards and inwards in a direction towards the navel, a reduction was soon effected, and all the symptoms of strangulation vanished.

Operation for it. If the operation for this variety of hernia be performed in the manner usually advised in bubonocele, that is, by dilating the hernial sac and stricture upwards and outwards, the epigastric artery will certainly be divided. It has therefore been recommended to alter the direction of the dilating incision to upwards and *inwards*, to avoid the epigastric artery, and, if the surgeon is certain as to the species of hernia, that is the safest plan. But if, in some instances, the operator is directed to make the incision in one way, and in others precisely the reverse, there will always be reason to fear some mistakes in practice, which would be attended with the most serious consequences; such mistakes, it is true, would hardly occur to a surgeon constantly in the habit of dissection, but to the greater number the distinguishing marks of the two species will not be sufficiently discriminative. It is therefore desirable to point out such a mode of operating as would ensure the safety of the patient, whatever kind of hernia was found. Such are the advantages possessed by the method of making the division directly upwards, opposite to the middle of the hernial sac, for in this direction the epigastric artery is certainly avoided.

The operation, therefore, is to be performed in the following manner:—The surgeon first makes an incision through the integuments, along the middle of the tumour, from its upper to its lower part, following the longitudinal direction of the tumour; so that if it has any inclination inwards towards the navel, the incision is to incline the same way. The fascia being thus exposed, is divided over the surface of the tumour from the abdominal ring down to its lower extremity. The hernial sac, which now comes in view, is then opened, from an inch below the ring down to the lower part of the sac, in the same cautious manner as has been formerly described. The surgeon then passes his finger into the sac, and feels for the stricture; if at the abdominal ring, he introduces the blunt-pointed bistory between the sac and the ring, slitting the latter directly upwards, till the aperture is large enough to allow of the return of the parts; if the stricture is above the ring, he follows it with the knife still in the same direction, and anterior to it, opposite the middle of the mouth of the sac, till the dilatation is sufficient to allow his finger to slip into the cavity of the abdomen; after which the hernia is to be pushed up, or, if not in a fit state for that purpose, to be treated as mentioned in a former chapter. The parts anterior to the sac above the ring, and divided by the knife, are the tendons of the transversalis and internal oblique muscles. If the stricture is within the sac, still the same direction is to be preserved, but the knife must then be passed into the sac itself.

In this way the epigastric artery will, with certainty, be avoided; which it cannot be if the division of the stricture is made outwards, and in the common hernia it will be divided by dilating inwards.

Some, however, have doubted of the possibility of the epigastric artery ever being divided, whatever may have been the direction of the incision; and, in support of this opinion, they adduce the great number of operations which have been performed by various practitioners, without the occurrence of this accident. However, this artery may actually have been divided, and produced the patient's death by pouring its contents into the cavity of the abdomen, without the surgeon being aware of the mischief which his knife has occasioned; and even when the accident has been known by him to have happened, the circumstance has been concealed from the public. In proof of the possibility of dividing this artery, I shall mention the two following cases. *Epigastric artery divided.*

A patient of Mr. Sterry's, Surgeon in Bermondsey Square, had been for three days labouring under the symptoms of strangulated hernia. The hernia was scrotal, and as it had resisted every attempt at reduction, Mr. S. requested me to see him, when the operation was agreed upon, and I performed it precisely according to the rule usually laid down, of dividing the mouth of the hernial sac; that is, upwards and outwards. As soon as the division was made, a quantity of arterial blood was seen flowing down over the intestine within the sac, and the bowel being immediately returned, a considerable stream of arterial blood flowed into the sac. Pressure was made upon the groin in the situation of the epigastric artery in order to prevent the hæmorrhage, and apparently with success; but four hours afterwards Mr. Sterry was sent for on account of a copious discharge of blood from the wound. He made a further pressure, but without success, and the man died in ten hours after the operation; becoming gradually faint after it, and the abdomen being distended with blood. *Case.*

For the following case I am indebted to my friend Mr. Davie, now unfortunately no more, who allowed me to insert it here.

" Daniel Pyson, a farmer's servant at Wingham, in the county of Kent, about twenty years of age, and
" of a healthy constitution, had been subject to an inguinal hernia from a child, which, at Christmas 1801,
" became strangulated, but had been reduced by Mr. Ferriar, surgeon of the place, by the application of ice.
" In August 1802, it became again strangulated, and, as I happened to be in the neighbourhood, I was sent
" for to him. I found that he had worn a truss, which had closed the sac of the original hernia; but another
" had protruded to the outer side of this, nearer to the spine of the ilium. *Case.*

" The tumour was scrotal, about the size of a hen's egg, and had all the characters of hernia, excepting a
" slight inequality near the ring. I tried the usual means of reduction without success, on which the operation
" was proposed, to which the patient readily consented.

" After making an incision from the upper to the lower part of the sac, I cautiously made an opening into
" it, and was surprised to find that it contained neither intestine nor omentum, but only about two ounces of
" water. It had no communication either with the abdomen or the tunica vaginalis testis, and had the appear-
" ance of an old hernial sac, and, as I did not then know that he had formerly had a strangulated hernia, I was
" at a loss to account for it. I continued the incision upwards, so as distinctly to expose the abdominal ring,
" and then saw a second hernial sac, about the size of the end of the thumb projecting through it, situated on
" the side of the other. Having opened this hernial sac, I found within it a fold of strangulated intestine,
" which was closely embraced by the ring. I passed a Pott's bistory between the tendon and intestine, and
" divided the tendon, which I could distinctly see. The sac was continued upwards under the tendon, and on
" introducing my finger within it, I found the stricture infinitely greater at this part, so that I long tried in vain
" to introduce the point of a curved bistory within the stricture. At last I succeeded in dividing this stricture;
" but unfortunately, though I was at that moment aware of the danger to the epigastric artery, I cut that vessel
" whilst dilating the stricture, of which I was immediately sensible, by perceiving a copious flow of blood *.
" The nature of the injury being clear, it only remained for me to stop the blood, for which I made many fruit-
" less endeavours, till after bleeding for an hour the patient fainted from the hæmorrhage. At this time a
" coagulum was formed over the wound, and he was ordered to bed, and to be kept cool. On recovering, it
" seemed as if the bleeding was entirely stopped; but at four o'clock on the succeeding morning a vomiting
" came on, and about four ounces of coagulated blood, which had been collected in the abdomen near the wound,
" being thereby forced out, a second bleeding took place, which, before I could reach him, had run through his
" bed to the floor. When I visited him at eight o'clock he had no pulse at the wrist, and seeing that his death

---

* Mr. Turner, one of my house pupils, was present at this operation, and informs me that Mr. Davie divided the abdominal ring upwards, and the stricture at the mouth of the sac inwards.

" was inevitable, unless something was done to stop the flow of blood, I determined to cut down upon the artery;
" but as I wished for the presence of some respectable surgeon at the time, I went to Mr. Wood, of Wingham,
" to request a consultation, having, before I left my patient, introduced a dossil of lint within the wound up
" towards the abdomen, and desiring a constant and considerable pressure to be kept up midway between the
" abdominal ring and the spine of the ilium. On my return I was rejoiced to find that there had been no external
" bleeding, and that his appearance was improved; it was therefore thought right to suffer the lint to remain in,
" and the pressure to be continued; which was accordingly kept up without intermission for four days, after
" which the lint was withdrawn without any further accident. The extreme degree of debility which followed
" the loss of blood, rendered his bowels so torpid as to prevent his having a stool before the third day, and it was
" then produced by calomel and colocynth, and by glysters. On the same account I was under the necessity of
" using a catheter to draw off his urine. However, at the end of five weeks, he had so completely recovered as
" to resume his usual occupation."

The hernia in the first of these cases must have been the variety I have mentioned, in the second it was a common hernia; but no one can now doubt of the possibility of dividing the epigastric artery in the common method of performing the operation; other testimonies might here be added, but without the permission of the surgeons who performed the operations, I should not think myself justified in mentioning the cases. However, in all the varieties that hitherto have been observed in the structure of these parts (excepting where the spermatic cord passes over the sac, when the dilatation must be made outwards) the division of the stricture directly upwards, opposite to the middle of the mouth of the hernial sac, will obviate every danger.

CHAPTER XVI.

Of Hernia in the Female.

The round ligament of the female, which arises from the fundus uteri, and is fixed in the fat and integuments of the pubis, preserves a course similar to the spermatic cord in the male; that is, it passes out from the abdomen midway between the symphisis pubis and spinous process of the ilium, under the edges of the internal oblique and transversalis muscles, above Poupart's ligament, and on the outer side of the epigastric artery. To confine the lower edge of the transverse muscle, a fascia similar to that in the male is sent upwards by the crural arch, which passes behind the muscles of the abdomen. Structure of parts.

The round ligament of the uterus, like the spermatic cord, takes an oblique course in its passage from the abdomen, before it emerges through the ring to be gradually lost upon the pubis; so that the opening immediately from the cavity of the belly is two inches to the upper and outer part of the abdominal ring. As this ligament is much narrower than the spermatic cord, the opening corresponding to the abdominal ring in the male is much smaller; being, in the female, not more than about half an inch in length, and a quarter of an inch in breadth. On this account inguinal hernia is a much less frequent disease in the female than the male.

The female inguinal hernia, as in the other sex, passes out of the abdomen midway between the ilium and pubis, under the edges of the internal oblique and transversalis muscles; both of which, but especially the latter, form a semicircle over it, being attached to Poupart's ligament on the outer side of the tumour, and after passing across it, are inserted into the pubis on its inner side. The facsia given off by Poupart's ligament runs directly upwards on each side of the tumour. The hernia, therefore, descends behind the tendon of the external oblique muscle to the abdominal ring, at which place it becomes less confined than before, and generally appears as a tumour about the size of a pigeon's egg in the upper part of the labium pudendi. Below the abdominal ring, this hernia receives a covering from a fascia given off by the tendon of the external oblique muscle, as in the male; and above the ring it is covered by the tendon itself. Course of the hernia.

The same symptoms characterize, and the same causes produce the disease in the female as in the male. The contents, also, are for the most part intestine and omentum; but sometimes, also, it happens that the hernia contains the appendages of the uterus.

This disease is little liable to be confounded with any other; for the round ligament is not subject to the same enlargement and diseases as the spermatic cord, and it is the diseases of the testis and its coats which occasion the principal difficulties in distinguishing hernia in the male. I have known, however, the inguinal hernia in the female mistaken for the femoral species, which is not unlikely to happen from the contiguity of the situation of the two. Diagnoses.

I was sent for last summer to a lady in the country, who had for several days been suffering under the symptoms of strangulated hernia, which had been supposed by her medical attendant to be inguinal, and had resisted all the means of reduction. I found it however to be a femoral hernia, and this mistake was the cause of the failure in the attempts to return it, as the means of reduction differ much from those necessary in the other species; so that, when known to be femoral, it was very soon reduced.

The way of distinguishing the one species from the other, is to feel with the finger the course of Poupart's ligament; if the neck of the tumour is situated above its edge, the hernia is inguinal; but if the tumour is below the ligament it is femoral.

This hernia, as in the former instances, may be considered in the three states of reducible, irreducible, and strangulated.

In the reducible state a truss must be worn similar to that used in the male, to prevent a future descent; but I saw about twelve months ago a case of this kind, in which the hernia was so large that it could not be supported by a common truss; and the method which the woman adopted to enable her to attend sufficiently to her domestic affairs, was to have a sling bandage passing over her shoulders and between her thighs, thus embracing the tumour and preventing it from increasing so much as to impede the motions of the thigh, which was continually Reducible.

happening before she used this contrivance. The springs by which this bandage was supported, were the spiral elastic wire springs now so generally worn by gentlemen across the shoulders.

Irreducible. If irreducible, this hernia can only be supported by a common T bandage; but the women that I have seen labouring under irreducible inguinal Hernia have generally preferred leaving the complaint to itself; and, excepting in the instance above related, where I had reason to suspect some mal-conformation and unusual enlargement of the opening into the abdomen, I have never seen the tumour grow to a very considerable size. If it is omental only, a spring truss may be worn.

Strangulated. When an inguinal hernia in the female becomes strangulated, reduction must be attempted by the taxis in the manner formerly described, the thighs being bent at right angles with the body, and brought very near to each other, the tumour is then to be embraced with one hand, and pressure made at the mouth of the sac with the other. If this does not succeed, the tobacco glyster, ice, and the other powerful means to assist reduction must be resorted to.

Operation. If the operation becomes necessary, it should be performed in the following manner:—The patient being prepared, and placed as in the male subject, an incision is to be made, beginning at the abdominal ring, and continued down to the lower part of the tumour, which seldom projects much below the ring. This divides the external pudendal artery, which is not so large in the female as in the male, and exposes the fascia which covers the hernial sac. The fascia being then cut through, the sac itself appears, which is to be carefully penetrated by a small incision, to allow of the contents being examined; after which a bistory is to be introduced between the sac and the abdominal ring, which last is to be dilated. If any stricture be felt higher up, this also must be dilated; which may be here done with equal safety, as far as our knowledge at present extends, either upwards, or upwards and outwards towards the spine of the ilium. The contents of the sac, if not mortified, are then to be returned.

If the operation be undertaken so early as to render it highly improbable from the symptoms that mortification has taken place, it may be performed without opening the sac, by dividing the integuments and fascia, and setting free the stricture at the ring, or higher up, as above described. The wound is to be closed with sutures, and all that has been observed in the after treatment of hernia in the other sex will equally apply here.

Small hernia. As in the male, the inguinal hernia of the female sometimes lies concealed under the tendon of the external oblique, not having yet forced its way through the ring, and in this state, if strangulated, the cause of the symptoms often remains unknown to the medical attendant.

Case. A woman was admitted into St. Thomas's Hospital for symptoms of inflammation of the bowels, and as she vomited frequently, and had no passage by stool, Dr. Blane, whose patient she was, enquired if she had no tumour at the groin or navel, to which she replied in the negative. She was bled, put into the warm bath, and various means were used to procure a passage by the bowels, but without success; and in two days she died. The Doctor still suspecting, however, that some concealed hernia might have been the cause of the symptoms, had the body examined; when a small fulness was seen on the right side, which being opened, proved to be a hernia, extending from the abdomen to about an inch below the abdominal ring. It contained a very small portion of intestine, which was strangulated by the pressure of the parts that surround the aperture through which the round ligament quits the abdomen. The preparation of this hernia is preserved in the Museum of St. Thomas's Hospital.

Operation. The operation on this small concealed inguinal hernia is the same as that required for the same disease in the male. An incision is to be made the length of the tumour, and the tendon of the external oblique exposed, which being next cut through, the hernial sac appears. This is to be opened, the stricture which surrounds its mouth set free, and the hernial contents returned.

That variety of inguinal hernia in the male which descends upon the inner side of the epigastric artery, I have never met with in the female.

CHAPTER XVII.

On the Congenital Hernia, or Hernia Tunicæ Vaginalis.

THE difference between this and the common inguinal hernia is, that the protruded parts are contained, not in a distinct sac given off by the peritoneum, but in the tunica vaginalis testis, in immediate contact with the testis itself. <small>Difference from the Inguinal.</small>

The origin of this disease is derived from the change of situation which the testis naturally undergoes during the fœtal state; for during the first seven months of fœtal life the testicles are situated within the abdomen upon the loins, whence, in the eighth or ninth month, they descend into the scrotum. <small>Change of situation in the testis.</small>

Previous to their descent each lies upon the psoas muscle, just under the kidneys, this being the most convenient situation for receiving the spermatic arteries from the aorta, and for returning the spermatic veins into the vena cava inferior, on the right side, and into the emulgent vein on the left. (See Plate IV.) The vas deferens at this time passes down from the testicle behind the bladder to terminate in the urethra. From the lower part of the testicle and epydimis arises a long ligament, called the gubernaculum, which passes into the scrotum in the same course that the spermatic cord takes after the descent of the testicle, and it seems designed to draw the testis down into the scrotum, or at least to direct it in the course which it is about to take.

The testicle, and the different vessels connected with it, are covered by peritonæum, every where except at the posterior side of the testicle where the vessels enter it, and the same may be observed of the gubernaculum through a part of its course.

At the eighth month the testis descends through the abdominal ring into the scrotum, bringing with it a peritoneum, which is previously somewhat looser at the lower part of the abdomen than elsewhere, and which becomes afterwards the tunica vaginalis testis. This descent is so gradual, that the peritoneum is not drawn out from the abdomen, nor is any part of this membrane within the belly displaced, but it falls down into the scrotum by elongation or slow increase of growth. The time at which the testes are usually found in the scrotum is at the ninth month, but this is liable to great variety, so that frequently one testicle appears in the scrotum at birth, and often neither. In some persons months and years elapse before they are descended. The abdominal ring appears to be the chief impediment, so that in persons in whom the testicles have not descended, these organs are usually found in the groin just above the ring. They are exposed to injury, and give a general form to the pelvis like that of the female. I saw, some months ago, a gentleman who had a tumour in each groin, which was the testicle. Sometimes, however, they remain entirely within the cavity of the abdomen. <small>Time of the descent of the testis.</small>

After the descent of the testicle, the opening through which it passed from the abdomen closes: but the time at which this takes place is liable to considerable variation. Professor Camper gives the following remarks on this subject from his own observation. In seventeen new-born children which he dissected, eleven had the cavity of the tunica vaginalis open to the abdomen; in three, it was obliterated on the left side, and in two, on the right. In one only it was entirely obliterated on both sides. When the cavity of the tunica vaginalis remains open at birth, the violent efforts which the child makes as soon as it begins to breathe, occasion a portion of the small intestines, which lie over this opening, and are in an empty state, to fall down into this cavity. This protrusion is the hernia congenita, and it is immediately perceived by the swelling of the scrotum during the efforts of crying. It is called by nurses The Windy Rupture. <small>Tunica vaginalis closes,</small>

The tunica vaginalis sometimes remains unclosed for many years after birth, though the testis has descended. I dissected a boy, six years of age, in whom both the testes were in the scrotum, where the opening of the tunica vaginalis was still so large, that I could pass a female catheter through it down to the testis. There was no appearance, however, of a hernia having yet formed, but when he had begun to labour hard, one of the congenital kind would probably have been produced. This explains the case of a man who underwent the operation for strangulated congenital hernia in St. Thomas's Hospital, and he assured me, after the operation, that he had never had any appearance of rupture till seven weeks before. <small>remains open,</small>

Sometimes the tunica vaginalis becomes closed at the ring, but remains open above it, in which case, if a <small>closed only at the ring.</small>

descent of the intestine occurs, a singular variety of hernia is produced; being congenital, but at the same time inclosed in a proper sac within the tunica vaginalis. I shall presently relate a case of this kind, which was furnished me by my friend and colleague Mr. Forster. A similar case is given in Mr. Hey's very excellent Surgical Observations.

Course of this hernia. The course of the hernia congenita must necessarily be the same as that of the spermatic cord, which descends from the abdomen under the edge of the transversalis and internal oblique muscles to the abdominal ring, through which it passes to the bottom of the scrotum. The tunica vaginalis, which contains both the cord and the hernia, is covered by the tendon of the external oblique muscle above the ring, and by the cremaster and fascia below it. The epigastric artery passes obliquely upwards close to the orifice where the tunica vaginalis first quits the abdomen, between it and the symphisis pubis. The spermatic artery in its whole course lies behind the hernia.

Distinctions. The distinguishing mark of the congenital hernia as it commonly occurs, is, that the testis, which is distinct from the hernial sac in the common inguinal hernia, is here involved in the contents of the hernia, so as to be with some difficulty distinguished from it. Besides, as the general appearance of this tumour resembles that of hydrocele, much care is requisite in attending to all the other characteristic marks of the two diseases. Sometimes water, collecting in the abdomen, descends along with the hernia, and as the lower part of the tumour is transparent, it gives the idea of the whole being a hydrocele. This complication of disease may be known by returning the whole contents into the cavity of the abdomen, when the patient is in a horizontal posture; then, by putting the finger against the abdominal ring, the water will slip by it and fall down into the scrotum, producing a transparent tumour or true hydrocele, after which, if the pressure of the finger is a little lessened at the ring, and the patient is desired to cough, the intestine and omentum will be felt falling down into their former situation.

Reducible. In the reducible state, the congenital hernia requires the application of a truss precisely in the same manner as in common inguinal hernia: when the tumour is small, the pad must rest midway between the symphisis pubis and spine of the ilium, but when large it should reach the upper part of the abdominal ring. In children, who are but just born, pressure can only be made by means of a compress of linen, or of a cushion filled with wool, and compressed upon the part by means of a bandage, and if the descent of the intestine is thus only for a few days prevented, the tunica vaginalis will generally close; but if it does not, a truss with a very weak spring, covered by oiled silk to prevent its being spoiled by moisture, may be applied. The earliest time at which I have known one worn has been at the period of three months after birth.

Hernia and testis at the ring. I have seen a congenital hernia complicated with an interruption of the descent of the testicle, which had only reached the abdominal ring. In such cases no truss should be applied, as the hernia is of use in forcing the descent of the testicle. When a truss has been worn for some time, it shuts the mouth of the tunica vaginalis at the abdomen, sometimes leaving an effusion of water in the tunica vaginalis below. If in these instances, by pressure at the abdomen, the tunica vaginalis also becomes closed immediately above the testicle, the portion intercepted between these two closures retains the effused water, forming a hydrocele of the spermatic cord.

Hydrocele of the spermatic cord. I lately operated on a child aged five years, who had a large watery tumour in the scrotum, extending down from the scrotum to the upper part of the testicle. The tumour being laid open the testis was found separated from it by a distinct adhesion, but the fluid appeared to be contained in the tunica vaginalis, and extended through the ring to the opening from the abdomen which was now closed. This boy had worn a truss for a congenital hernia.

Operation for the congenital hernia. When the hernia is strangulated, the same means are to be employed for its reduction as in the inguinal hernia; but if these do not succeed the operation becomes necessary, which in some respects differs from that for the common inguinal. The incision should begin at the upper part of the abdominal ring; and in large herniæ should extend to a little above the testis. This lays bare the fascia and cremaster muscle, which cover the tunica vaginalis. This latter membrane is then to be cautiously opened, and divided in the same direction as the first incision, to within an inch of the abdominal ring upwards; but downwards no lower than the upper part of the testicle, as a sufficient quantity of the tunica vaginalis should be left to cover this organ. The finger being passed within the tunica vaginalis, which is here the only sac of the hernia, the seat of the stricture should be felt for, and, if at the ring, the dilatation should be made by insinuating the knife between the sac and the ring.

If the impediment to the return of the hernia is formed by the transversalis muscle, the knife, (still in the anterior side of the sac), is to be carried up to it through the ring; but if the stricture is in the tunica vaginalis itself at its orifice into the abdomen, the knife must be introduced within it, and the strictured part cautiously divided.

The injunction usually given of dilating upwards and outwards towards the ilium, to avoid the epigastric artery, is always safe in this hernia, because that artery passes on the posterior and inner side of the tunica vaginalis; but it is equally safe to dilate directly upwards, opposite the middle and superior part of the tunica vaginalis; and therefore, to preserve an uniformity in the mode of performing the operation, it is better to pursue this direction in the dilatation.

If the congenital hernia is large, and more especially if it has been for any length of time irreducible, I should advise the return of the parts without inspection, if the stricture can be removed without opening the tunica vaginalis. In Plate XI, Fig. 3, will be seen a long-existing congenital hernia, which had been of very large size, and the abdomen much contracted: in the attempt to return the intestine, it burst, the fæces were discharged through the opening, at which the bougie was introduced, and the man survived only a few days. But there is a still greater reason for reduction without opening the tunica vaginalis, if the intestine has contracted an adhesion to this membrane. I know of no operation in surgery so difficult as that of detaching a congenital hernia which is closely agglutinated to the tunica vaginalis. The adhesions are too short to be safely cut through, the tunica vaginalis cannot be returned into the cavity of the abdomen, nor can any portion of it be cut away at its posterior part, without endangering the spermatic vessels. All these difficulties are removed by dividing the abdominal ring and transversalis muscle without opening the tunica vaginalis; or if this proves insufficient, which is rarely the case, the tunic should only be opened at the abdominal ring, or at the upper orifice into the abdomen, wherever the stricture exists, and dissected so as to set free the strangulation, after which the edges of the wound should be brought together and united by the first intention. The strangulating compression being thus removed from the viscera, they still remain in the same situation, and irreducible, and must afterwards be permanently supported by a bag truss.

Large congenital hernia.

I shall conclude this chapter with the following singular and interesting case, which Mr. Forster has been so kind as to permit me to insert.

Variety of congenital hernia.

DEAR SIR,

As you communicated to me your intention of publishing a work on the varieties of Abdominal Herniæ, I flatter myself that the subjoined case, which came under my care in January 1801, will prove a valuable addition to your collection, as it appeared upon dissection to be connected with circumstances so very unusual, that I have never seen or read of a similar case[*]. It is accompanied with drawings, which I executed whilst the parts were in a recent state, of which I made a preparation, now in my possession.

I am, Dear Sir,

Your most obedient humble servant and colleague,

Southampton Street, Bloomsbury Square.

THOMPSON FORSTER,

Senior Surgeon of Guy's Hospital.

" William Chadwick, a shoemaker, aged thirty-one years, of a spare habit, was admitted into Guy's Hos-
" pital, under my care, on the 31st of January 1801. He complained of great pain in his right groin, which
" was tense and painful to the touch; he had great anxiety of countenance, singultus and subsultus tendinum.
" I learnt that, thirty-six hours previous to his admission into the Hospital, during a fit of coughing, he was
" seized with an acute pain in the groin, and on examination I discovered a small tumour just below the ab-
" dominal ring, and extending about three inches into the scrotum. I adopted every plan my experience could
" suggest for the reduction of this tumour, but all my efforts proved fruitless; and as the symptoms were of the
" most urgent nature, and the life of my patient in such imminent danger, I considered any further delay as
" improper, and proposed an operation as being the only probable means of saving his life; to this, however, he
" objected, and he died the following day.

Case.

[*] Mr. Hey's book was not then published.

" On dissection, the following were the appearances. When the scrotum was divided the tumour was brought "in view, taking the course of the spermatic cord, evidently involved with it, and much contracted at the ring. " On investigating further, and cutting carefully through the tunica vaginalis of the cord near the ring, a fluid " escaped. I then continued the incision to the bottom of the scrotum, through the tunica vaginalis of the " cord, and the tunica vaginalis testis, which I now found to be one cavity, the edges of which being turned " back on either side, exposed a hernial sac pendent from the ring, and descending towards the testicle.

" From hence it evidently appeared that the hernial sac, and its contents, were contained in the tunica vagi- " nalis of the spermatic cord, which formed only one cavity up to the ring. On opening the hernial sac, it was " found to contain a portion of small intestine, of a claret colour, and in a mortified state."

Formation.

The idea which I have formed of the nature of this case, is, that the tunica vaginalis, after the descent of the testis, became closed opposite the abdominal ring, but remained open above and below it. That the intestine descended into the upper part, and elongated both the adhesion and tunica vaginalis, so as to form it into a bag, which descended into the tunica vaginalis below the adhesion, and becoming narrow at its neck, though wide at its fundus, it received a portion of intestine, which was too large either to be returned into the abdomen, or to retain its functions whilst it continued in the sac.

Appearance of.

This disease does not appear like a hernia of the tunica vaginalis, as the testis is not involved in it, but can be distinctly perceived below it. Some embarrassment will be produced in the operation, if the surgeon does not open the tunica vaginalis very freely, so as to completely expose the parts. The strangulation arises from the contracted state of the mouth of the hernial sac, which may be very safely divided upwards.

THE END.

PLATE I.

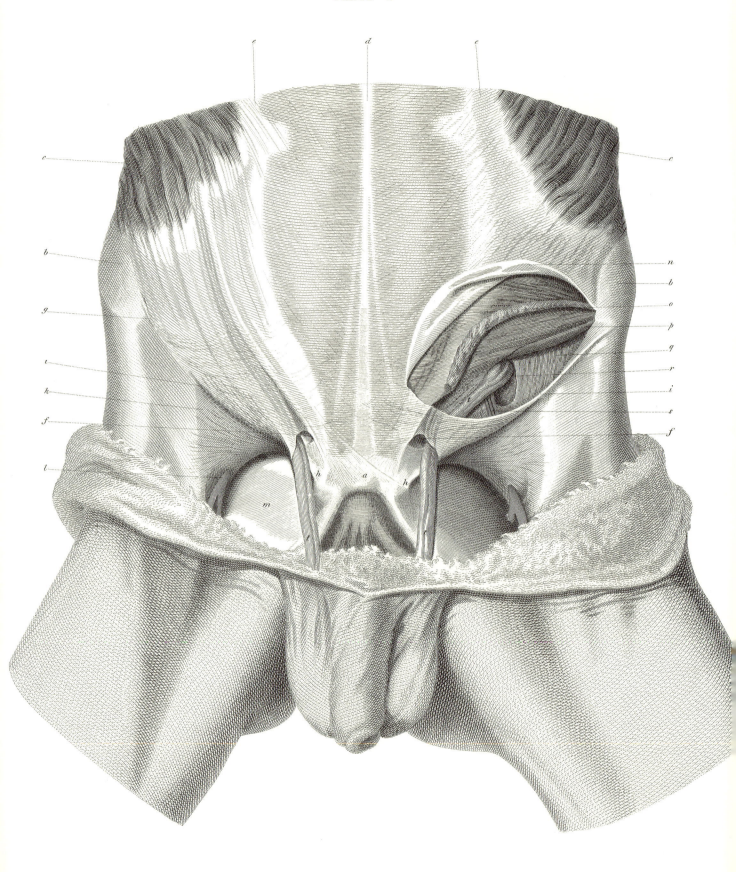

London Published as the act directs July 1.st 1803. by T. Cox, St Thomas's St Boro.

EXPLANATION OF PLATE THE FIRST.

This Plate is intended to shew the insertions of the external oblique muscles, the formation of the abdominal rings, and of two of the fasciæ which are connected with Poupart's ligament, as well as the course of the spermatic cord under the edges of the internal oblique and transverse muscles, before it reaches the abdominal ring.

a. Symphisis pubis.

b b. Anterior and superior spinous process of the ilium.

c c. External oblique muscles.

d. Linea alba extending down to the symphisis pubis, and formed by the union of the tendinous fibres of the two oblique and transverse muscles.

e e. Lineæ semilunares, formed by the union of the tendinous fibres of the external and internal oblique and transverse muscles.

f f. The abdominal rings, formed by the separation of two columns of tendinous fibres; the upper inserted at *a* into each pubis; the lower inserted into the pubis at *h.* after passing behind the spermatic cord.

g. The origin of some tendinous fibres which proceed from the anterior spinous process of the ilium, and crossing the columns of tendon, assist in uniting them above the abdominal ring.

i i. Poupart's ligament, or the crural arch, which is extended from the anterior spinous process of the ilium at *b*, to the pubis at *h*, receiving the lower column of tendon, which forms a part of the abdominal ring, and which passes behind the cord to be inserted from the spinous process to the crest of the pubis.

k. The fascia lata of the thigh, which is continued from Poupart's ligament, and seen turning in under the femoral vessels near the middle of the fore part of the thigh.

l. Is the saphæna major vein of the leg going through the fascia to enter the femoral vein.

m. Another part of the same fascia which arises from Poupart's ligament, and joins with the fascia lata, which it assists in forming.

n. The tendon of the external oblique muscle cut open to shew the parts which are situated behind it.

o. The internal oblique muscle, its lower edge which arises from Poupart's ligament, is raised and turned to shew the parts behind it. It is inserted into the pubis behind the upper column of tendon which forms the abdominal ring.

p. The transversalis. Its lower edge also arises from Poupart's ligament, but is here raised and turned up. It in its natural state runs over the cord to be inserted into the pubis behind the abdominal ring, which it serves as a valve to close behind.

q. A fascia, connected with Poupart's ligament, which runs upwards to the transversalis, and unites itself to the posterior part of the transverse muscle and its tendon, and thus prevents the bowels from slipping between the lower edge of the muscle and Poupart's ligament, or between the fibres of the muscle itself.

That portion of the fascia which is placed between the spinous process of the ilium at *b*, and the hole *r* is strong; but that between the hole *r* and the pubis, is often little more than condensed cellular membrane, as that part is strengthened by the tendon of the transversalis, and by the epigastric artery.

A portion of the fascia i s fixed in the pubis, and another part of it passes behind Poupart's ligament to unite with the femoral vessels.

r. The place at which the spermatic cord goes into the abdomen. The fascia situated on its outer side and lower part, is of considerable density, but becoming thin upon its inner side, so as to shew the epigastric artery and vein behind it; from the edge of the fascia a thinner is sent off which unites itself to the spermatic cord, which fascia in this dissection has been removed.

s. The epigastric artery and vein, situated behind the fascia, at first on the inner side, and afterwards behind the spermatic cord.

t t. The spermatic cord, near two inches of which is above and to the outer side of the abdominal ring, and still not in the abdomen; it is also seen below the ring, running to the testicle.

PLATE II.

EXHIBITS an internal view of Poupart's ligament, the origin and course of the fascia, which it sends upwards to unite the transversalis muscle to Poupart's ligament, and the origin and course of a second fascia which passes over the iliacus internus muscle; also the course of the spermatic cord through the first of these fasciæ, and the situation and course of the epigastric artery and vein; with their origin from the iliac artery and vein.

- *a.* Symphysis pubis.
- *b.* Anterior spinous process of the ilium.
- *c.* Articulation of the ilium with the sacrum.
- *d.* Spinous process of the ischium.
- *e.* Foramen ovale.
- *f.* The muscles of the abdomen.
- *g.* The rectus muscle.
- *h.* United tendons of the internal oblique and transverse muscles passing behind the rectus.
- *i.* Semicircular insertion of Poupart's ligament into the pubis.
- *k.* Tendon of the transversalis which is inserted into the pubis behind the abdominal ring, and which prevents the abdominal ring from being seen.
- *l.* A white tendinous line from which the fasciæ proceed which shut up the lower part of the abdomen.
- *m.* The anterior fascia, which is separated to allow of the passage of the spermatic cord. This fascia begins at *l*, and runs upward on the inner side of the transversalis muscle, and adheres to the linea semilunaris.
- *n.* The other fascia which passes upon the iliacus internus muscle, and unites to the inner part of the crista of the ilium.
- *o.* Iliac artery.
- *p.* Iliac vein.
- *q.* Internal iliac artery.
- *r.* Internal iliac vein.
- *s.* Spermatic artery and vein.
- *t.* Vas deferens.
- *v.* Epigastric artery.
- *w.* Epigastric vein.

These vessels passing two inches upwards before the peritoneum, are then continued between the rectus muscle and the tendon behind it.

PLATE II

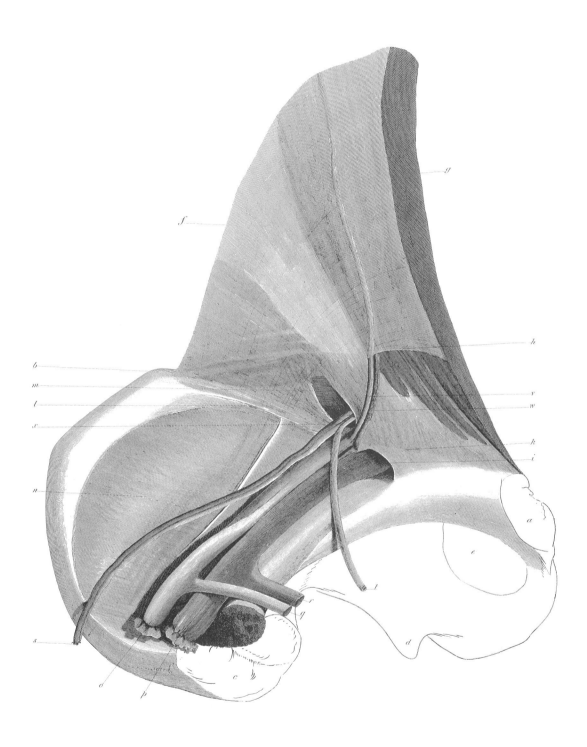

PLATE III

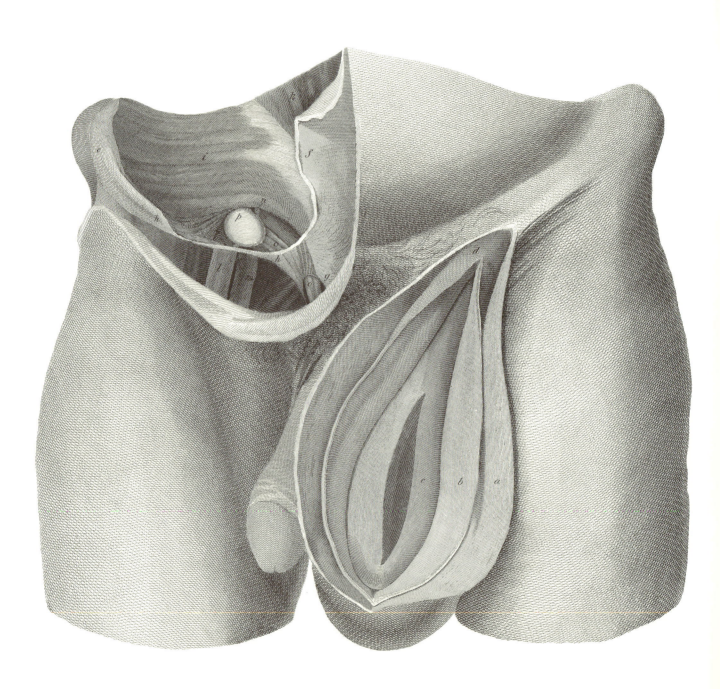

PLATE III.

SHEWS two inguinal herniæ. That on the left side, having existed many years, has descended into the scrotum, and become of great magnitude. That on the left side, is in an incipient state, and shews the distance from the abdominal ring, at which it first protrudes from the abdomen.

a. Common integuments cut through and turned back.

b. The fascia, which is extended from the external oblique muscle over the spermatic cord, in the healthy state; and over the hernial sac, when it descends into the scrotum. To the inner side of this fascia the cremaster muscle adheres.

c. The hernial sac cut open.

d. Abdominal ring, concealed in some degree by the fascia which passes over it.

e. Anterior and superior spinous process of the ilium.

f. Tendon of the external oblique muscle.

g. Abdominal ring on the right side.

h h. Poupart's ligament.

i. Internal oblique muscle passing above the hernial sac.

k. The rectus muscle.

l. Femoral artery.

m. Femoral vein.

n. Epigastric artery passing behind the hernial sac.

o o. Spermatic cord above and below the abdominal ring.

p. Sac of an incipient inguinal hernia, situated as usual, below the edges of the internal oblique and transverse muscles, and above the middle of Poupart's ligament.

PLATE IV.

Is an internal view of the preparation contained in the former plate. It exhibits the orifices of the two herniæ in the abdomen, and shews the change of place which the mouth of the sac undergoes as it enlarges, by approaching nearer than at its first descent to the symphisis pubis. The origin and course of the vessels connected with the disease are shewn.

a. Situation of the symphisis pubis.
b. Spinous process of the ilium.
c c. c c. Abdominal muscles drawn downwards.
d d. The thighs.
e e. The psoas muscle upon each side.
f. The spine.
g g. The kidneys.
h h. Aorta.
i i. Iliac arteries.
k k. Epigastric arteries, arising from the iliac arteries, and passing between the mouths of the hernial sacs and the symphisis pubis, but still near to the inner side of the mouth of each sac.
l l. Spermatic arteries, arising from the aorta, and passing out of the abdomen behind the hernial sacs.

m m. Inferior cava.
n. Iliac vein.
o o. Epigastric veins accompanying the epigastric arteries.
q q. Spermatic veins arising upon the right side from the inferior cava, on the left, from the emulgent vein.
r r. Emulgent veins which in part cover the emulgent arteries.
s s. Ureters.
t. Urinary bladder.
v v. Vasa deferentia passing to the posterior part of the bladder.
x. Incipient inguinal hernia; its mouth seen midway between the spine of the ilium and symphisis pubis.
w. Mouth of the large inguinal hernia extended towards the symphisis pubis, and occasioning an unnatural curve in the epigastric artery.
y y y. The peritoneum.

PLATE IV

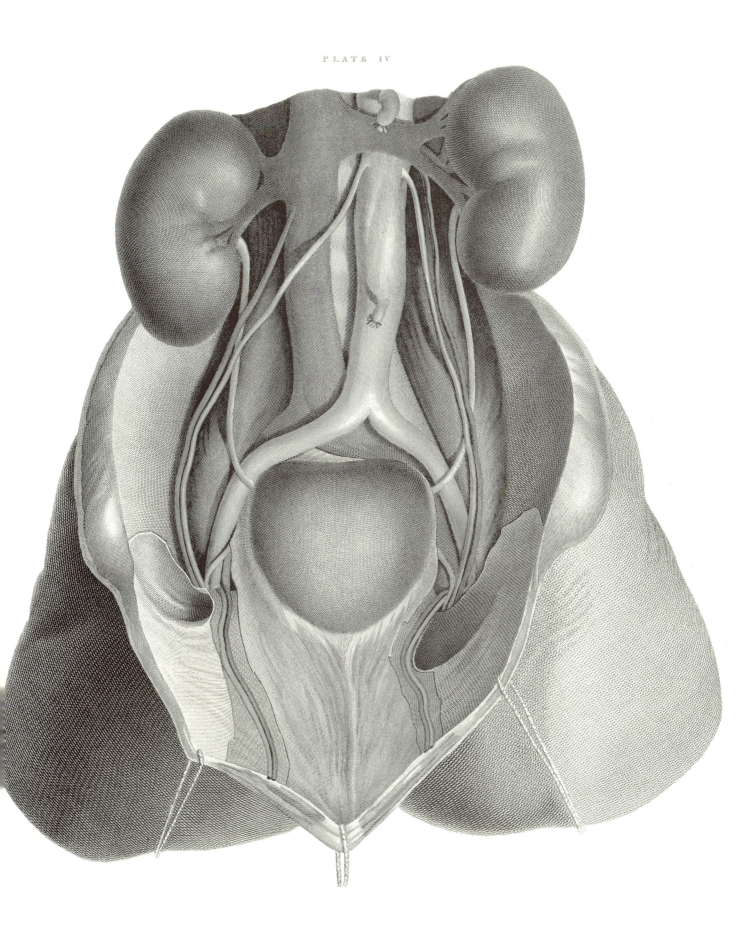

PLATE IV.

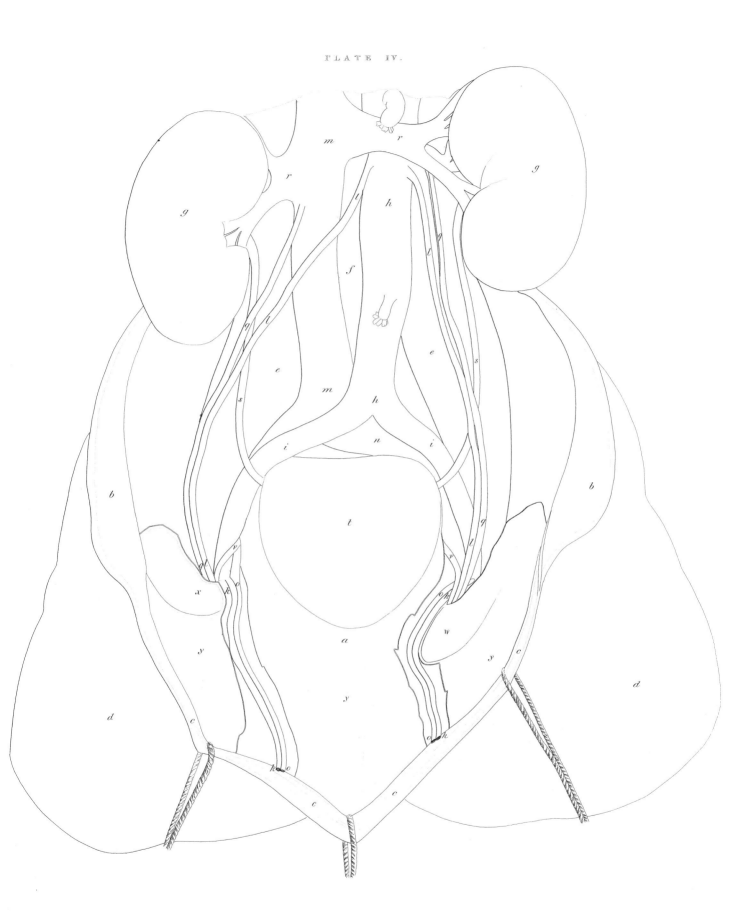

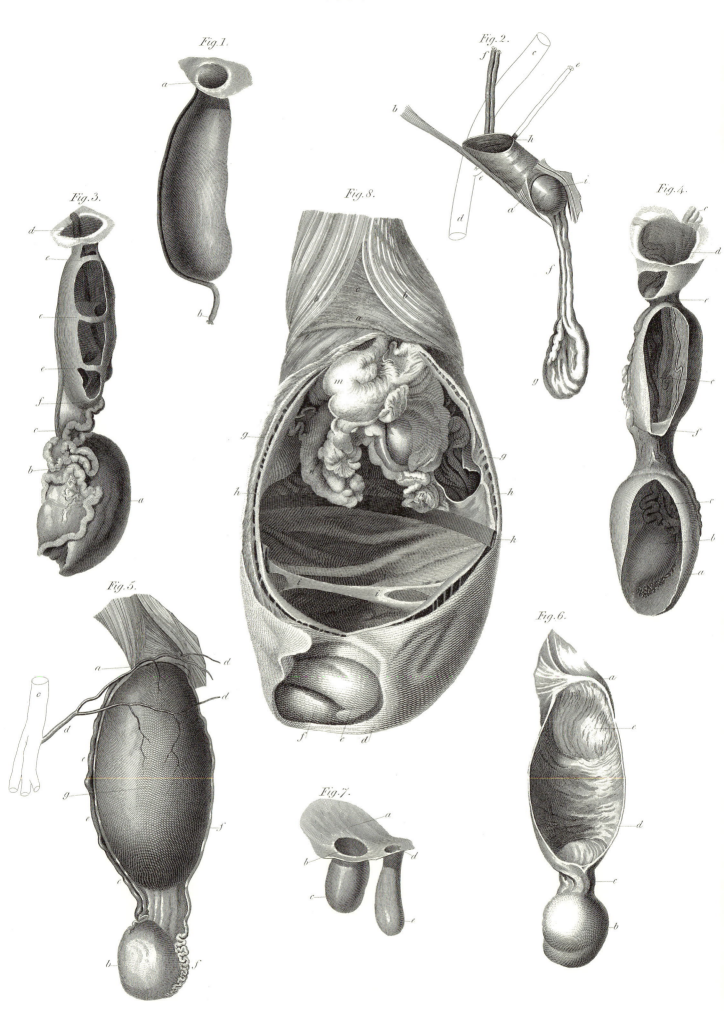

PLATE V.

PLATE V.

FIG. 1. Shews a sac taken from the body of a person who laboured under an inguinal hernia.
    a. Its mouth.
    b. The course of the vas deferens behind it.

FIG. 2. This gives a view of a hernial sac, which has passed no further than the abdominal ring, so that the whole of this sac is included between the abdominal ring and the place at which the spermatic cord quits the abdomen.
    a. Abdominal ring.
    b. Poupart's ligament.
    c. Iliac artery, *d* femoral artery.
    e e. Epigastric artery passing behind the mouth of the sac.
    f f. Spermatic cord passing behind the sac, and through the abdominal ring, to the testis.
    g. The testis.
    h. Mouth of the hernial sac.
    i. The fundus of the sac which just reaches the abdominal ring.

FIG. 3. Shews the hernial sac divided by several septa.
    a. The tunica vaginalis testis.
    b. Spermatic vessels.
    c. Vas deferens.
    d. Mouth of the hernial sac.
    e e e. Septa seen in the sac, with small apertures in them.
    f. The fundus of the sac.

FIG. 4. Shews a hernial sac closed opposite to the abdominal ring, but open above the ring to the abdomen. This arises from improperly wearing the truss at the abdominal ring, instead of the mouth of the hernial sac.
    a. Tunica vaginalis testis.
    b. Testis.
    c c. Spermatic vessels.
    d. Mouth of the sac.
    e. The place at which the sac is closed, which is opposite to the situation of the abdominal ring.
    f. The fundus of the sac.

FIG. 5. A hernial sac, in which the spermatic cord has been divided by it, so as to place the spermatic artery and vein on one side, and the vas deferens upon the other.
    a. Abdominal ring.
    b. Testis.
    c. Femoral artery.
    ddd. External pudendal artery.
    e. Spermatic artery and vein.
    f. Vas deferens.
    g. Hernial sac.

FIG. 6. Hernial sac shut at the abdominal ring by adhesion, leaving a circumscribed bag, in which water was collected.
    a. Sac shut at the ring, but it was open towards the abdomen above the ring.
    b. The testis.
    c. Spermatic cord.
    d. Sac cut open.
    e. Part at which the sac was closed by adhesion.

FIG. 7. Shews two sacs, one by the side of the other; the one contracted by wearing a truss so as to be no longer capable of receiving the viscera; the other larger, and forming by the side of the first.
    a. The peritoneum.
    b. Mouth of a newly formed sac.
    c. Its fundus.
    d. Contracted mouth of an old hernia.
    e. Its fundus.

FIG. 8. An omental and intestinal hernia irreducible from adhesion; and membranous bands extending across the hernial sac.
    a. Abdominal ring.
    b b. Columns of tendons forming the ring. *c* Transverse tendinous fibres passing to the two columns.
    d. Tunica vaginalis.
    e. Epidydimis.
    f. Testis.
    g g. Fascia coming from the abdominal ring to cover the sac.
    h h. Hernial sac.
    i i. Membranous bands crossing the sac.
    k. A piece of whalebone to keep the sac extended.
    m. Intestine adhering to the sac.
    n n. Omentum also adhering to the sac.

PLATE VI.

Fig. 1. A small inguinal hernia just quitting the abdomen. Dissection of the muscles, tendons and fascia.
    a. Pubis.
    b. Spinous process of the ilium.
    c. External oblique muscle.
    d. Abdominal ring.
    e. Tendon of the external oblique muscle turned up to shew the parts behind it.
    f. Same tendon turned down to shew Poupart's ligament posteriorly.
    g g. Fascia proceeding upward to the transversalis muscle. This fascia which passes off from Poupart's ligament, shuts the abdomen between the ligament and the transversalis muscle, which it also lines.
    h h. Internal oblique muscle and its tendon.
    i i. Transverse muscle shewn by raising the internal oblique muscle, its tendon passing to the pubis.
    k. Testis.
    l. Spermatic cord below the ring.
    m. Spermatic cord above the ring, and to its outer side.
    n. A small hernia just quitting the abdomen, and separating the vessels of the spermatic cord in an unusual manner.

Fig. 2. A view of a strangulated portion of the ilium.
    a. Strangulated portion.
    b. Hole in it from mortification at that spot.
    c. Seat of the stricture upon the intestine.

Fig. 3. Single spring truss.

Fig. 4. Double spring truss.

Fig. 5. Single truss, applied at the proper place, for an incipient inguinal hernia.

Fig. 6. Double truss, applied for an incipient inguinal hernia on each side.

Fig. 7. Back view of the truss, shewing the buckle by which the truss is adjusted.

    In large herniæ the truss should press upon the abdominal ring, as well as upon the mouth of the hernial sac, but it should never press upon the pubis.

PLATE VI.

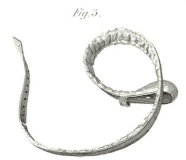
Fig. 3.

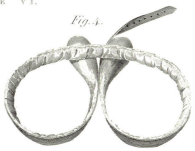
Fig. 4.

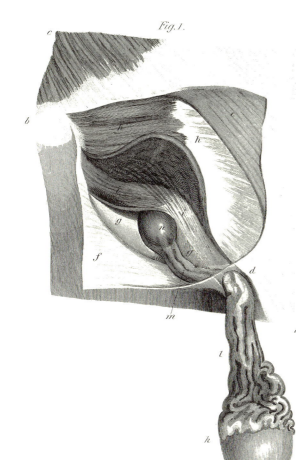
Fig. 1.

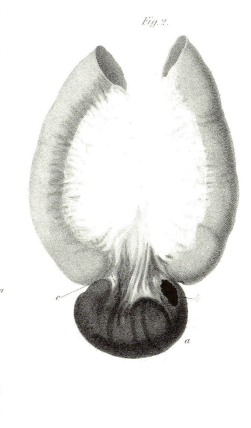
Fig. 2.

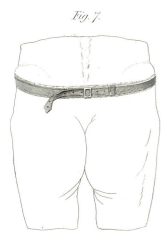
Fig. 7.

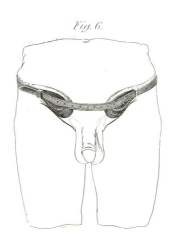
Fig. 6.

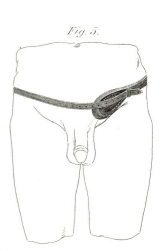
Fig. 5.

London Published as the act directs July 1ˢᵗ 1805, by T. Cox, Sᵗ Thomas's Sᵗ Boro'.

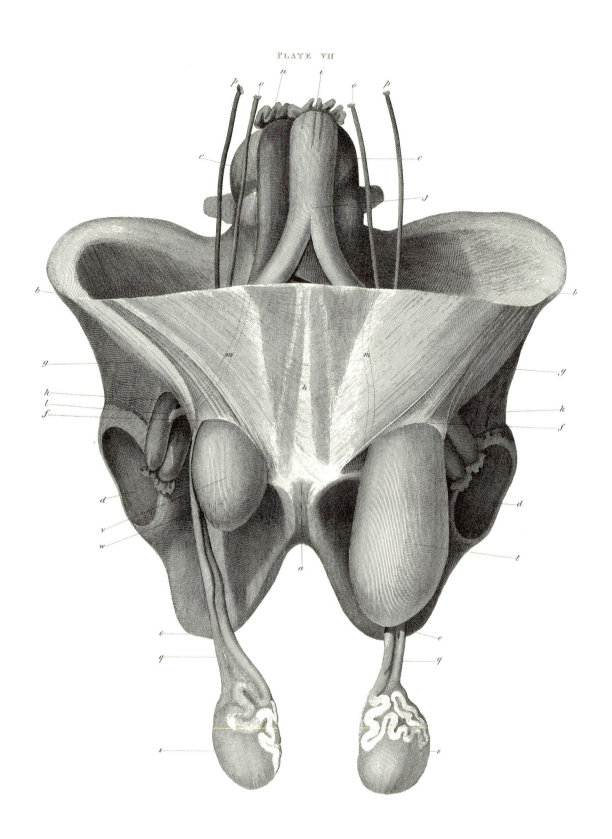

PLATE VII.

In this Plate a common inguinal hernia is shewn upon the left side, taking its course through the abdominal ring on the outer side of the epigastric artery, between that artery and the spine of the ilium. The hernia upon the right side is that variety of the inguinal hernia which passes from the abdomen on the inner side of the epigastric artery, or between that artery and the symphisis pubis.

a. Symphisis pubis.
b. Anterior superior spinous process of the ilium.
c c. The spine.
d d. The acetabula.
e e. Tuberosities of the ischia.
f f. Abdominal rings.
g g. Poupart's ligaments.
h. Linea alba.
i. Aorta.
j. Bisurcation of the aorta.
k k. Iliac and femoral arteries.
l. Origin of the epigastric artery on the right side.
m m. Course of the epigastric artery on each side, marked by dotted lines; the left side passing on the inner, the right, on the outer side of the hernial sac.
n. Vena cava inferior.
o o. Spermatic arteries.
p p. Spermatic veins.
q q. Spermatic cords.
s s. Testes.
t. Hernial sac upon the left side, which is a common inguinal hernia, situated on the outer side of the epigastric artery.
v. Hernial sac upon the right side, which is the less frequent species, placed upon the inner side of the epigastric artery.
w. The spermatic cord passing on the outer side of the hernial sac, on that side on which the variety exists; whilst it is seen on the posterior part of that on the opposite side.

PLATE VIII.

An internal view of the same preparation as that of the former Plate, shewing the orifice of the hernial sacs, with the relative situations of the epigastric and spermatic vessels.

- *a.* Symphisis pubis.
- *b.* Anterior superior spinous process of the ilium.
- *c.* The spine.
- *dddd.* Abdominal muscles drawn downwards to shew the cavity of the pelvis.
- *e.* The bladder.
- *f.* The rectum.
- *g.* Bifurcation of the aorta.
- *h.* The inferior cava.
- *i i.* Spermatic arteries.
- *k k.* Spermatic veins.
- *l.* Vas deferens.
- *m m.* Epigastric arteries and veins.
- *n n.* Origin of epigastric artery on each side.
- *o o.* Peritonæum.
- *p.* Mouth of the hernial sac upon the left side, taking the usual course of inguinal hernia.
- *q.* Mouth of the hernial sac on the right side, situated upon the inner side of the epigastric artery.

By this Plate it will be at once seen, that the division of the sac upwards, and opposite the middle of its orifice, will be in both species of hernia perfectly safe.

PLATE VIII.

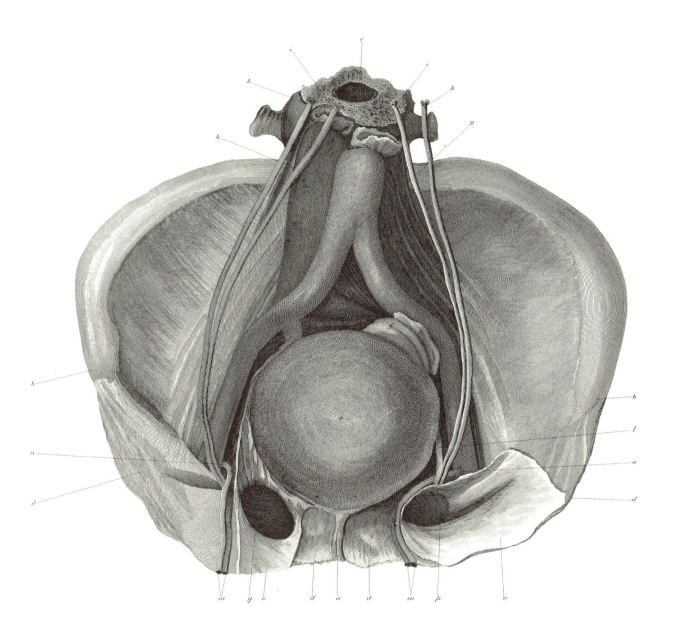

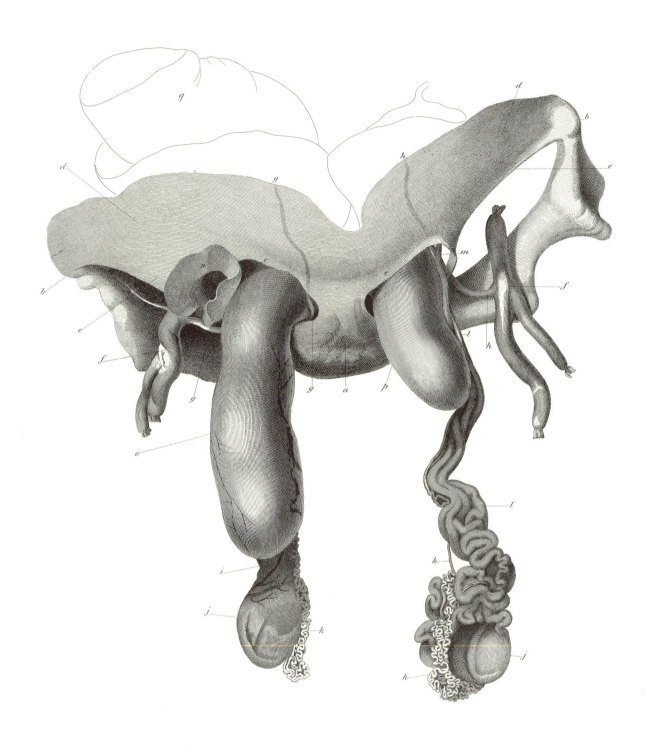

PLATE IX.

On the right side is seen an inguinal hernial sac in the common situation, upon the anterior part of the spermatic cord. On the outer side of this hernia appears an artificial anus, formed from a second protrusion of intestine on the side of the former: at this opening the ilium had prolapsed, but in making the preparation it was returned into the abdomen. Both of these herniæ had passed through the abdominal ring, and were situated on the outer side of the epigastric artery, which has an unusual curve, produced by the long continued pressure of the hernia. On the left side a hernial sac is seen, which has passed down on the inner side of the epigastric artery and spermatic cord.

a. Symphisis pubis.
b. Anterior superior spinous process of the ilium.
c c. Abdominal ring.
d d. Abdominal muscles.
e e. Poupart's ligaments.
f f. Femoral arteries.
g g. Course of the epigastric artery upon the right side.
h h. Origin and course of the epigastric artery on the left side.
i i. Spermatic cord on the right side.
j j. Testes.
k k. Vasa deferentia.
l. Spermatic vessels on the left side in a varicose state.
m. Spermatic and epigastric arteries crossing upon the outer side of the left hernial sac.
n. The artificial anus, by which for eleven years the fæces were discharged.
o. The sac of the inguinal hernia, which was the first which had descended in this man.
p. Hernial sac on the inner side of the epigastric and spermatic vessels, which will be found to have an inclination inwards and upwards towards the pubis, and not as in the common inguinal hernia, towards the ilium.
q. The colon.

PLATE X.

This Plate shews six hernial sacs, which were taken from a patient of Mr. Weston's, surgeon, Shoreditch, who laboured under a difficulty in discharging his urine, from a stricture and stone in his urethra. Two of the sacs upon each side were placed between the umbilical and epigastric arteries; and one on each side is situated between the remains of the umbilical arteries and the pubis. They passed between the tendinous fibres of the transversalis, which they had separated, and entered the abdominal rings, after which they were covered, as usual, by the fascia, which is extended from the external oblique muscle over the spermatic cords.

a. Situation of the symphisis pubis.
b. The muscle removed from the anterior superior spinous process of the ilium.
c. Abdominal muscles lined with peritoneum.
d d. Spermatic cords.
e e. Testes.
f f. Remains of the umbilical arteries.
g g. Epigastric arteries and veins.

h i. Two hernial sacs on the left side, formed between the epigastric and umbilical arteries.
j. Hernial sac formed between the umbilical artery and symphisis pubis.
k l. Two hernial sacs formed between the epigastric and umbilical arteries on the right side.
m. Hernial sac between the umbilical artery and the pubis on the right side.

PLATE X.

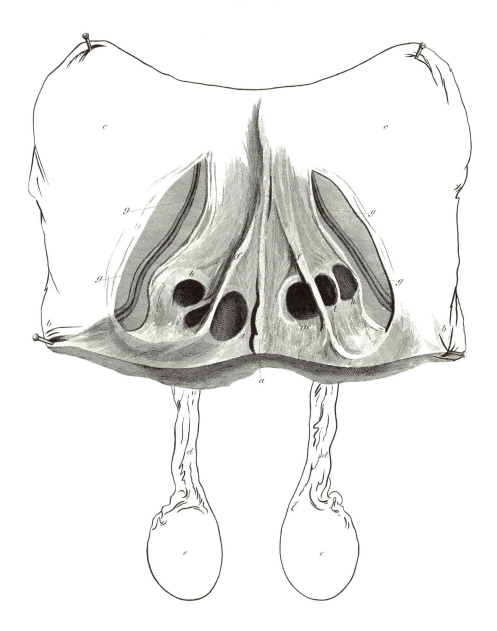

PLATE XI

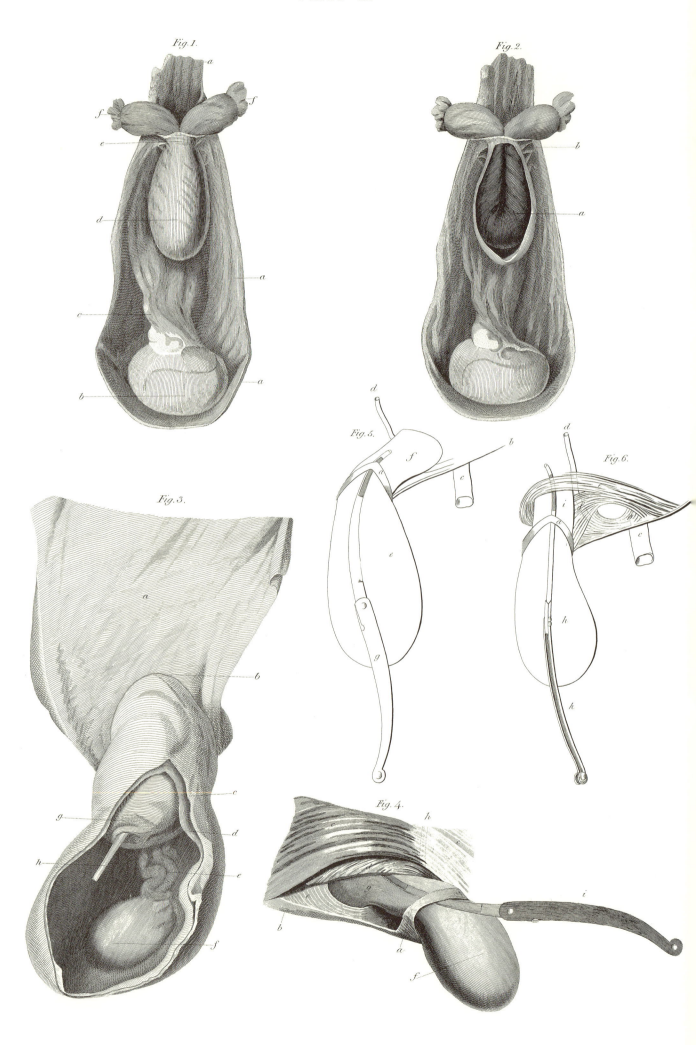

PLATE XI.

This Plate shews the hernia congenita under its usual appearance; also the variety of congenital hernia taken by Mr. Forster from a patient in Guy's Hospital. The other figures shew different views of preparations of the inguinal hernia, intended to shew the mode of operating on each variety.

FIG. 1. *aaa.* Tunica vaginalis.
    b. Testis.
    c. Spermatic cord.
    d. Hernial sac within the tunica vaginalis.
    e. Mouth of the sac, which has been produced by an adhesion of the tunica vaginalis, opposite the abdominal ring.
    ff. Intestine going within it.

FIG. 2. *a.* Hernial sac cut open to shew the strangulated intestine.
    b. The adhesions of the tunica vaginalis to the mouth of the sac.

FIG. 3. Hernia congenita.
    a. Abdominal muscles.
    b. Abdominal ring, and cremaster muscles.
    c. Fascia upon the tunica vaginalis.
    d. Tunica vaginalis testis.
    e. Spermatic cord.
    f. Testis.
    g. Strangulated intestine.
    h. Bougie within it.

FIG. 4. Inguinal hernia in the females, strangulated at the aperture into the abdomen.
    a. Abdominal ring.
    b. Poupart's ligament.
    c c. Internal oblique muscle and its tendon.
    d. Transversalis passing over the hernial sac.
    e. Fascia passing up to the transversalis.
    f. Hernial sac below the abdominal ring.
    g. The sac passing under the transversalis into the abdomen.
    h. Dotted lines marking the direction of the epigastric artery as it runs under the muscles.
    i. Knife placed with its side upon the sac, the edge of which is to be turned forward to divide the transversalis and internal oblique muscle at *d*. Cutting upwards toward *h* would endanger the epigastric artery.

FIG. 5. Common Inguinal hernia.
    a. Abdominal ring.
    b. Poupart's ligament.
    c. Femoral artery.
    d Epigastric artery.
    e. Hernial sac below the ring.
    f. Hernial sac above the ring.
    g. The sharp part of the knife introduced between the ring and the sac, with its side placed towards the sac; its edge is to be turned forwards to divide the ring.

FIG. 6. Hernia on the inner side of the epigastric artery.
    a. Abdominal ring.
    b. Poupart's ligament.
    c. Femoral artery.
    d. Epigastric artery.
    e. Internal oblique and transverse muscles passing over the sac.
    f. Tendon of the transverse muscle passing under it.
    g. Fascia from Poupart's ligament, from which the cord has been withdrawn to shew the place through which it passes.
    h. Hernial sac.
    i. Hernial sac above the ring.
    k. Knife introduced to shew the manner of dilating the stricture, which is to be always done forwards and upwards opposite to the middle of the mouth of the hernial sac, in all the varieties of inguinal hernia, excepting when the spermatic cord is on the anterior part of the mouth of the sac, when the division should be made outwards.

    Cutting upwards is necessary in the variety shewn in Fig. 6, as dividing outwards towards *e* would divide the epigastric artery.

THE ANATOMY

AND

SURGICAL TREATMENT

OF

CRURAL AND UMBILICAL

HERNIA,

&c. &c.

By ASTLEY COOPER, F.R.S.

HONORARY MEMBER OF THE MEDICAL AND PHYSICAL SOCIETIES OF EDINBURGH; LECTURER ON ANATOMY AND SURGERY,
AND SURGEON TO GUY'S HOSPITAL.

ILLUSTRATED BY PLATES.

PART II.

LONDON:

PRINTED FOR LONGMAN, HURST, REES, AND ORME, PATERNOSTER ROW; AND
FOR E. COX, ST. THOMAS'S STREET, BOROUGH;

AND SOLD BY

MESSRS. JOHNSON, ST. PAUL'S CHURCH YARD; MURRAY, FLEET STREET; HIGHLEY, FLEET STREET; PHILLIPS, GEORGE YARD; CALLOW, SOHO;
A. CONSTABLE AND CO. AND W. CREECH, EDINBURGH; MESSRS. DUNCANS, GLASGOW; AND GILBERT AND HODGES, DUBLIN.

1807.

T. BENSLEY, PRINTER, BOLT-COURT.

TO

ALEXANDER MONRO, SEN.ᴿ M.D.

PROFESSOR OF ANATOMY

IN

THE UNIVERSITY OF EDINBURGH,

𝕿𝖍𝖎𝖘 𝖂𝖔𝖗𝖐

IS DEDICATED, AS A TESTIMONY OF RESPECT AND GRATITUDE,

BY HIS FRIEND AND PUPIL,

THE AUTHOR.

PREFACE.

In the following work I have pursued the same general plan of description as in the former, beginning with the structure of the parts, to which succeed the symptoms and causes of the disease, its anatomy, and the treatment which it requires; and to these I have added occasional cases in illustration.

I feel much diffidence in giving to the public my description of the structure of the parts connected with Crural Hernia. They are extremely complicated in their nature, are subject to some varieties, and are so intimately connected and blended with each other, as not to be fully unravelled without a very minute and tedious dissection. I am therefore apprehensive that the description of these parts may sometimes want that conciseness and perspicuity, which should be a chief object in every scientific work.

It may be thought by some that I have been too minute in the anatomical description, and have dwelt too much upon the subdivisions of fascia and other parts apparently of inferior importance. To this however I must answer, that a right conception of these parts is of great moment; for though in their natural state these fascia and membranous processes are often extremely delicate in their texture, and closely approaching to the nature of common cellular membrane, yet when they have long been subjected to the pressure of herniæ, they become condensed, tough, and not unfrequently of a firmer and thicker texture than the sac itself. Hence arises the common and most embarrassing uncertainty in the operation in distinguishing the hernial sac from its covering. Hence the frequent pauses in the operation, and the hesitating appeals to the judgment of the bye-standers, whether the membrane immediately under the knife is or is not the sac, which every one must have observed, when the operation is undertaken by Surgeons not familiar with this complicated anatomy, and which are only relieved by a gush of serum, when this fluid is fortunately interposed between the intestine and its coverings.

I must also request the reader not to consider the events of the cases of crural hernia here given as a fair average statement of the general success of the operation, when performed without delay, as soon as all reasonable attempts at reduction have failed. From a conviction of the great and often superior utility of relating unsuccessful cases, I have given both those that have occurred to myself, and such as I have observed in the practice of other Surgeons, wherever I have had an opportunity of verifying and explaining the peculiar circumstances by subsequent dissection. In general little utility arises from the relation of successful cases, beyond the mere description of the mode of operation, unless some peculiar circumstance arises; but the dissection of a fatal case is both a warning to future practice, and often establishes some important principle in the treatment of the disease, by accounting for anomalous appearances which have occurred during its progress. In by far the greater number of unsuccessful cases, the failure has appeared to be owing to delay in resorting to the operation, which delay is still more dangerous in the crural than in the inguinal hernia, inasmuch as the orifice through which the hernia descends in the former species, is much smaller, and less yielding, and hence the strangulation is more complete.

The preparations from which the plates are taken are all preserved; and I shall be always happy to shew them to any one to whom the representations here given are not satisfactory. The preparations which are the subjects of Plates V. XI. XII. XIII. XIV. and XVI. are in the collection at St. Thomas Hospital: those of Plates IV. VI. VII. IX. X. XIV. and XVII. are in my possession: one of Plate V. is in Guy's Hospital: that of Plate VIII. is in the cabinet of Dr. BARCLAY: and one of Plate XI. belongs to Mr. CUTTLIFFE of Barnstaple.

I should be ungrateful to Mr. SAUNDERS, our Demonstrator of Anatomy, if I were not to acknowledge his kindness in putting aside for my examination every specimen of hernia which has been of late years brought into the dissecting-room; and I have to thank my numerous medical friends for the zeal they have shewn in assisting me in my object, by giving me an opportunity of examining every case of this disease which has fallen under their observation.

In the relation of the case with which I was favoured by Mr. NORRIS, (See Part the First, page 17,) an error has arisen from a cause which his letter will explain, and I have, therefore, introduced it here in its corrected state.

The following is his Letter on this subject.

DEAR SIR,

I THINK it is nearly two years ago that you reminded me of a case of *bursten intestine* which I had mentioned to you, and shewn you the preparation; and you expressed a wish to have the particulars in writing, which I soon after furnished you with. A mistake having happened in the communication of that case in your work on Hernia, it must equally be your desire and mine that it be rectified. In our first conversation on this subject, I had mentioned the case of a bursten intestine, and another of a *lacerated intestine* in a man who had an *hernia*; and I shewed you both the preparations, which are still in my possession. The former of these cases was what I understood you to have asked for; and as I had not an opportunity of seeing a proof-sheet, the printer, by the omission of a whole sentence, has altered the meaning of the paper. I therefore request the insertion of the inclosed (which I believe to be a literal transcript of the paper I gave you) in the second part of your valuable work. Annexed are the particulars of the case of hernia.

" A middle aged man who had been many years afflicted with a scrotal hernia and had not worn a truss,
" received, on the neck of the tumour, a very violent push from the pole of a coach. Within an hour after the
" accident I saw him. His countenance was that of a dying man; his pulse was quick and feeble; he vomited
" very frequently, and complained of extreme pain all over the abdomen. In the part which received the stroke,
" there was not, externally, any wound, and it was, comparatively, without pain. The tumour was now larger
" than it had ever before been, but quite free from that tension that accompanies a strangulated intestine. I had
" no difficulty in returning the contents into the abdomen, from which, however, he obtained no relief; very soon
" after removing the pressure of my hand the tumour became as large as before. In consultation with an emi-
" nent physician, various purgatives were prescribed, and occasionally, opium, to quiet the stomach and allay
" pain; but nothing that we could devise had the effect, during the three days that he survived, of either pro-
" curing a passage or in any degree alleviating his torture.

" The examination of the body was commenced by opening the hernial tumour, the whole contents of which
" were now found to be blood: the sac did not appear to have sustained any injury. The abdomen contained at
" least three quarts of extravasated blood, which was found to have proceeded from a lacerated wound of the
" Mesentery and Intestine Ileon. It seems probable, that between those parts and the hernial sac there had
" been adhesions which were separated by the accident. The intestine was torn from the mesentery to the ex-
" tent of about five inches."

The following is the Case of *bursten* intestine.

" In the night of February 23, 1802, ... SERJESON, a young man of a spare habit, running at a
" quick pace, and turning the corner of a street, came suddenly and violently against a post. About the middle
" of the abdomen was the part that received the shock, from the effects of which the man soon appeared to have
" recovered; but after proceeding a little farther he felt great pain and became very faint, which obliged him to
" sit down on the steps of a door, from whence after remaining there ten minutes, he was able with difficulty to
" crawl home, a distance of about two hundred yards. I saw him early the next morning, and received the fore-
" going account. There was not the slightest appearance of injury on the part that had received the stroke, but
" in the course of the spermatic vessels on the left side and extending into the scrotum, there was ecchymosis
" with enlargement equal to that which a moderately sized hernia might be supposed to produce. He was very
" sick; he vomited frequently and with great straining; his pulse was quick and extremely feeble; his coun-
" tenance was pale and expressive of the greatest anxiety; and he complained of acute pain all over his belly.
" The abdomen, however, was quite soft, and the contents of the tumour in the groin were easily returnable into

" the abdomen, but quickly came down again when pressure was removed. I repeated this so often, and so
" minutely examined the parts as to be perfectly sure that the swelling was caused merely by an extrava-
" sated fluid.

" The abdomen was fomented, and a solution of Epsom salt in mint water was ordered to be taken every
" fifteen minutes until a passage should be procured. In the course of the day he swallowed four ounces of the
" salt without effect; the same symptoms continued with the most torturing pain; and in the morning, he
" died.

" Having some years before seen a man, who, in consequence of an accident had his intestine torn from
" the mesentery (in an old hernia) with a laceration of the gut itself, in whose case the symptoms were exactly
" similar to those of the present, I ventured to predict that we should find a wound in some part of SERJESON'S
" intestines. Having obtained permission to examine the body, Dr. YELLOLY and I met for that purpose, the
" day after death.

" The tumour was then larger than before, was discoloured, and contained air, clearly discoverable by the
" touch; and being opened was found to contain water, blood, and air. On opening the abdomen, a fluid of
" the same kind, to the quantity of about a quart, was there effused. Not the least appearance of injury or dis-
" ease was discoverable in any part of the contents of the abdomen, except an irregular aperture in the ilion, which
" readily admitted my finger, and through which every thing that descended from the stomach easily found its
" way into the general cavity.

" Such accidents, it is to be feared, will be almost necessarily fatal, principally on account of the circular
" fibres of the intestines drawing, as in this case, the lips of the wound asunder."

The size of this work has been objected to, and I am very ready to acknowledge its inconvenience, but I hope that this will be counterbalanced by the advantage of having all the parts exactly of their natural size, which gives a facility for making measurements, and ascertaining the relative position of parts, with as much accuracy as could be done by reference to the dead body.

With respect to the execution of the plates, I should think it unworthy of the importance of the subject, and (let me be allowed to add) of the pains which I have bestowed upon it, if I had had the paltry ambition of being the editor of *splendid* plates. My only object has been to give accurate and perspicuous engravings, such as may convey to the reader, as exactly as the pencil can do, the precise form and size of the parts which are exposed by the knife of the anatomist, and I shall consider myself as fully repaid for the attention which I have given to this subject, if my labours prove useful to those who, by being placed in less favourable circumstances than myself for actual observation, have not had the same opportunity of becoming acquainted with this disease in the living, or in the dead.

MARCH 20, 1807.

CONTENTS.

Chapter 1. Of the Structure of the Parts concerned with Crural Hernia, ... Page 1
2. Of the Symptoms and Dissection of Crural Hernia, ... 6
3. Of the Reducible and Irreducible Crural Hernia, ... 11
4. Treatment of Strangulated Crural Hernia and Operation, ... 14
5. Of the Varieties of Crural Hernia, ... 20
6. Of the Operation inwards, ... 22
7. Cases of Crural Hernia, ... 23

Chapter 1. Of the Symptoms and Causes of Umbilical Hernia, ... 35
2. Of the Reducible and Irreducible Umbilical Hernia, ... 39
3. Of the strangulated Umbilical Hernia, ... 41
    Cases of Umbilical Hernia, ... 44
    Of the Ventral Hernia, ... 58
    Of the Pudendal Hernia, ... 62
    Of the Vaginal Hernia, ... 65
    Of the Perinèal Hernia, ... 67
    Of the Thyroideal Hernia, ... 70
    Of the Cystic Hernia, ... 72
    Of the Ischiatic Hernia, ... ib.
    Of the Phrenic Hernia, ... 76
    Of the Mesenteric Hernia, ... 82
    Of the Mesocolic Hernia, ... 84
    Of the Strangulated Intestine, ... 85

*_{*} The word *Femoral* may be always substituted for *Crural*, without altering the sense.

All the drawings are exact copies of the preparations, excepting that of Mr. CUTCLIFFE, to which I have taken the liberty of adding the right vesicula seminalis, as it is naturally connected with the posterior part of the bladder, otherwise the relative situation of the sac could not be completely understood.

ERRATA.

Page 7, line 3, from the bottom, read " protrudes " instead of " penetrates."
7, ... 6, instead of " ever since," read " since."
8, ... 1, for " behind," read " upon."
8, ... 1, for " arises from," read " attached to."
8, ... 23, for " Surgeon to the Universal Dispensary," read " Apothecary to the Universal Dispensary, Ratcliffe Highway."
21, ... 31, for " it will be found," read " for I suspect it will be found."
22, ... 3, from the bottom, for " but is situated at some distance from its anterior part," read " but is situated at some distance from the common seat of the stricture at its anterior part."
29, ... 6, for " Mr. WHITE," read " Mr. SMITH."
31, ... 30, for " it might be returned," read " it might be first sewn and then returned."
32, ... 13, from the bottom, for " and if they did not succeed, would have the operation performed," read " and if they did not succeed after a judicious trial of the taxis, would have the operation performed."
54, ... 3, from the bottom, for " after the evacuation," read " after an evacuation."
55, ... 3, read " Exomphalos," instead of " Exempholos."
56, ... 12, from the bottom, in Dr. HAMILTON's case, instead of " . And " read " , and "
63, ... 7, for " pubis ischium," read " pubis and ischium."
80, ... 8, from the bottom, read " Emphysema," instead of " Emptrysema."
81, ... 6, " Expiration," instead of " Expiation."
87, ... 10, instead of " under which," read " under which adhesion."

Plate I. *h*. read " tendinous " instead of " tendonous."
..... I. *y*. read " on the pubis " instead of " in the pubis."
..... IV. In the note to this plate, instead of " several years," read " three years."
..... XI. Fig. 3, *m*. read " was not," instead of " is not."
..... XVI. *b*. read " sygmoid " instead of " sygmord."
.... for " Mr. WARDROPER," read " Mr. WARDROP."

IN the preface to my former work there is an error which I am anxious to correct. In the sentence which alludes to the time at which I first advised the operation *upwards*, it is stated that I recommended the division of the stricture in that direction from the period at which I first began to give Surgical Lectures. But I find that at first I described the operation as directed by my friend Mr. CLINE, viz. by making the incision *upwards and outwards* in the common inguinal hernia, and *upwards and inwards* in that variety of it which descends on the inner side of the Epigastric Artery. But afterwards finding that it would be extremely difficult in the living subject to distinguish the one species from the other, I advised the operation *upwards* as the most likely mode of avoiding the artery under each situation of the disease. When my first part was published I had chiefly practised this operation on the dead subject, and afterwards dissected the parts to ascertain its safety with respect to the Epigastric Artery. I had also recommended it to others when I have been a by-stander at an operation. I have since several times performed it on the living subject, and the result has been such as to lead me to believe not only that it will be always found safe, but that it will do away those apprehensions which a doubt of the true nature of the disease will always create in the mind of the operator.

I HAVE given no other Index than the marginal, as I conceived that this with the table of contents would be sufficient.

OF CRURAL HERNIA.

CHAPTER I.

Of the Structure of the Parts concerned with Crural Hernia.

It will be necessary previous to the description of the symptoms and treatment of Crural Hernia, to give as accurate a view as I am able of all the parts directly and indirectly concerned in this intricate and difficult part of Anatomy; and to shew what are the means that nature has adopted to prevent the contents of the lower part of the abdomen from quitting their natural position, and how it happens that these means sometimes fail in producing the desired end.

The anatomy of the bones is as follows. Bones.

The distance between the symphysis pubis and the anterior superior spinous process of the ilium is from five and a half to six inches; and if a line be drawn from one of these points to the other, the space beneath it will be bounded at its lower part for about half its length by the pubis and half by the ilium.

About an inch and a quarter from the symphysis pubis (in the dried bone) upon its anterior and upper part is situated the tuberosity of the pubis, or (as it has been improperly called) its Spinous Process. A line is seen to extend along the upper part of the pubis as far as its juncture with the ilium, and is continued to the side of the sacrum. This is called the Linea Ileo-pectinea, and it forms the superior edge of the brim of the pelvis.

About an inch and a quarter from the tuberosity of the pubis is a natural depression, formed for the lodgement of the crural artery and vein, which, upon its outer side, is bounded by the beginning of the ilium, forming a projection over the acetabulum.

On examining that part of the ilium which forms the outer part of the space that has been just mentioned, it will be found that two inches below the anterior superior spinous process of the bone, is situated another process, called the anterior and inferior spinous process; and that between the two is a small depression about an inch and a quarter in extent: immediately below the latter process is the acetabulum, and an inch anterior to it is a flat surface, extending to the beginning of the pubis.

It will be seen upon dissecting the soft parts which fill up the space between the ilium and pubis, that they are wonderfully and beautifully constituted for the purpose for which they are designed; but it must be acknowledged that they are parts of all others the most difficult to investigate and to describe with perspicuity.

The pubis is covered by a ligamentous substance, which forms a particularly strong production above the linea ileo-pectinea, extending from the tuberosity of the pubis outwards, and projecting beyond the bone above that line. Into this process the external oblique muscle is inserted, as will be seen in Plates II, and III. To see this clearly in dissection, the fascia covering the pectineus muscle and the muscle itself must be cut away. Ligament of the pubis.

The lower tendinous edge of the external oblique muscle has generally been called *Poupart's Ligament*, but is now more commonly named the *Crural Arch*. This arch is stretched from the anterior superior spinous process of the ilium to the tuberosity of the pubis, into which a part of it is fixed, whence it proceeds forwards to the symphysis pubis, where the remainder is inserted. Crural arch.

Above the tuberosity of the pubis is the External *Abdominal Ring*, which is bounded above and below by two columns of tendon; the one forming an insertion into the tuberosity of the pubis, the other into the sym- External oblique muscle.

B

physis. These two columns are joined at the upper and outer part of the ring by transverse tendinous fibres. The external oblique muscle, besides terminating in the symphysis and tuberosity of the pubis, is also inserted by strong tendinous fibres into the ligament of the pubis near an inch outwards from the tuberosity, whence it is extended inwards behind the tuberosity into the upper part of the pubis towards its symphysis, and outwards to the spinous process of the ilium, forming a thin and sharp edge, which is turned towards the abdomen, and makes the *posterior edge* of the crural arch. From the anterior superior spinous process of the ilium to the tuberosity of the pubis, is stretched the anterior rounded edge of the crural arch, and it thus forms an arch over the crural artery and vein, the psoas and iliacus internus muscles and the anterior crural nerve. It appears then that the lower part of the tendon of the external oblique muscle has three distinct insertions; first, into the symphysis pubis, and this forms the superior column of the external abdominal ring; secondly, into the tuberosity of the pubis, which forms the lower column of the ring; and thirdly, into the ligament of the pubis over the linea ileo-pectinea. This last portion by its conjunction with the ligament of the pubis forms a crescent-shaped edge, which is turned towards the crural vein, but situated about the distance of five-eighths of an inch from it.

Superficial fascia.

The parts below the crural arch are constructed in the following manner. When the skin is removed from the crural arch and fore part of the thigh, a thin fascia will be seen to extend over the tendon of the external oblique muscle, and to adhere firmly to the edge of the arch, whence it passes downwards upon the absorbent glands of the groin, where it is usually said to terminate, but erroneously, since it may be traced down the thigh, covering and supporting the absorbent vessels, their glands, and the superficial veins. The strongest fibres of this facsia are transverse; and though in its natural state it is so thin as easily to escape observation, yet when it has been long pressed upon by a hernia, particularly in a subject loaded with fat, it becomes of considerable density. The covering which this gives to the hernial sac, with the attachment which it has to the lower edge of the external oblique muscle, will be seen in Plate IV.

Fascia Lata.

To the lower edge of the external oblique muscle is attached a much stronger fascia, called the *Fascia Lata*. It may be said to have two attachments or origins. One part of it rises from the rounded edge of the crural arch, between the tuberosity of the pubis and the anterior superior spinous process of the ilium. This covers the femoral artery and vein, the femoral part of the iliacus internus and psoas muscles, and the anterior crural nerve, and its breadth at its origin is from four to five inches in the adult. The other part of the fascia lata arises from the ligament of the pubis at the insertion of the external oblique muscle, extends over the pectineus and triceps muscles, and afterwards unites with the first mentioned part under the saphena major vein. The united portions then form the fascia lata which extends down the thigh, embracing the muscles and supporting them in their actions.

When the fascia lata is first laid bare, it appears to be turned in under the femoral artery and vein; but on removal of the fibres which are at first exposed, is found to form a sharp crescent-shaped edge; a part of this fascia has been called by Mr. HEY the *Femoral-ligament*.* It has been well described by Mr. ALLAN BURNS of Glasgow, (in the Edinburgh Medical and Surgical Journal), and is called by him the *Falciform Process*. This fascia passes over the crural vessels, and its principal use is to cover the femoral artery and vein, and thus strengthen the sheath in which they are contained. Its *lunated* edge, covered by some tendinous fibres, will be seen in Plate I, of my former part, and the whole of the edge in Plate II and III of this work.

When the fascia lata is dissected away, the muscles are exposed on each side, and the anterior crural nerve is laid bare, but the femoral artery and vein still remain enclosed in a sheath.

Fascia transversalis.

The anterior part of this sheath is formed by a thin fascia that appears, at first sight, to arise from the crural arch, but may be detached from it by passing the finger behind the arch, where it will be found to be a continuation of the fascia which lines the transversalis muscle; but as it passes under the posterior edge of the arch it closely adheres to it. This fascia is particularly described in the former part of this work, (page 5 and 6,) as passing upwards to form the internal abdominal ring, and it also passes down behind the crural arch adhering to it, and uniting to the femoral artery and vein. Some fat will be generally found between this fascia and the fascia lata of the thigh. The whole of this fascia will be distinctly seen in Plate II and III, detached from its juncture with the crural arch, and it will appear that it might be described as arising from the crural arch

---

* Mr. HEY's plate does not do justice to his ideas; for, from a conversation which I have had with that excellent Surgeon, I find he does not mean to confine the term *femoral ligament* to the outer fascia alone, but extends it to the portion of the sheath behind the crural arch.

and dividing into two portions; one, ascending to the transversalis muscle, the other, descending to form the crural sheath. The anterior part of the sheath in which the crural vessels are contained, is joined to the fascia transversalis, and when it is removed the crural artery and vein are laid bare.

Crural arch.

These fascia and the crural arch are rendered extremely tense by extending the thigh, and are much relaxed by bending it, and by throwing the knee inwards.

Through the inner side of the crural sheath next to the pubis, pass the crural absorbent vessels into the abdomen. In the male subject I have seen them enter the sheath in a cluster, through a single hole in this fascia; but in both male and female the fascia is generally cribriform, and these vessels pass through a variety of openings, but still if the sheath is cleanly dissected, and the finger thrust into it from the abdomen, the cellular membrane and absorbent vessels are pushed out through one of these holes which is larger than the rest. Some of the absorbent vessels also pass between the artery and the vein, and on the outer side of the artery, entering by two small holes in the anterior part of the sheath. See Plate I.

Absorbent vessels.

When the sheath is cut open the crural artery and vein are exposed. These vessels pass down within the sheath for about two inches, after which they carry with them a closely investing fascia, derived from the fascia lata, which accompanies them in their course down the thigh. The sheath is therefore formed like a funnel; it is large above, but contracted around the artery and vein below. The crural artery is situated on the outer side of the vein: its distance from the symphisis pubis is about three inches.

Contents of the sheath.

Crural artery and vein.

The epigastric artery arises from the anterior part of the external iliac artery, where it terminates in the crural, and passing inwards is continued obliquely upwards to the rectus muscle. In its course inwards, it approaches to from half to three quarters of an inch of the aperture by which the crural absorbent vessels enter the abdomen. This vessel is subject to some variety in its origin; for although it generally arises at the mouth of the sheath, yet I have seen it arise an inch below its usual place; and when its origin is lower than usual, it passes proportionally nearer to the crural hernial sac. It is always accompanied by one, and often by two veins. This vessel is drawn down into the sheath by extending the thigh.

Epigastric artery.

The spermatic cord in the male, and round ligament of the uterus in the female, enter the internal abdominal ring from a quarter to half an inch to the outer side of the epigastric artery, and descend to the external ring through the inguinal canal. In this course they become placed before the epigastric artery, behind the tendon of the external oblique muscle, and just above the crural arch.

Spermatic cord and round ligament.

The arteria circumflexa arises from the external iliac artery, nearly opposite, but a little below the epigastric artery, and passing into a small space situated at the junction of the fascia iliaca and fascia transversalis, it is continued towards the inner part of the superior spinous process of the ilium.

Arteria circumflexa ilii.

The vena saphena major enters the crural sheath about an inch below the crural arch, and terminates on the inner side of the femoral vein.

Saphena major.

Of the Parts which shut the Abdomen from the Thigh.

When the peritoneum is dissected off the inner side of the abdominal muscles from the symphysis pubis to the anterior superior spinous process of the ilium, the distance, which is usually from five and a half to six inches, will be found to be occupied in the following manner.

From the spinous process of the ilium to the external iliac artery, a fascia is attached to the posterior edge of the crural arch, and extends from thence over the iliacus and psoas muscles. It is fixed in the inner labium of the crista of the ilium, and a process from it extends behind the iliac artery and vein, to be fixed in the linea ileo pectinea, and into the ligament of the pubis. Another portion also of this fascia descends behind the crural artery upon the upper and middle part of the thigh, which sends a process forwards to pass between the artery and vein. This fascia then shuts up the space behind the crural arch on the outer side of the iliac vessels, and prevents any descent of the viscera to the thigh in that direction. It has been particularly described by GIMBERNAT, and should be called from its situation, the *fascia iliaca*.

Fascia iliaca artery.

Anteriorly to the crural arch is situated another fascia, which may be divided into two portions, the one being placed a little before the other. Its outer portion is attached to the greater part of the posterior edge of the crural arch, from as far as the spinous process of the ilium, and the inner labium of that bone, and it ascends

Fascia transversalis.

to the posterior part of the transversalis muscle on the outer side of the spermatic cord, where that cord first quits the abdomen: the inner portion is thinner than the former, but is strengthened in its fore part by the tendon of the transversalis muscle; it is also slightly attached to the crural arch, but is more firmly fixed to the ligament of the pubis, and is extended over the pubis into the cavity of the pelvis; it rises to the tendon of the transversalis muscle on the inner side of the spermatic cord, and is firmly attached to the linea semi-lunaris.

This anterior fascia, which is described in the first part of this work, should be called the *fascia transversalis*; it lines the posterior part of that muscle, and there prevents the viscera from descending between the fibres of the abdominal muscles, but leaves an opening for the passage of the spermatic cord and round ligament, which I have ventured to name the *internal abdominal ring*. This fascia sends a process before the external iliac artery and vein, and another between them, which unites with one passing from the fascia iliaca, and these vessels are thus united to the crural arch. A process of fascia extends from the inner side of the vein to the ligament of the pubis, in which there is an aperture for the passage of the absorbent vessels.

Crural sheath. Each of these fasciæ sends down a portion of its substance under the crural arch, to form the crural sheath for the artery and vein. The fascia iliaca sends the posterior part, the fascia transversalis the anterior, and by the union of these on each side the lateral portions of the sheath are produced.

Contents of the sheath. The crural sheath contains, when examined from the abdomen, the crural artery, which is situated on the outer side of the sheath, the crural vein, which is placed in the centre, and the absorbent vessels, which are found principally on the inner side of the vein, where they enter an absorbent gland; but some absorbents enter the abdomen between the artery and vein. The fascia which is united to the iliac artery and vein is firm and resisting; but that which invests the absorbent vessels and lines the crural ring is of looser texture.

Crural ring. The space called the crural ring is situated between the crural vein, which forms its outer part, and the crescent-shaped edge of the insertion of the external oblique muscle into the ligament of the pubis, anteriorly by the inner edge of the crural arch, and posteriorly by the pubis and the ligament which covers it. It is lined by the fasciæ which form the sheath, and unless the fascia transversalis, and the internal oblique and transversalis muscles are removed, the insertions of the external oblique are not seen. When that fascia is detached from the posterior edge of the crural arch, an oval space appears, which contains the crural artery, vein, and an absorbent gland, and which extends from the edge of the third insertion of the external oblique muscle into the pubis to the junction of the fascia iliaca with the posterior edge of the crural arch.

If the finger is pressed upon the crural ring, it may be passed from half to three quarters of an inch towards the thigh within the sheath. But there is no other aperture at this part if the sheath remains, except the minute cribriform holes for the absorbent vessels, or a single one if they enter in a cluster. When the finger is thrust down through the crural space, the lunated or semilunar edge of the fascia lata may be distinctly felt.

There is a depression at the junction of the two internal fasciæ, which tends towards the crural ring, and there is a similar depression and tendency from the crest of the pubis to the same part.

Difference of structure in the male and female. The difference in the structure of these parts in the male and female, which chiefly conduces to the production of crural hernia, is well explained by Dr. Monro, Jun. in his Observations on Crural Hernia. The oval space forming the orifice of the crural sheath is larger in women than in men. The distance from the spine of the ilium to the symphisis pubis is greater, and consequently the crural arch is longer. The third insertion of the external oblique muscle is not so deep in the male as in the female. The psoas and iliacus internus muscles occupy less space in the female than in the male. I have generally found this disease in women who have a very large pelvis, in whom the ilia and pubes project more than usual.

Measurement. The following measurement of the parts I have described was made from subjects which appeared to be well formed, and although the precise distance will vary according to the size of the person, the relative proportion of the parts will be still preserved.

MALE.

	Inches.
Symphisis pubis to the anterior spinous process of the ilium	$5\tfrac{3}{4}$
.... to the tuberosity of the pubis	$1\tfrac{1}{8}$
.... to the inner margin of the external abdominal ring	$0\tfrac{7}{8}$

	Inches
Symphysis pubis to the inner edge of the internal abdominal ring	3
.... to the middle of the iliac artery	$3\frac{1}{8}$
.... to the middle of the iliac vein	$2\frac{5}{8}$
.... to the origin of the epigastric artery	3
.... to the course of the epigastric artery on the inner side of the internal abdominal ring	$2\frac{3}{4}$
.... to the middle of the lunated edge of the fascia lata	$3\frac{3}{4}$
Anterior edge of the crural arch to the saphena major vein	1
Symphysis pubis to the middle of the crural ring	$2\frac{1}{4}$

FEMALE.

Symphysis pubis to the anterior superior spinous process of the ilium	6
.... to the tuberosity of the pubis	$1\frac{3}{8}$
.... to the inner margin of the external abdominal ring	1
.... to the inner edge of the internal abdominal ring	$3\frac{1}{4}$
.... to the middle of the iliac artery	$3\frac{3}{8}$
.... to the middle of the iliac vein	$2\frac{3}{4}$
.... to the origin of the epigastric artery	$3\frac{1}{4}$
.... to the course of the epigastric artery on the inner side of the internal abdominal ring	$2\frac{7}{8}$
.... to the middle of the lunated edge of the fascia lata	$2\frac{3}{4}$
Anterior edge of the crural arch to the saphena major vein	$1\frac{1}{4}$
Symphysis pubis to the middle of the crural ring	$2\frac{3}{4}$

CHAPTER II.

Of the Symptoms and Dissection of Crural Hernia.

Symptoms.   The first symptom of the disease is pain produced on straightening the thigh, which extends to the stomach, and produces nausea; and when the thigh is examined, an absorbent gland may be more distinctly felt in that groin than in the other, and gives considerable uneasiness even on slight pressure. The first time this pain is perceived is generally at night, when the patient, after stooping to undress, suddenly rises and straightens the limb; and it continues some time after he is in bed, obliging him to lie with the knees elevated, which posture soon relieves him. The cause of the pain on stretching the limb is the extension of the fasciæ of the thigh and the pressure which they make on the tumour.

The first distinct external mark of crural hernia is a general swelling of the part easily returnable by pressure, descending in the erect, and ascending in the recumbent posture, and which at first seems to be only the dilatation of the sheath that contains the crural artery and vein. The next appearance is that of a small circumscribed tumour, about the size of the finger's end, situated under the crural arch, about an inch on the outside of the tuberosity of the pubis, and lying in the hollow between this process and the crural artery and vein. As the tumour enlarges, instead of falling downwards like the inguinal hernia, it passes forwards and often turns over the anterior edge of the crural arch, this being the direction in which there is the least resistance. As it proceeds, the swelling increases more laterally than upwards or downwards, so as to assume an oblong shape, the longest diameter being in a transverse or horizontal direction. In the female it is generally very moveable, and being soft, and the skin not being discoloured, it has the appearance merely of an inguinal tumour of one of the absorbent glands; but in the male the skin is generally not so loose, the swelling not so distinctly circumscribed, and the tumour appears buried more in the substance of the thigh.

Size.   The largest size to which I have seen the tumour arrive, was in cases of which I have given Plates in this work. The one was in the male, the other in the female; they were each of them about the size of the fist, and each occupied the whole of the hollow from the anterior superior spinous process of the ilium to the tuberosity of the pubis. But my friend, Mr. Thompson, Professor of Military Surgery at Edinburgh, mentions a case of a woman labouring under an old irreducible crural hernia, in whom the tumour extended half way down the thigh. In this case the parietes of the abdomen were so thin, that the peristaltic motion of the intestine could be distinctly perceived.* Upon the whole, however, it is unquestionable, that the crural hernia is comparatively smaller than the inguinal, and on this account it is more dangerous.

Direction.   The direction in which the crural hernia passes is obliquely inwards and forwards, and, excepting at first, very little downwards, so that in cutting into this tumour the incision is made into its fundus. This is the general situation of the tumour; but it sometimes happens, that instead of crossing the thigh in the direction of the crural arch, it extends downwards along the edge of the crural vein and the vena saphæna major.

Dissection.   The crural hernia, when dissected, presents the following appearances: when the skin is removed, the superficial fascia of the external oblique muscle is laid bare, which, though it is of a delicate texture in its common state, when pressed upon by a hernia becomes extremely thickened and very distinct, more especially in a subject loaded with fat. Under this covering there is generally another fascia, precisely of the form of the hernia itself, and which it very closely embraces. A thin fascia naturally covers the opening through which the hernia passes and descends on the posterior part of the pubis. When the hernia therefore enters the sheath it pushes this fascia before it, so that the sac may be perfectly drawn from its inner side, and the fascia which covers it left distinct. The fascia which forms the crural sheath, and in which are placed the hole or holes for the absorbent vessels, is also protruded forwards, and is united with the other, so that the two become thus consolidated into one. If a large hernia is examined, this fascia is only found to proceed upwards as far as the edge of the orifice on the inner side of the crural sheath by which the hernia descends, but in a small hernia it passes into the abdomen as far as the peritoneum and forms a pouch, from which the hernial sac may be with-

---

* See a very clear and ingenious Essay on Crural Hernia by Mr. William Wood, Surgeon, at Edinburgh.

drawn leaving this, forming a complete bag over the hernia. In a small hernia the fascia is thicker than the sac itself, but by being gradually extended it becomes thinner and less distinct, and in one example of this kind from the female subject (which forms the subject of one of my Plates), this and the superficial fascia have coalesced into one. I first observed this fascia in dissecting a male subject brought into St. Thomas's Hospital in the year 1800, who had a strangulated crural hernia on the one side, and a reducible one on the other: I next saw it in the operation performed upon Mrs. Bispham hereafter to be mentioned, and have ever since demonstrated it in preparations whilst delivering my lectures on crural hernia. This fascia will be seen in almost all the plates, and in one of the drawings of Plate IV very distinctly, as the hernial sac is removed from its inner side. It may be termed the *Fascia Propria* of the crural hernia. When this fascia is divided, a quantity of adipose membrane is found between it and the sac, and when this is cut through, the peritoneal sac itself is exposed. Behind the hernial sac is the fascia lata, and the sac rests in the hollow between that part of it which covers the crural vessels, and that which passes over the pectineus and triceps muscles, so that the fascia lata is situated posteriorly to the hernia. Fascia propria.

The form of the sac in crural hernia differs from that of the inguinal: the shape of the latter is pyriform, but the fundus of the crural bears a very large proportion to its orifice, and the form of the sac when inflated and dried is generally that of the following outline. Form of the sac.

The orifice of the sac is surrounded by a fascia or cellular membrane, much condensed by an adhesive process which forms with the fascia below a complete bag, out of which the hernia may be drawn and the bag left behind perfect. Between the orifice of the hernial sac and the tuberosity of the pubis is situated the insertion of the external oblique muscle into the linea ileo-pectinea, and ligament of the pubis. Behind it, is the pubis covered by its ligament and fascia iliaca; anterior to it, is the beginning of the posterior edge of the crural arch, and below this the lunated edge of the fascia lata and part of the crural sheath; and on its outer side is a thin process of fascia, which passes between it and the iliac vein. Indeed, it is according to the size of the hernia that there is more or less remaining of the original fascia, which extends from the insertion of the external oblique to the iliac vein. If the hernia is small, a process of this fascia remains round the orifice of the sac; but if it is large, the orifice of the sac occupies the whole space between the insertion of the external oblique and the crural vein; excepting that a thin portion of fascia still remains between the vein and the sac. This vein runs on the outer side of the hernial sac, about half an inch from the center of its orifice, and half an inch beyond the vein; and exterior to it is the center of the external iliac artery: the epigastric artery arises from the external iliac, about three quarters of an inch from the center of the sac, and as it passes forwards and upwards it approaches this point about a quarter of an inch nearer. The general distances of the different parts are as follows. Seat of its orifice.

MALE.

	Inches.
From the symphysis pubis to the center of the orifice of the sac	2
...... the center of the orifice of the sac to the external iliac artery	1
...... the center of the orifice of the sac to the center of the external iliac vein	$0\frac{1}{2}$
...... the center of the orifice of the sac to the origin of the epigastric artery	$0\frac{1}{4}$
...... the center of the orifice of the sac to the inner edge of the internal abdominal ring	1
...... the tuberosity of the pubis to the center of the orifice of the crural hernia	1

Measure of distances.

FEMALE.

Each measure is from one-eighth to one-fourth of an inch more where the pelvis is large and well formed.

The spermatic cord of the male, and the round ligament of the uterus of the female, pass about half an inch anterior to the mouth of the hernial sac, being first situated to the outer side, and afterwards crossing its fore part. Spermatic cord.

When the opening through which the hernial sac has passed is examined anteriorly, it will be found that the sac, after descending a little way into the crural sheath, turns inward and penetrates the inner part of this sheath where the absorbent vessels pass. The hernial sac is here placed between two columns of fascia of the crural sheath; the one proceeds from the anterior part of the insertion of the external oblique muscle into the Direction of the sac.

pubis, is reflected behind the crural vein, and passes over the neck of the sac: the other arises from the point of insertion of the external oblique into the linea ileo-pectinea and ligament of the pubis, is continued behind the neck of the sac, and is at last undistinguishably blended both with the fascia that covers the crural vein, and with that part of the fascia lata which passes over the pectineus muscle. See Plate II and III.

Diagnosis. The same general symptoms characterize crural as inguinal hernia; it appears in the erect, and disappears in the recumbent posture; it dilates when the patient coughs, is elastic and uniform to the touch when it contains intestine, and then gives a guggling noise when it returns into the abdomen. When it contains omentum the surface is less equal, it feels doughy, and gives no particular sound when it returns into the abdomen.

The crural hernia is less liable to be confounded with other diseases than the inguinal, because tumours of the groin from other causes, are much less frequent than those of the scrotum, but still great care is required to prevent the practitioner from mistaking the disease, and persons have, to my knowledge, lost their lives from such errors, or from the swelling being altogether overlooked.

Enlarged gland. It would scarcely be supposed that crural hernia could be mistaken for a glandular enlargement of the groin, yet such a mistake has been made, as the following instance will shew: A man who was sent into Guy's Hospital for this complaint by a surgeon in considerable practice, had been poulticed for three days for what was supposed to be a venereal bubo, and when the operation was performed the intestine was found mortified. Also in the case which I have detailed on the authority of Mr. BETHUNE, a crural hernia was opened under the idea of its being a suppurating gland, the stools were discharged at the opening, and the patient soon after died. Now such mistakes as these must arise from inattention to the patient's account of the progress of the case, to the circumstance of the tumour appearing in the erect, and disappearing in the reclined posture, and especially being dilated on coughing, together with a general irregularity of the bowels, costiveness, eructation, and vomiting. The following case, however, will serve to shew the necessity of minute attention in cases of this *Case.* kind. I was called to a lady, aged fifty-five years, by Mr. OWEN, Surgeon to the Universal Dispensary, who had laboured from Wednesday the 12th of November, to Friday the 21st, 1806, under symptoms of strangulated hernia. She had been attended by a physician and apothecary for *ileus*, but had not mentioned to them her having a tumour in her groin. Mr. OWEN discovered a swelling in the right groin, which he told me was extremely hard, and did not feel to him like a hernia; yet he supposed from the symptoms it could only be that disease. Upon examination I found a gland enlarged to the size of a pullet's egg and very moveable, but upon feeling behind this gland I could perceive an elastic tumour distinct from the swollen gland. I pressed upon it for about seven minutes, when a part of the tumour suddenly slipped into the abdomen, and in about three minutes more the remainder returned with a guggling noise. Fifteen minutes afterwards she had a stool, and had several others in the evening, when all the symptoms of strangulation had ceased. The glandular tumour still remains. This case struck me as important, both for the duration of the symptoms of strangulation, which was ten days, as well as from the combination of the two diseases.

Psoas abscess. The psoas abscess and crural hernia have some symptoms in common, and therefore a surgeon may be deceived by this disease. The seat of the tumour when first perceived is nearly the same, it dilates when the person coughs precisely as hernia does, and it is rather fuller in the erect than the recumbent posture. The distinguishing marks of the two diseases are, that the psoas abscess is preceded by pain of several weeks duration in the loins, that though the posture makes a sensible difference in the fulness of the tumour, it rarely entirely returns into the abdomen; a sense of fluctuation also may generally be felt; and its situation, though nearly that of crural hernia, is generally rather more towards the spinous process of the ilium. It is also unconnected with an interrupted state of the bowels; and lastly, the enlargement of the tumour, when it has appeared in the thigh, is much more rapid than that of an hernia. Fatal errors, however, are not so liable to occur, from confounding these diseases as the former, because the psoas abscess requires no immediate active attention on the part of the surgeon, and sufficiently distinctive marks will arise whilst he is waiting for the further progress of the disease.

But the error which is the most frequent, and by far the most dangerous, is that of mistaking crural for inguinal hernia. It is dangerous during the operation of the taxis, as the direction of the pressure should be entirely different in the two diseases; and it is extremely dangerous in the operation, particularly if the surgeon's usual habit of operating in inguinal hernia is to make the incision upwards and outwards towards the *Mistaken for inguinal.* spinous process of the ilium. Several instances of such mistakes have come to my knowledge. I once went with a physician into the country to operate, as I was told, on a case of inguinal hernia, but when I examined the patient, I found that the hernia was crural, and had been three days strangulated, during which time repeated attempts had been made to reduce it by pressing the tumour towards the spinous process of the ilium. It was reduced in five minutes by employing pressure proper for the crural hernia.

A Surgeon who had operated on a crural hernia sent his patient afterwards to London, to request that a proper truss might be procured for her, and in his letter stated, " that, during the operation, he had found the stricture in this case at the abdominal ring." He was fortunate in having escaped destroying his patient. Another Surgeon in operating in a supposed *inguinal hernia* had a venous hæmorrhage arise, which delayed the operation fifteen minutes, and which he found it was difficult to stop. It was a crural hernia, and it was probably the crural vein which he had injured, as he cut towards the spinous process of the ilium. This dangerous mistake is liable to happen without considerable attention, particularly as the crural hernia, after descending into the thigh, often turns before the crural arch. The marks of distinction, as far as I have been able to observe, are the two following: first, that the neck of the inguinal hernia is situated above the tuberosity of the pubis, but that of the crural below it and to its outer side; and secondly, if the sac is drawn down in the crural hernia, the crural arch may be traced above it. If these two circumstances are carefully attended to, the disease will not be confounded by those who have studied the natural structure of these parts.

An enlargement of the crural vein may be mistaken for a crural hernia. Mr. Hosegood, Surgeon in the Borough, requested me to see a patient of his who had a tumour in the groin, which dilated when she coughed, disappeared in the recumbent, and reappeared in the erect posture, and which he informed me had been supposed to be a hernia. It was easy to detect the nature of the case, for, although it disappeared in the recumbent posture, it was immediately reproduced, although she continued in that posture, by pressing on the vein above the crural arch, and retarding the return of blood. She died of a stricture in the colon; and, upon inspecting the body, I found that I could readily thrust my finger into the crural vein, but that she had no hernia. *[margin: Varicose crural vein.]*

I lately dissected a person whose case is detailed hereafter, and who had an artificial anus in consequence of the operation for hernia, in whom I found on the left side a steatomatous tumour occupying exactly the place of a crural hernia. It appeared that this woman had laboured under crural hernia, that the sac had gradually contracted, for a very small portion of it remained in the crural orifice, and that the space had not only been occupied by fat, but that this had grown into a tumour of considerable size. I have made a preparation of this tumour, but it did not come into my possession until it was too late to include it amongst the plates. *[margin: Steatomatous tumour.]*

Dr. Monro, jun. mentions an instance of an hydatid tumour which was removed from the upper and inner part of the thigh, which might easily be mistaken for a hernia; and he gives another example of it from Dessault, who found it transparent when a candle was brought near to it, and that he could draw it from the crural arch so as to leave a space between the tumour and abdomen, which proved that it was not formed from it. *[margin: Hydatid tumour.]*

Two herniary sacs have been stated to pass behind the same crural arch; but, although I would not be understood to deny their existence, I have not seen an example of sacs having two separate orifices into the cavity of the abdomen; but I have known one hernial sac descending into the sheath for the crural vessels and crossing the anterior part of these, and another portion of it quitting the sheath and extending in the usual direction upon the thigh. *[margin: Plurality of sacs.]*

Crural hernia occurs more frequently on the right side than on the left, and, probably, because the greatest exertions are generally made on the right side. On dissection, however, I have generally found that if there was a large hernia on one side, a small one could be detected on the other, though, for the most part, not such as had been discovered during life. *[margin: Occurs most in the right side.]*

Crural hernia occurs more frequently in the female than in the male, which arises partly from the difference which has been described in the parts behind the crural arch; and partly because the orifice for the spermatic cord in the male is so much larger than that of the round ligament in the female, that inguinal hernia is a more frequent occurrence in the male, which has a tendency to prevent the crural. I have, however, known both inguinal and crural hernia exist on the same side in the same subject; but only in two examples. Sometimes crural hernia is found on one side, and inguinal on the other; and an example will be found in one of the Plates of a crural and inguinal hernia (the latter of which had been cured by adhesion), on one side, and on the other side an inguinal hernia still remaining open. Of this specimen I have given two different views, as it conveys a very clear idea of the relative situation of parts in both these species of hernia. Women who have borne children are more subject to this disease than others, and, probably, because the extension of the *[margin: Most frequently the female. Crural and inguinal in the same subject.]*

abdominal muscles, during gestation, leave after delivery the parts under the crural arch in a state of relaxation.

Contents. The crural hernia most frequently contains intestine only, and generally the ilium, sometimes both intestine and omentum; but I have seen only two instances of its containing merely omentum. The cæcum is sometimes in the hernia of the right side. The ovaria have also been found in crural hernia, and in one of my Plates the uterus will be seen drawn to the orifice of the hernial sac.

Age. The youngest period at which I have known the disease to occur was seven years of age. The patient was a girl who was very much weakened by scrophulous complaints: she had worn a truss about half a year. I have also seen it at eleven years; and next in point of age was a lady of nineteen years, on whom I performed the operation. (*See the Cases.*) The frequency of this disease is proportionate to the age of the person, and one reason independent of the relaxation of age, that old persons are so much more subject to crural hernia than the young, is, that the psoas and iliacus internus muscles, in consequence of the more sedentary habits of advanced years, become of less size than at an earlier period of life; and as they occupy less space behind the crural arch, there is more room for a dilatation of the crural sheath. The fasciæ also in age are much weakened by absorption.

Causes. The causes which produce crural hernia are nearly the same as those that occasion the inguinal, and which have been already detailed in the former part of this work. They are, in general, whatever increases the pressure of the viscera and lessens the resistance of the parietes of the abdomen. But there is one circumstance in which they differ, for I have never known the crural hernia produced by a blow; this disease being the effect only of gradual pressure and extension of parts, for they are so constructed as scarcely to allow of laceration without extreme violence. The term *rupture*, therefore, is peculiarly inapplicable to this species of hernia.

During the enlargement of the uterus in pregnancy, crural hernia generally disappears; but I saw with Mr. RICHARD PUGH of Gracechurch Street, a large crural and umbilical hernia in a lady between five and six months gone with child.

CHAPTER III.

Of the Reducible and Irreducible Crural Hernia.

The crural hernia is found in the three states of reducible, irreducible, and strangulated.

As the opening through which this hernia passes is of very small diameter, the subject of it is in great and constant danger of losing his life by obstruction in the bowels; and though when it is reducible it returns into the abdomen during the night, yet this is done with less facility than in inguinal hernia, and symptoms of strangulation are liable to occur on any distended state of the bowels, and irregularity in the digestive functions. Dangerous state of the patient.

The reduction by the taxis or manual skill, is also much more difficult in this than the other species of hernia, and in consequence of the smallness of the opening through which the intestine descends, and the direction which it takes, a different management is required in this operation. The method is the following: the position of the patient is to be such as to relax the abdomen as much as possible, for which purpose the shoulders should be elevated, and the thighs bent at right angles with the body; but even this posture produces but little effect, unless the knees at the same time are brought together. If the parts are dissected directly with the view of observing what difference it made in the relative tension of parts in the dead body, it will be found that when the thighs are extended, the crural arch and all its fasciæ are upon the stretch; when the thighs are bent, but the knees turned outwards, the fasciæ are somewhat relaxed; but when the thighs are bent and the knees brought together, the crural arch and its fasciæ are all extremely loosened, and still more are the parts loosened by throwing one thigh, when bent, across the middle of the other. When the body is in the recumbent posture, the thighs bent, and the knee thrown inwards, the Surgeon is to place himself over the body of the patient, and putting both his thumbs on the surface of the tumour, he is to press gently directly downwards, as if he were endeavouring to press the tumour into the thigh rather than towards the abdomen. If this pressure is steadily kept up for some minutes till the surface of the tumour is brought even with the line of the crural arch, the hernia may then be pressed towards the abdomen and will return into that cavity. I am convinced that much of the difficulty found in returning this species of hernia often depends on the improper direction given to the pressure; for if the tumour is pressed at first towards the abdomen, it turns over the crural arch instead of passing under it, and then the utmost degree of force which may be applied will only endanger the bursting of the intestine, but cannot contribute to its reduction. Taxis. Direction of the pressure.

The same general precautions that were mentioned, when treating of inguinal hernia, apply to the reduction of the crural, so that when the position of the patient and the direction of the pressure are correct, the reduction is to be attempted by long continued and gentle pressure, avoiding all kind of violence, which can be of no service in accomplishing the end in view, and may be productive of much and very serious mischief; examples of which I have given in my former volume, and others equally impressive I have since seen in the form of the disease of which we are now treating. Pressure gentle, and continued, not forcible.

A spring truss is the only method of preventing the danger to which this disease exposes the sufferer, and the observations made in the former volume on the application of this instrument in inguinal hernia, will apply (with some few exceptions) to the crural. Indeed, if the hernia is small, precisely the same truss should be applied for crural hernia as that which is constantly worn for the inguinal; but it must be placed rather lower than for the inguinal hernia; but though this answers the purpose in a small hernia, a truss of a different kind is required if the hernia is large, because the orifice of the hernial sac is proportionably more extended. Truss.

The distance between the crural ring and the upper abdominal ring is just an inch; and between the lower abdominal ring and the middle of the crural hole is also about an inch; and this aperture is from half to three quarters of an inch below a line drawn from one abdominal aperture to the other. It is, therefore, necessary that the bearing of the pad of the truss should be from half to three quarters of an inch lower down than in inguinal hernia, and should also press on the upper part of the thigh. For this purpose it is best that the pad of the truss be bent somewhat downwards, and not, as in the inguinal truss, continued nearly in a line with Distance of the apertures.

the spring. It will then rest in the hollow at the upper part of the thigh on the outer side of the tuberosity of the pubis; and as it lies upon the crural arch, the motions of the thigh will have no tendency to displace a truss thus constructed, which, with an inguinal truss pressed downwards to cover a large crural hernia, is an inconvenience constantly felt on every violent exertion. In the Plate which shews inguinal and crural hernia on the same subject, the truss will be seen bent as much as is ever required for crural hernia, and between this and that which is there seen and applied for inguinal hernia all the varieties will be comprehended.

Permanent cure unfrequent. A truss thus formed and regularly worn will have the effect of preventing the descent of the hernia, and may in process of time entirely obliterate the mouth of the sac. But I must say, that, as far as I have had an opportunity of observing, this effect is not so frequently produced in the crural as in the inguinal hernia; for I have known persons wear a truss for a great length of time, yet as soon as it was discontinued the hernia has descended with very little diminution of its original size. The reason of this, I believe, is, that when once a hernia has been formed, and the crural hole consequently dilated, the opening into it from the abdomen becomes nearly perpendicular when the body is erect, and the pressure of the contents of the abdomen, on this account, *Why.* is always the greatest and most direct at the time when pressure operates with the greatest force. Whereas in the inguinal hernia the direction of the upper part of the sac is oblique; the abdominal viscera press together the sides of that part of the canal which lies between the two rings, and thus it becomes more easily contracted, so long as the passage into it maintains some degree of its original obliquity. Another reason of the comparative infrequency of the cure of crural hernia by pressure, is, the constant variation in the tension of the crural arch on every motion of the body, which must as constantly alter the pressure of the truss, and destroy that uniformity of action on which the gradual obliteration of the opening into the sac may be supposed to depend.

Whether this be the true explanation or not, the fact is that this hernia is more liable to reappear, so that the truss must be worn night and day, and continued for some years before it will be safe to leave it off and make a trial of the effect which it has produced.

Mode of measuring for a truss. The mode of measuring a person for a truss in crural hernia is the following: place him in a recumbent posture, return the hernia, and then putting the finger upon the orifice of the hernial sac, desire him to rise, and if the hernia does not descend, carry a piece of tape from under the finger round the pelvis, midway between the trochanter major and the spine of the ilium, and bring it round to the point from which the measurement began. Any intelligent instrument-maker from this measure will be able to make a truss of a proper length. The angle which the pad of the truss is to form with the spring, should be somewhat more than a right angle for the largest hernia, and gradually approaching to that for the inguinal in the smallest.

Hernia large and descending. If the crural hernia extends far down on the thigh, instead of turning upwards towards the crural arch, it is owing to the aperture on the side of the crural sheath being very large, and under these circumstances there is great difficulty in keeping the intestines within the abdomen. In this case it is necessary that the pad of the truss should be of great length, and the spring unusually strong; and it will also be useful to carry a strap from the lower part of the pad round the upper part of the thigh, to prevent the pad from rising out of its proper place.

Double truss. When a hernia exists on both sides a double truss will be required, which is to be constructed upon the same principles as the single truss, and is to be made to buckle behind, so that it may be easily adjusted to the shape of the wearer.

Whalebone truss. I have lately seen an ingenious person from Scotland of the name of HINCHLIFFE, who shewed me trusses, the spring of which was made of whalebone instead of steel; and if its elasticity is not affected by the heat of the body or change of climate, this must prove a great improvement on the common truss, as the steel of the latter will rust, and the spring will sometimes give way in situations in which another cannot be readily procured.

More simple the better. With respect to variations in the form of trusses, which every man, whether he knows any thing of the structure of the parts or not, thinks he has a right to make, I shall only observe, that the less complicated a truss is the better; first, because it answers the purpose more completely of keeping the hernia in the abdomen; and secondly, because if it is out of order, which it is very apt to be, it is more difficult to get it repaired, and a person with a complicated truss, whilst it is repairing, is constantly exposed to the danger of having his hernia strangulated. There is no difficulty in applying a proper truss if the seat of the aperture is known.

Of the Irreducible Crural Hernia.

As far as I have had an opportunity of observing, there are three causes by which the crural hernia is rendered irreducible; the one, the formation of adhesions between the omentum or intestine, and the inner side of the hernial sac; another, so great a growth of parts that they become too large to repass into the cavity of the abdomen; and the third, a contraction of the hernial sac. <small>Causes of.</small>

With regard to the first of these causes, I must observe that I have very rarely seen the intestine adhering, and that I do not believe it is so frequent an occurrence in the crural as in the inguinal hernia. I have, however, twice seen it adhering in cases in which the operation was performing; in the first, the adhesions were of recently effused lymph which could be readily torn through; and in the second, they had existed long, and formed firm membranous bands which required a division by the knife. I have also in the dead body seen a very firm adhesion of the intestine to the inner side of the sac, leaving no space between the inner side of the sac and the surface of the intestine. <small>Intestine adheres.</small>

The omentum is often found adhering to the sac; but this is a circumstance of little importance in the operation: whereas an adhesion of the intestine increases much the difficulty of the operation, and adds greatly to its danger. <small>Omentum adheres.</small>

Adhesion of the intestine to the inner side of the sac, is sometimes followed by ulceration, of which the following case, which Mr. JOHN KENT, Surgeon, in the Borough, has communicated to me, is a good example. Mrs. B, the wife of a butcher in the Borough, had a crural hernia in the right side, which had existed twenty years. When Mr. KENT was called to her, she had complaints which indicated a diseased state of the abdominal viscera, and accidentally mentioned a swelling in the right groin. Upon examining this he found it ulcerated to about the extent of a shilling, and fæculent matter was frequently discharged at the orifice, though the fæces still, in part, passed by the anus. She suffered a long time under this disease, and at length died dropsical. <small>Ulceration of intestine.</small>

The growth of the protruded parts, the second cause which I have mentioned as rendering this hernia irreducible, arises from neglecting to wear a truss; so that the omentum having for a long time remained unreturned increases with the bulk of the body, dilates the sac on each side, and becomes at last so bulky, that it can no longer be returned through the small orifice through which it originally descended. (*See Plate* V.) <small>Growth of parts.</small>

Under these circumstances it becomes highly desirable that pressure should be made upon the hernia, so as to prevent its increase; and I have had the pleasure of observing that under this treatment the increase of the swelling is entirely prevented, and even a gradual absorption of the protruded parts has taken place, so as to prevent the troublesome bulk of the swelling, and to make it almost entirely disappear. The intestine, however, must be first carefully reduced. <small>Treatment of.</small>

Mr. GASELEE, of High Street, Borough, requested me to accompany him to see a gentleman who had long suffered under an irreducible crural hernia. I tried to pass it back into the abdomen, but without success. I then ordered a truss for him of the usual form of that used for hernia, but hollowed out so as to embrace the surface of the swelling, by the use of which the swelling very soon lessened and ceased to become troublesome, and in a few weeks it had almost entirely disappeared. I prefer a hollow truss to one of the usual make, as the pressure which it exerts is easier to the patient, and may be worn without pain for a sufficient length of time. <small>Case.</small>

But if the hernia is intestinal the pressure of a truss, even thus constructed, cannot be borne in the crural hernia; for I applied one on the intestinal crural hernia of a lady whom I attended with Mr. PUGH, and it gave her so much pain that it was obliged to be discontinued after a few hours. <small>Pressure cannot be borne in the intestinal.</small>

The contraction of a portion of the hernial sac is another cause that renders hernia irreducible; an example of which I have in my possession in a large hernia, in which the contraction was situated an inch below the orifice of the sac, and had been occasioned by the pressure of the lunated edge of the fascia lata; but generally this contraction is at the mouth of the sac, and is more frequently found there than in the inguinal hernia. <small>Contraction of sac.</small>

CHAPTER IV.

Treatment of Strangulated Crural Hernia and Operation.

Symptoms and causes of strangulation.

As the symptoms of strangulation have been detailed in the account of the inguinal hernia in the former part of this work, it is unnecessary to repeat them here. The same may be observed of the causes of strangulation, which are generally the same, viz. sudden distension of the abdominal viscera; great exertion of the abdominal muscles, more especially in lifting a heavy weight in a stooping posture; flatulent vegetable food, or any food difficult of digestion.

Three seats of the stricture.

With regard to the seat of the strangulation in crural hernia, it will be found in three different situations.

First, in the crural sheath, and semilunar or lunated edge of the fascia lata.

Secondly, at the posterior edge of the crural arch.

Thirdly, in the mouth of the hernial sac, and fascia which covers it.

Orifice of the crural sheath, and semilunar edge of the fascia.

With respect to the first of these, it will be found that a portion of the crural sheath remains below the crural arch, which forms a strong circular band by which the hernial sac is surrounded. When the sac is drawn from the sheath in the male, the orifice by which it has passed will be found to be formed by two strong columns of fascia, one passing above, and the other below the sac, and meeting on the inner side at the posterior insertion of the external oblique muscle into the ligament of the pubis, and on the outer side at that part of the sheath which covers the crural vein. In the female these columns are not equally strong, still a portion of the sheath surrounds the hernial sac. (See Plate II and III.) If the hernia is large, it reaches to the semilunar edge of the fascia lata, and is compressed by it.

Posterior edge of the external oblique.

The second place at which the stricture is found, and which requires division in large crural herniæ, is the posterior edge of the external oblique muscle and the fascia transversalis, which pass before the mouth of the hernial sac, and which extending inwards to be inserted into the pubis, form also the inner boundary of the sac at this part, whilst a small process of fascia on the inner side of the vein forms its outer boundary. Thus then there are two seats of stricture, one the edge of the aperture in the crural sheath, and the other about half an inch above it, formed by the posterior edge of the external oblique muscle.

Mouth of the hernial sac.

The mouth of the hernial sac is the other seat of the stricture.

This aperture is very generally small when compared with the size of the hernial sac, and being much pressed upon by the posterior edge of the crural arch it undergoes a slow process of inflammation, which thickens very much the fascia in which it is inclosed. If the sac is removed with the fascia which incloses it, its mouth will be found to form a dense and compact substance, which firmly resists any attempt to dilate it by pressure.

The anterior edge of the crural arch, or POUPART's ligament, does not form the stricture, or require any division, excepting in very large herniæ.

Small size of the tumour.

The possibility of crural hernia being the cause of symptoms of strangulation, renders it even more than in inguinal hernia necessary for a physician called in on account of symptoms of ileus, to inquire whether there is any tumour in the groin, or the upper part of the thigh, for in crural hernia the tumour is smaller and less prominent than in the inguinal, and more liable to be overlooked. These tumours are sometimes so small that it is not without hesitation that the Surgeon determines with respect to the operation; for they are, when small, generally covered with an absorbent gland, and with so much difficulty distinguished, that I confess I have more than once began the operation with much doubt about the nature of the tumour, making it rather the means of determining with certainty, than being assured that it was the disease which I suspected. I have already given two examples, one of the disease being overlooked, and the other of its being mistaken. Those who doubt the possibility of their being thus deceived, ought to read a case published by Mr. ELSE, in the Medical Observations and Enquiries, Vol. X. p. 355. It may be also here observed, that the patient is sometimes unacquainted with the existence of the disease, and often entirely unsuspicious of its being the cause of the symptoms.

The treatment which this hernia requires when strangulated, differs but little from that of the inguinal: the mode of using the taxis is, as I have explained in a former chapter, different, but still the same general treatment is to be pursued, such as bleeding, opium internally, the warm bath, topical applications of cold, and tobacco glysters; but as far as my observation extends, these means are less frequently effectual here than in the inguinal hernia, which is probably owing to two causes, viz. to the nature of the parts through which the hernia descends, and the smallness of the aperture forming the mouth of the sac. In the inguinal hernia the parts are so connected with muscles, that any relaxation brought on in these, affects the aperture through which the hernia descends; but in the crural hernia the seat of the stricture is in parts less connected with the action of muscles, and general relaxation has but little effect on them. To this cause then, and to the smaller size of the aperture through which the crural hernia descends, may be attributed the more frequent failures of the means employed for reduction. *The treatment.*

The delay of the operation, which I lamented and condemned when speaking of inguinal hernia, is to be still more deprecated in the crural; for death very generally happens earlier in the latter disease than in the former. *Danger of delay.*

A female servant to Mr. HERVEY, Coppersmith, in Houndsditch, aged forty-one years, who had long a crural hernia on the left side, and who had been employed in her usual manner all the day, was at half past eight o'clock in the evening of Tuesday the 6th of January 1807, seized with symptoms of strangulated hernia. She vomited almost incessantly; her countenance was sunken, and pain excessive both in the tumour and in the stomach. Mr. ROBINSON, Surgeon, in Mansell Street, Goodman's Fields, was sent for on Wednesday morning, who employed the means usually had recourse to in these cases, but nothing afforded her any relief; but seeing her danger, he promised to call early in the evening. At four o'clock in the afternoon she became very feeble, being unable to speak, but still the vomiting continued, and she died at six o'clock, having lived only twenty-one hours and an half after the accession of the symptoms. The event of this case was certainly unusually rapid; but I have twice known the operation performed only forty hours after the accession of the symptoms of strangulation, and the parts so much altered as not to be in a fit state to be returned into the cavity of the abdomen. This rapid progress to mortification arises from the small size of the hernia, and the narrowness of the aperture through which the intestine protrudes, so that a very great degree of compression is accumulated upon a small portion of the intestine. I should, however, observe, on the other hand, that I have known the operation successfully performed eight days after the accession of the symptoms of strangulation, as will be seen in the case of Mrs. SHEFFIELD, at the concluding part of this subject. But in this case there was a large hernia, and a large quantity of omentum protruded along with the intestine, which formed a kind of cushion around it, and prevented the pressure upon it from being so complete as if the hernia had consisted solely of intestine. *Case.*

When the parts have proceeded to mortification, the skin over the tumour is red and very painful to the touch, and it is in some degree an indication of a state of intestine very unfavourable to the success of the operation. However, I may observe, that in a large hernia, where the covering of the sac is very thin, I have known the skin become red and œdematous, yet the hernia was returned by the taxis, and the patient recovered. *Mortification.*

If the intestine mortifies, and the parts covering the hernia become inflamed and proceed to slough, the intestine will also separate, and an artificial anus will follow. And sometimes the fæces will, after a time, resume their natural course, the wound will heal, and the patient be completely restored. See Part I. Case from Mr. COOPER of Wootton-under-Edge, p. 33. *Artificial anus.*

Of the Operation for the Crural Hernia.

THE patient is to be placed upon a table three feet six inches in height, the body lying in a horizontal posture, but with the shoulders a little elevated; the legs as high as the knees, hanging over the edge of the table; and the thighs a little bent, in order to relax the abdominal muscles. The bladder must be emptied, and the diseased side shaved. *Situation of the patient.*

The incision is to be begun an inch and an half above the crural arch, in a line with the middle of the tumour, and extended downward to the center of the tumour below the arch. A second incision nearly at *First incision.*

right angles with the other is next made, beginning from the middle of the inner side of the tumour and extending it across to the outer side; so that the form of this double incision will be that of the letter T reversed. The advantage of this form of the incision is, that it gives an opportunity both of examining the parts distinctly, and of turning them aside to give a view of the orifice by which the hernia has descended, and of the parts which form the external portion of the stricture.

For want of this precaution I have known great difficulties occur in the operation, the incision, when single, being too small to give a sufficient view of the parts, and the depth at which the hernia is situated not allowing the Surgeon to have a distinct view of the progress of the operation.

The longitudinal incision sometimes occasions a slight bleeding from the division of the external pudental artery, and it is better to secure the vessel before any thing farther is done.

<small>Superficial fascia.</small>

The first incision exposes the superficial fascia, which is given off by the external oblique muscle, and which covers the anterior part of the hernial sac; but if the patient is thin, and the hernia has not been long formed, this fascia escapes observation, as it is then slight and delicate, and adheres closely to the inner side of the skin.

When this fascia is divided, the tumour is so far exposed that the circumscribed form of the hernia may be distinctly seen, and a person not well acquainted with the anatomy of the parts would readily suppose that the sac itself was now laid bare. This, however, is not the case, for it is still enveloped by a membrane, which is the fascia that the hernial sac pushes before it as it passes through the inner side of the crural sheath. This

<small>Fascia propria.</small>

membrane, the fascia propria, is to be next divided longitudinally from the neck to the fundus of the sac; and if the subject is fat, an adipose membrane lies between it and the sac, from which it may be distinguished by seeing the cellular membrane passing from its inner side to the surface of the sac. This is, in my opinion, the most difficult part of the operation, for the fascia propria is very liable to be mistaken for the sac itself; so that when it is divided, it is supposed that the sac is exposed and the intestine is laid bare; following up this idea, the stricture is divided in the outer part of the sac, and the intestine, still strangulated, is pushed with the unopened sac into the cavity of the abdomen. I have given a Plate, from an excellent preparation now in my possession, of an undivided sac returned into the cavity of the abdomen, and containing the strangulated intestine, and the particulars of the disease at the end of this part of the subject.

It must be remembered, however, that in large herniæ the fascia propria of the sac is sometimes inseparably united to the superficial fascia, so that the same incision divides both.

<small>Hernial sac opened.</small>

The hernial sac being exposed is to be next opened; and to divide it with safety, it is best to pinch up a small part of it between the finger and thumb, to move the thumb upon the finger by which the intestine is distinctly felt, and may be separated from the inner side of the sac; and then to cut into the sac, by placing the blade of the knife horizontally. Into this opening a director should be passed, and the sac opened from its fundus to the crural sheath. A small quantity of serum usually escapes when the sac is opened, which is either transparent or sanious according to the length of time that the strangulation has continued. The intestine or omentum, or both, then become exposed.

<small>Fluid in the sac.</small>

It often happens, however, that there is no fluid contained in the sac of femoral hernia, even although no adhesion exists between the sac and its contents; a circumstance which probably may be attributed to the small size of the sac and its contents, and the very limited secreting surface which it affords, for when there is much unadhering intestine, there is always a notable quantity of serum. If the strangulation has continued for many hours, the intestine is also covered with a coating of coagulable lymph, but not otherwise.

<small>First stricture divided.</small>

The next part of the operation consists in the division of the stricture; for this purpose the finger is to be pushed gently into the sac, and the omentum and intestine separated from its anterior part, the probe-pointed bistory which I have recommended, which does not cut near its point,* is to be pushed into the crural sheath at the anterior part of the sac, and the sheath is to be cut as far as the anterior edge of the crural arch, or Poupart's ligament. In a small hernia this division, which does not exceed half an inch, will be sufficient for the reduction of the parts. This was all that was done in Cases II, IV, and V. and the intestine was easily returned by this incision.

<small>Second stricture.</small>

But when the sheath has been thus divided, if the intestine, when slightly compressed, cannot readily be

---

* I have used this instrument several times, and can now recommend it still more strongly than formerly, on account of its safety in not injuring the intestine within the abdomen.

emptied, the finger must be passed at least half an inch higher, and then the posterior edge of the crural arch and the fascia that covers it will be felt, forming a sharp edge, strongly compressing the mouth of the hernial sac. To divide this edge the knife must be carried within the stricture, and being inclined obliquely inwards and upwards at right angles with the crural arch, a cut may be very safely made in that direction sufficient for the purpose of liberating the intestine from pressure.

The two incisions which I have directed being made from the interior of the sac, any stricture arising from the contraction of the sac itself will be at the same time removed, and the protruded parts be thus completely liberated. Third sac.

If the hernia is large and any pressure has been made on its contents by the semilunar edge of the fascia lata, the first incision will divide that edge.

Much danger will arise from any forcible attempt to press the intestine into the abdomen after the dilatation of the opening of the crural sheath; for if the stricture is at the second part, viz. at the posterior edge of the crural arch, this makes so firm a pressure on the parts, that the intestine will rather give way than the stricture will yield, and I am induced to believe, that this seat of the stricture has not been generally understood; yet in several of the cases in which I have operated, it has been situated there. Mr. JOHN PEARSON, also informed me that he lately operated upon a crural hernia, and divided all the parts which he could at first feel forming the stricture; but still an impediment existed to the return of the protruded parts, and he was obliged to divide the stricture much higher up before he could return them. No considerable pressure made after the division of the first stricture.

Surgeons talk very carelessly upon the subject of dividing the stricture; they say that the finger must be put into the sac, and wherever the stricture is felt that it should be divided. Again, it is said, the stricture is situated on the inner side of the sac, and derived from the pressure of the insertion of the tendon of the external oblique, or what they call GIMBERNAT's ligament. They do not consider that a stricture is a circle produced in the same way as if a cord were tied round the protruded parts, and that the division might be made at any part excepting the posterior, where the bone is placed, if other circumstances did not prevent it. The stricture may be divided on the inner side of the sac, that is, towards the pubis; but to this there are strong objections, which I shall make the subject of a future chapter. It cannot be divided directly outwards, for there the crural vein must necessarily be injured, and if the division is made upwards and outwards, towards the spinous process of the ilium, the epigastric artery is much endangered. However this artery is not so liable to be cut in the crural hernia as has been imagined; for it does not approach nearer than half an inch of the upper and outer part of the sac, and an incision of half an inch is more than is usually required to liberate the protruded parts in crural hernia. The stricture may be safely divided upwards, but the mode of doing it, in which there is the greatest security, both as respects the blood vessels and the protruded intestine, is to pass the bistory into the middle and anterior part of the mouth of the hernial sac, and to cut the stricture upwards, and with a slight obliquity inwards. Circumstances to be attended to in dividing the stricture.

Crural vein.

Epigastric artery.

Mr. HEY, whose name should be never mentioned but with respect, who is not contented with the mere practice of his profession, but who studies to improve it, advises that the knife should be introduced on the inner side of the sac, and the division be made directly upwards. Division upwards.

In the female, if the hernia is large, it will be sometimes, though very rarely, necessary to cut through the anterior edge of the crural arch, or POUPART's ligament, and this may be done from the inner side of the hernial sac by cutting obliquely inwards and upwards. But in a large hernia in the male subject, when the division of the crural arch is required, a different operation becomes necessary to prevent the spermatic cord from being injured. When the parts have been laid bare, and are found to be too large to be liberated by the division of the sheath and posterior edge of the crural arch, an incision should be made through the tendon of the external oblique muscle over the mouth of the hernial sac, about a quarter of an inch above the crural arch, which will expose the spermatic cord. This being drawn up by the finger, or by a curved probe, and removed from the direction of the incision, the Surgeon carries his finger into the sac with the bistoury upon it, and the anterior edge of the crural arch is cut without the smallest risk to the spermatic cord. See Plate relative to the operation, where a view is given of the parts in which this operation has been performed. Large herniæ.

Spermatic cord how avoided.

Mr. ELSE proposed that after an incision had been made above the crural arch, a director should be thrust behind it, and the arch divided upon the director to free the strangulated parts. But the reflection of the fascia transversalis renders it impossible, without considerable violence, to force a director thus into the crural sheath, and a friend of mine, Mr. Borrett, Surgeon, at Great Yarmouth, who performed this operation, told me, that he found great difficulty in passing the director under the arch.

<small>Treatment of the mortified intestine.</small>

When the stricture has been divided, and the protruded parts liberated from pressure, the state of the intestine must be examined, and if the circulation returns in it, if the dark colour produced by the constriction disappears or is much diminished, and if on drawing down the intestine, the part at which it had been girt by the stricture appears uninjured, it may be then returned into the cavity of the abdomen. If the intestine is mortified, that portion of it is to be cut away, and the ends of the intestine joined; and I would advise, that instead of leaving an opening in the intestine for the escape of the fæces, after the contents of the intestine have been evacuated at the wound, four ligatures should be applied, so as to shut the bowel in the whole of its circumference; and my reasons for differing in this respect from the opinion I gave in my former work are, that I have found in one case, that, by leaving a small opening, an artificial anus followed, and in another that where the upper part of the ilium had been mortified, that by the small aperture that was left, every thing the woman swallowed was so speedily discharged at the wound that it afforded no sustenance, and she died in four days after the operation. The stricture must be very freely dilated when the restoration of the canal is attempted, or the fæces will not pass through the intestine; and if after twelve hours no fæces have passed by the anus, and the vomiting continues, one of the stitches must be cut, and the chance of sustaining life by an artificial anus must be given.

Two cases have also occurred, since writing my former Part, of mortification in the intestine, in which, after opening the hernial sac, I left the process of separation to the efforts of nature, applying a poultice only: one of these patients died in two hours, and the other in twenty-one hours.

If after the symptoms of strangulation have continued for some time, and the external parts become mortified, it is best to leave them to slough, without attempting to assist nature by an operation; in proof of which I will again refer the reader to the case in the first part of this work sent me by Mr. Cooper, of Wootton-under-Edge, Gloucestershire. See p. 33.

I should still have great fears of returning the intestine into the abdomen after sewing it, notwithstanding the experiments which were made by Mr. Thompson and myself, and since confirmed by Mr. Smith, in his Inaugural Dissertation, which proved that an intestine may be returned into the abdomen after being secured by ligatures. But it is to be recollected that, in the disease before us, the intestine is highly inflamed, and that ligatures ulcerate so quickly in inflamed parts that there would be great danger of the escape of the fæces into the cavity of the abdomen; for in a case in which I left the intestine within the sac, after securing it by ligatures, the intestine burst open on the third day and an artificial anus was produced. (See Cases of Mortification.) I therefore think it safer to carry the intestine to the mouth of the hernial sac and there to fix it by its mysentery.

If the intestine is mortified, it requires great care in the operation to prevent the portion within the abdomen from being torn from the mortified part, which if the finger is forcibly introduced into the sac will undoubtedly happen, and the fæces escaping into the abdomen will destroy the patient in a few hours. To prevent this, after exposing the intestine, and finding it mortified, the finger should not be put into the mouth of the sac, but the bistory only be passed into the stricture; and when this is divided, the intestine is to be gently drawn down into the sac to expose the part at which it has been girt.

<small>Adhesion of the intestine.</small>

If the intestine adheres to the sac, extraordinary caution is required, both in the division of the stricture and in separating the adhesions. It is best to begin with gently separating the adhesions with the finger rather than with the knife, which can generally be effected without doing violence to the parts; but if the adhesions are short and very firm, portions of the sac must be cut away and returned into the abdomen with the intestine to which they adhere; the stricture too must be divided fibre by fibre with extraordinary care.

With respect to the omentum, if it adheres, its adhesions may be safely torn through with the finger; and if more of it has descended than can be easily returned, or if it has become hard and knotty, it must be cut away. I have done this in inguinal, crural, and umbilical hernia, and have seen it done by others without any bad consequences ensuing. It must be cut through where it is sound, which it will be known to be by the vessels bleeding, and this is to be the criterion of its being done sufficiently high up; and the vessels are to be secured by ligatures, and the omentum returned only to the mouth of the hernial sac.

Putting a ligature around the whole of the protruded omentum is either useless or dangerous: if it is placed upon the mortified part, it is obvious it must be useless, as the sloughing process will go on above it: if it is placed upon the healthy part of the omentum, why divide the stricture, as another is made immediately by the thread which is applied around it. Ligature on the omentum useless or dangerous.

Leaving the omentum in the hernial sac to slough appears to me unadvisable, because it is unnecessarily preserving a discharge for a length of time and protracting the cure. I have never seen this intentionally done, but in a patient in Guy's Hospital (*see the former Part, p.* 32); the omentum which had been returned into the abdomen redescended into the sac on the sixth day from the operation and gradually sloughed, keeping up during the time a very offensive discharge, and a great degree of constitutional irritation. A circumstance somewhat similar happened in the case of Mrs. CULF, which is mentioned under the head of Umbilical Hernia. Omentum sloughing.

When the protruded parts have been returned into the cavity of the abdomen sutures are to be made upon the integuments, and the wound closed as carefully as possible by lint, adhesive plaister, and bandage.

CHAPTER V.

Of the Varieties of Crural Hernia.

It is by no means common to meet with deviations from the usual structure of crural hernia. Those which have occurred to me are the following:

<small>Rupture of the superficial fascia.</small> The fascia which usually covers the hernial sac has given way, so as to allow of a portion of the tumour to pass before it; thus dividing the tumour into two parts, with a sort of hour-glass contraction between them. A variety of this kind would embarrass a person who was not aware of its nature, but it adds little to the real difficulty of the operation to one who understands well the anatomy of the parts; for as soon as the fascia is divided by the knife the hernia reassumes its usual appearance. See Case III.

<small>Hernia within the crural sheath.</small> Another variety is when the tumour does not quit the sheath for the crural vessels. The appearance of this disease is that of a general swelling of the fascia on the inner side of the femoral vein, but without its producing any circumscribed tumour. The part swells whenever the patient coughs or uses any considerable exertion, but the swelling diminishes, though it does not entirely subside, when he stands at rest. I have given a Plate of this disease from a dissection which I made, and believe it to be not an unfrequent variety, as I have met with it three times in the dead body, and it existed on both sides in each. In this case the hernial sac descends as usual on the inner side of the femoral vein; but instead of passing out of the sheath at the place at which the absorbents enter, it is continued downwards within the sheath, passing anteriorly to the femoral vein, and descends as far below the crural arch as the sheath will allow, the distance being in general from two to three inches.

This species of hernia is very easily reducible, and, I believe, is little liable to become strangulated, as the mouth of the sac is of considerable size. A truss should be applied in this hernia, both to prevent its increase, and to obviate the danger of its passing out of the sheath, in the usual manner. This species of hernia may also give rise to another variety of hernia, by passing out of the sheath at the opening by which the external cluster of the absorbent vessels enter it. The cause of this hernia within the sheath is the entire want of the process of fascia which passes on the inner side of the crural vein, so that the hernia turns before the vein instead of descending by its side.

If the variety of herniæ above described were to become strangulated, the operation would be attended with some difficulty, as the parts are more concealed. The superficial fascia must be first cut through, and the crural sheath laid bare, and the latter being then divided longitudinally, the hernial sac will be exposed, and is to be opened in the usual manner, and the stricture being felt for with the finger, is to be divided in the same direction as in the common crural hernia. The difficulty therefore arises from the depth of the situation of the hernia, and this circumstance will often make the Surgeon more than usually doubtful of the real nature of the disease. The stricture in this case must be always at the posterior edge of the crural arch See Plate VIII.

<small>Hernia in part in the sheath, in part out of it.</small> A third variety of crural hernia which I have met with is that in which the hernia is formed in part within the sheath, and also in the common way. I have given a view of the inflated sac of a case of this kind, which was taken from the body of a patient of Dr. Marcet's, in Guy's Hospital, who died of an aneurism of the aorta, and who had, at the same time, a crural hernia on the right side. In dissecting this case I directed one of the Students to pass his finger down into the sac whilst I cut upon the swelling. After dividing the superficial aponeurosis I laid bare several absorbent glands which were dissected away, and the femoral sheath exposed, which being cut open the hernial sac came into view. I removed the parts in order to preserve them, and on examining the femoral sheath I found that its inner side had given way, and a small hernial sac had been produced through the opening by which the absorbent vessels usually pass; whilst the greater part of the sac was stretched across the crural artery and vein, and had in consequence extended the sheath in which these vessels were contained. See Plate IV.

I have thought it right to mention this variety, although it would make little difference in the operation; as the part the most likely to be strangulated is that which passes out of the sheath in the usual manner, and not that which remains within it.

In one of the Plates the umbilical artery, which usually passes on the inner side of the sac by the side of the bladder, will be seen to pass on its outer side, and before its neck. It is probable, that it is in these cases the bladder protrudes into the hernial sac, but I could not ascertain it in this instance, as the omentum only remained down, but the bladder was very capacious, and laid over the orifice of the hernia. Umbilical artery on the outer side of the sac.

The last and most curious variety of crural hernia which I shall mention, is one in which the obturator artery passes round the neck of the hernial sac. Variety of the obturator artery.

I am indebted for the specimen of this variety to Dr. BARCLAY, Teacher of Anatomy at Edinburgh, and well known to the public for a valuable work, in which he has attempted to improve the language of anatomy, by substituting a philosophical and classical nomenclature for the perplexed and unmethodical set of terms now in use. This preparation (which Dr. BARCLAY was so kind as to send me for my inspection from Edinburgh) was taken from the body of a young woman, whose history was unknown. Dr. Barclay's case.

On examining the situation of the hernial sac, it was found taking its common course under the crural arch, and situated, as usual, on the upper part of the thigh; but on examining the neck of the sac, it was observed that the epigastric and obturator arteries had arisen by a common trunk, and that they had passed anterior to the sac before they divided; after which the epigastric artery proceeded upwards to the rectus muscle, and the obturator artery passed backwards on the inner side, and close to the neck of the sac, to the obturator foramen, through which it usually passes. The obturator artery, indeed, very frequently deviates from its natural course, and instead of arising separately from the internal iliac artery, it derives its origin from the external iliac in common with the epigastric. But in all the cases which I have myself dissected, where this variety existed with crural hernia, the obturator has passed into the pelvis on the outer side of the neck of the sac, entirely out of the reach of any injury by the knife, as will be seen in two of the Plates. In twenty-one preparations of crural hernia, I found six out of the twenty-one had this variety in the origin of the obturator artery.[*] When therefore this artery passes before to the sac (as in the case observed by Dr. BARCLAY), the arterial trunk common to it and to the epigastric is of unusual length; for when the trunk is short, the obturator passes behind the sac. A hernia thus situated is surrounded by blood-vessels, except at its posterior part, which might seem to render it advisable to deviate from the usual mode of operation to prevent this blood-vessel from being wounded. This however is not so liable to happen where the division of the stricture is made upwards, or a little upwards and inwards; for it will be found that the greatest distance between the artery and the hernial sac is at its anterior part. It is impossible to feel this artery before the introduction of the knife, for the finger cannot be passed behind the posterior edge of the crural arch, beyond which this artery is placed, until the stricture has been divided. The sac therefore is to be carefully divided anteriorly; but even supposing the artery to be wounded in the operation, it may be asked, what other direction of the wound would afford greater facility of tying the bleeding vessel? For by slitting up the crural arch, and drawing down the mouth of the hernial sac, the vessel would be brought into view, and might be secured.

My friend Mr. WARDROPE, of Edinburgh, has communicated to me two cases of a similar kind taken from each side of the same subject. His words are, in explanation of a sketch which he favoured me with, that " the " peritoneum is thrown aside, and the parts underneath exhibited without any further dissection. The epigas- " tric and obturator arteries come off from the iliac in one branch, and the accompanying veins divide in the " same manner. The obturator artery creeps close on the muscle, and completely surrounds, or rather passes " over the mouth of the hernial sac. The sac is extremely small, and its orifice is blocked up with a very " large lymphatic gland." Mr. Wardrope's case.

---

[*] The obturator artery arises more frequently from the epigastric than I have here mentioned, but is found to do so in less proportion in crural hernia, because this situation of the artery has some tendency to prevent a protrusion by passing over the crural aperture.

CHAPTER VI.

Of the Operation inwards.

Reasons for it.

The division of the stricture inwards in the operation for strangulated crural hernia, was first published by Gimbernat, in his treatise on this disease. The author having dissected the parts with great care, and finding that the firmest part of the stricture was on the inner side, and that the blood-vessels covered the orifice of the hernial sac on the outer and on the anterior parts (the crural vein and the epigastric artery lying in the former direction, and the spermatic cord on the latter), was led to believe that the operation inwards was the safest mode of dividing the stricture. If anatomy only directed my judgment I should concur in this opinion; but it appears to me that the danger in crural hernia is not derived from the vicinity of these vessels, but from the chance of wounding the intestine. Nor does this operation entirely prevent even the danger of hæmorrhage.

Difficulty of the operation increased by it.

The objections which I have to urge against this operation are the following: First, It very much increases its difficulty; for the crural hernia lies buried deep within the thigh, and the orifice of the sac is proportionally difficult to be reached. Even where the stricture is divided anteriorly, the instrument must be passed down to some depth before it can be introduced within the stricture; but if the division is made inwards, the bistoury must be buried so deep as to be entirely obscured by the surrounding parts. Having tried both these modes of operating, I can assure those who have not had an opportunity of making a comparative trial, that the latter operation is much the most difficult to perform.

Danger to the ntestine.

Secondly, in Gimbernat's method a danger is incurred of wounding the intestine in two different ways. In looking for the seat of the stricture on the inner side, the intestine (which in crural hernia descends inwards) is obliged to be drawn very much to the outer side, to allow of the finger, or of a director, to be passed to the orifice of the stricture. In doing this the intestine is much stretched at the strictured part, and if it has been long strangulated it readily tears through at this place, and the fæces are discharged at the wound. This I have reason to believe, in one of the cases which will be detailed, was the cause of the laceration of the intestine and consequent death of the patient.

The other mode in which the intestine becomes injured, is by its being cut in passing the knife. The stricture is too small entirely to admit the finger, and the surgeon, fearful of bruising the intestine by attempting to force his finger up the stricture, introduces a director to guide the incision, or the knife without a director; in doing which, a fold of intestine gets before it, and in the way of the knife, within the mouth of the sac, or still higher, above the sac within the abdomen; but when the incision is made from the anterior part of the sac the intestine is entirely behind the knife. If this accident be immediately discovered, the patient has some chance of recovery with an artificial anus, which may either last only for a time, or continue during life, according to the treatment pursued; but if the intestine is within the abdomen at the time the injury is received, the strangulated portion is returned into the cavity without the wound being suspected, and the patient dies in a few hours, after suffering violent pain, and having the fæces escape through the wound. In such cases, on examination after death, the abdomen is found violently inflamed, owing to the escape of bile into the peritonæum. See Plate relative to the operation.

This division insufficient.

Thirdly, there is another strong objection to the operation inwards, which is, that if the hernia is large this mode of dividing the stricture is not sufficient to allow of the return of the protruded parts, for it gives but little additional room, so that great force must be used to reduce the hernia; and often, after all, the parts behind the crural arch must be divided in the usual way, and the whole operation rendered unnecessarily complex.

Obturator artery endangered.

Fourthly, the obturator artery, which, in the usual operation, is only endangered when it varies from its natural course, will be in much greater hazard in the inward incision, as this artery under this variety of course closely embraces the sac on the inner side, but is situated at some distance from its anterior part; and, moreover, if it is cut during the operation inwards, it will be scarcely possible to secure it, which it might be, when the anterior incision is employed.

CHAPTER VII.

Cases of Crural Hernia.

CASE I.

Mrs. Clark, aged forty, a patient of Mr. Brickenden's, of Horsleydown Lane, had, in August 1799, a strangulated crural hernia on the left side, of an oval form and considerable size, occupying almost the whole of the groin, and extending from the tuberosity of the pubis near to the spinous process of the ilium. Symptoms of strangulation had taken place forty-eight hours before I saw her, and during the last six hours she had frequent hiccough. I immediately attempted to reduce the hernia by the hand, but without success; and believing that no time was to be lost, I advised the operation, to which she very readily consented. The first incision was three inches long, and nearly midway between the pubis and crural artery, which, after dividing the fascia that covered the hernia, left the surface of the sac exposed; a very small puncture was made into the sac, and a director being passed up to the crural arch, I laid open the whole of the anterior part of the sac. This exposed both omentum and intestine; the latter of which was of a coffee colour, and the omentum adhered strongly to the inner part of the sac. I then passed a director into the mouth of the sac, carrying it about half an inch behind the crural arch, and as the hernia was large, I cut not only the mouth of the sac, but also Poupart's ligament, or the anterior edge of the crural arch, in the direction upwards and inwards.

The intestine was then particularly examined to observe whether it began to recover its natural colour, and its veins were pressed to see if the blood returned into them with freedom, which being the case, and no livid spots appearing, the intestine was passed into the abdomen.

The omentum being hard and thickened, all that had protruded was cut away, except a small portion which was left with a view of filling the mouth of the sac, and thereby lessening the probability of a future descent.

The edges of the wound were then brought together and closed by three sutures, and upon her being put to bed thirty-five drops of Tincture of Opium were given to her. In two hours she had two evacuations, and in the course of the evening had several others. The wound looked well on the following day, and she was free from constitutional disorder. However opiates were still required, as the stomach remained irritable, and she had vomited several times. On the next day this symptom disappeared and she seemed to be doing well. The wound was perfectly healed in about three weeks.

She was afterwards obliged to wear a truss, as the tumour became rather larger than before the operation, so that no advantage was derived in this case from leaving a portion of omentum with the view of closing the hernial orifice, which I attributed to her being suffered to rise without a truss before the wound was healed, or time had been given for the omentum to adhere.

CASE II.

Mrs. Bisphan, a patient of Mr. Holt's, of Tottenham, had for many years laboured under a crural hernia. In the summer of 1801, it became very painful, but without interrupting the regular functions of the bowels; however she kept her bed, chiefly on account of the extreme pain she suffered in attempting to put her leg to the ground, which was probably owing to the fascia pressing upon the tumour during the extended position of the thigh. She had remained in this state for several days when Mr. Holt requested me to see her. I made several unsuccessful attempts to reduce the hernia, and as the pain and inability to move continued, I advised the operation, which Mr. Holt performed. A longitudinal incision was made over the middle of the tumour at right angles, with Poupart's ligament, which exposed the aponeurotic expansion of the external oblique muscle: this being cut through, what was supposed to be the hernial sac was laid bare; but when the fascia that then appeared under the knife was opened, the sac itself was found beneath it. This being carefully cut through, instead of intestine, there appeared at first a large clot of coagulable lymph slightly tinged with blood, which being removed, there was found a small portion of intestine (not the whole of its cylinder) about three quarters of an inch in length and half an inch in breadth, of which a portion at the orifice of the sac, about the size of the little finger, was inflamed, but not deeply discoloured. This being carefully separated from its adhesions, was particularly examined. It was situated about half an inch below the crural arch, which was lying loose before it, for on taking hold of the arch I moved it forwards and backwards without affecting the stricture on the intestine, so that the constriction was derived from the opening in the crural sheath. The orifice of the sac was then very slightly dilated upwards with the probe pointed bistoury, and the intestine easily returned into the cavity of the abdomen. The sac was afterwards removed by an incision through its neck, and a ligature was passed through it and brought out at the external wound, (See page 43 of the First Part of this work) and the wound was closed by sutures. On the sixth day the ligatures came away, and on the tenth the wound was healed, but the hernia returned in a month as large as before, and a truss was continually required.

CASE III.

Mrs. SHEFFIELD, a patient of Mr. WESTON, Surgeon, in Shoreditch, had long laboured under a large crural hernia, which became strangulated on the 28th of November 1804. The symptoms had continued for seven days, but did not appear sufficiently urgent to justify an operation; but on the eighth day the vomiting becoming more frequent, and the pain very severe, I was sent for at eleven o'clock at night, and finding the hernia large and irreducible, I immediately proceeded to the operation.

I first made an incision downwards at right angles with the crural arch, beginning opposite the middle of the upper part of the tumour and extending it to its fundus, and another at right angles with the first in the direction of the longer axis of the tumour, so that the united incisions were of the form of the letter T reversed ⊥.

This exposed a portion of the tumour which had projected through a hole in the superficial fascia of the thigh, and which had been burst by the pressure of the hernial swelling. I next opened the anterior part of the sac and exposed a large portion of omentum, behind which was placed a fold of intestine much less discoloured than I have seen it in other cases in forty hours after the commencement of strangulation. Next passing my finger into the sac I found that it was divided into two cavities; the anterior was separated from the posterior part by a sort of hour-glass contraction, which was formed by the aperture in the superficial fascia. I therefore passed a director into this opening, and divided the superficial fascia upwards, and afterwards did the same below; the hernial sac was next completely opened below the crural arch. Passing my finger into the hernial sac to its orifice at the crural sheath, I divided the sheath upwards, and then pressing upon the intestine attempted to return it into the abdomen, but found that it would not pass. I again introduced my finger and felt the posterior edge of the crural arch pressing upon the mouth of the sac. The probe-pointed bistoury I have recommended was carried upon my finger under this edge and within the sac, and this portion of tendon cut obliquely inwards and upwards. The intestine was next drawn down to examine if it had suffered much at the strictured part, and finding that it had not, it was returned into the cavity of the abdomen, having first gently pressed upon it to evacuate its contents into the portion of the intestine above the stricture.*

As the omentum, of which a large portion had descended, adhered to the inner part of the sac, I cut it away, and it was found by Mr. WESTON to weigh two ounces and six drachms. I made pressure on the vessel, and left the divided surface of the omentum at the orifice of the hernial sac, after which the edges of the wound were brought together by adhesive plaister. On the following day she was free from pain, the vomiting had ceased, and she had two stools. Her recovery, however, was rendered slow by a portion of the integument which had been extremely thin over the sac prior to the operation, having turned livid and sloughed away. A poultice was applied, healthy granulations arose from the surface of the omentum, and the cure was completed in six weeks.

* It is of great consequence both to draw it down and to press out its contents, as it exposes that part of the intestine which had been girt by the stricture, and assists in restoring the course of the fæces through the intestine.

CASE IV.

Mrs. DEARLE, aged fifty-nine, a patient of Mr. EVANS, in Old Street, had been afflicted with a crural hernia on the left side for twenty years. On Monday, March 31, 1806, she had symptoms of strangulation, which continued till Thursday, April 3, at two o'clock, when I performed the operation.

As the swelling was of considerable length in the direction of the crural arch, I made my first incision over the middle of the tumour in the direction of the anterior edge of the arch, without making any cut at right angles with it, and cutting through the aponeurotic expansion of the external oblique muscle, I laid bare the fascia which immediately involves the hernial sac. Between this and the sac a number of small vessels could be distinctly seen embedded in a quantity of fat. This fascia being cut through and the sac exposed, I pinched up a small portion of it between my finger and thumb, and moving the thumb upon the finger I pushed the intestine from that part of the sac, which last I opened by a horizontal incision, and afterwards dilated it upon a director.

The protruded omentum and intestine were thus exposed, neither of which were in so material a degree discoloured as to render the propriety of returning them into the abdomen at all doubtful; and, therefore, I passed my probe-pointed bistoury into the mouth of the hernial sac, and cut directly upwards towards the crural arch. A very small dilatation of the stricture was required, and the intestine returned without difficulty by slight pressure.

The omentum being hard and adherent, I cut away all that had descended, compressed for a few minutes the small vessels which were bleeding till the hæmorrhage was stopped, after which I returned it into the cavity of the abdomen. Three sutures were made on the external wound, and lint was laid over it. She had several stools in the course of the evening, had no bad symptoms afterwards, and in a fortnight the wound was perfectly healed.

CASE V.

Miss........., aged 19, a patient of Messrs. SHUTERS', of Gainsford Street, Horslydown, on Saturday, April 19, 1806, was seized with violent pain in her stomach, a painful tumour appeared in the left groin, and she attributed these symptoms to her having used a degree of bodily exertion to which she was not accustomed.

She immediately sent for Mr. SHUTER, who gave her an opening medicine, which her stomach was unable to retain. Glysters were also administered, which produced some evacuation, but without affecting the size of the tumour. Frequent attempts were made to return the hernia; but though the swelling appeared to lessen, and she expressed herself somewhat easier after each attempt, the symptoms returned with all their former violence. Fomentations were tried, but they only gave a temporary relief.

On Sunday morning, April 20, the vomiting, costiveness, and tumour still continuing, Mr. SHUTER gave her a dose of Opium, and came for me.

When I saw her, which was about half past ten o'clock, the pain was somewhat relieved by the Opium; but she was still sick, the tumour painfully tense, and the whole abdomen becoming tender.

Having made an unsuccessful trial at reduction, and finding that an immediate operation was now the only chance for preserving life, I performed it at eleven o'clock.

My first incision through the integuments was in the form of an inverted T, (⊥) and the corners of the skin were turned back. Then dividing the aponeurosis of the external oblique muscle by a second incision, the fascia propria of the sac by a third, and the sac itself by a fourth, the last of which was assisted by a director, in the way already described, the contents of the hernia came in view. On opening the sac a small quantity of fluid was discharged, and after this a clot of coagulable lymph was squeezed from its inner part. The intestine was of a brownish red colour. Passing my finger into the sac, I carried it to the stricture, but could not enter it; I then introduced the knife blunted near the end, rubbed it from side to side to press every portion of intestine away from its blunt edge, and then pushing it forwards brought its cutting edge against the stricture which was in the crural sheath, and divided it upwards. The intestine then returned into the abdomen on gentle pressure, though the division which the knife had made was so small, that I could not pass my finger through it into the abdomen. The wound was then sewed in the usual manner.

Monday 20, she was much better; no vomiting had occurred after the operation, and the pain soon ceased, but she had no stool till this morning, which, when it occurred, entirely relieved the general irritation which the operation had occasioned.

Wednesday, she was quite free from pain, and in every respect doing well. She was ordered to keep her bed, as I much wished the omentum at the orifice of the sac to adhere. The ligature came away in ten days, and in three weeks the wound was healed. A truss was applied before the cure was completed, with the hope that this would produce adhesion of the sides of the sac whilst the process of inflammation was proceeding.

The following case is given to shew the danger of returning the hernial sac into the abdomen without opening it, and I hope I shall be excused for not entering more fully into its circumstances.

CASE VI.

A. B. had a crural hernia in the right side, which became strangulated at nine o'clock in the morning, which she attributed to having taken some bacon and potatoes for her supper the night before.

On the fourth day of the symptoms the following operation was performed. The incision was made to the fascial covering of the hernial sac, it was separated by the finger from the surrounding parts, and a cut being made into it, the hernial sac was supposed to have been opened, and the intestine exposed; but, as it afterwards appeared by dissection, the sac remained undivided. The crural arch being next freely cut, the sac containing the intestine was pushed into the cavity of the abdomen with much difficulty; and its fascial covering was also passed through the same aperture.

Fifth day—She has had no stool since the operation; the vomiting continues; the abdomen is tense, and sore upon pressure. She was ordered to be fomented, and glysters were prescribed to be frequently injected; but no medicines to be given whilst the irritable state of the stomach continued. In the evening a blister was ordered to the abdomen.

Sixth day—She has had no stool; the vomiting continues; the pulse is small and frequent; the belly tense and tender to the touch.

Seventh day—I was requested to see her by the Surgeon who performed the operation. I found her countenance flushed; her lips parched; her tongue covered with a brown fur; her eyes sunk, and opening with difficulty, and her countenance highly anxious. She was scarcely able to speak, but her mind was still collected; the pulse was small, fluttering, and frequent: she has had no stool; the abdomen was tense, and tender upon pressure; the vomiting continued, and she had a frequent hiccough. She drank frequently; but every liquid was soon rejected.

The fomentations were ordered to be continued, and a stimulant glyster to be injected.

Eighth day—She still has had no stool, and the vomiting continued; the tension and soreness of the belly remain: she did not suffer so much pain; but she was much weaker. She died at three o'clock in the afternoon.

DISSECTION.

Upon cutting through the integuments at the groin, the sac and its covering were entirely gone from thence; but behind the crural arch appeared a large aperture, by which they had been returned into the abdomen. The cavity of the abdomen was next opened, and as soon as a small incision was made into it, the intestines, which were much inflated, pushed through the opening. They were reddened by inflammation; adhered to each other by their sides, and anteriorly to the peritoneum which lines the abdomen; but the coagulable lymph, which thus united them, was of very tender texture, and when they were separated, red lines, extending along the intestine, marked the adhering surfaces. Looking at the right groin, from within the abdomen, the peritoneum was seen pushed upwards, to the extent of two inches on the iliacus internus muscle; and, upon examining this part, I found the hernial sac included in its fascial covering, and containing the intestine strangulated by a stricture at the mouth of the sac, and by the fascia covering it.

I have preserved the parts as I found them in the subject, and have given a Plate of them as they appeared on dissection.

This case strongly points out the necessity of being acquainted with the existence of the fascia propria.

The following case is related to explain the mode of operating which is required in large crural herniæ in the male.

CASE VII.

Joseph Falbrook was admitted into Guy's Hospital, Nov. 4, 1805, for a crural hernia on the left side, with which he had been afflicted for some years. He had before been a patient in the Hospital for a strangulated state of the same hernia, but the taxis had then succeeded.

The hernia had now been strangulated about forty hours, and the symptoms were more than commonly urgent. The vomiting was frequent, the constipation complete, and hiccough had existed for several hours; his countenance was pale, sunken, and anxious; and, above all, the abdomen was sore and tender to the touch.

The usual means of reduction having failed, though the taxis was employed for a considerable time, it was judged that the violence of the symptoms rendered the further delay of the operation very hazardous; and even then I thought it very probable that it might not save his life; but as it afforded the only chance for his preservation, and as I have seen persons recover who appeared to be dying at the time of the operation, it was thought right to perform it. The tumour had no appearance of inflammation on its surface, it moved to and fro under the skin like an enlarged absorbent gland, and was turned before the crural arch.

I made my first incision in the form of an inverted T, as already described, and after cutting through the fasciæ the hernial sac was opened, when a very small quantity of fluid made its escape; and on slitting up the sac, a portion of strangulated and highly discoloured intestine became exposed. As this portion of intestine was large, I could not make sufficient room for its return, without dividing the anterior edge of the crural arch, or Poupart's ligament; and being apprehensive of injuring the spermatic cord, I first made a small incision about half an inch above the arch to expose the cord, and then directing my dresser to draw this upwards with his finger, I passed the bistoury within the mouth of the hernial sac, and divided it and the arch with the greatest ease.

Although the intestine was much discoloured, no livid spots appeared upon it, and I therefore returned it into the cavity of the abdomen, but I expressed my fears to the students at the time, that the operation had been delayed too long.

On the following day I found that the operation had so far relieved him, that his pain was much less than before; but he still vomited, and his bowels were constipated, which made me apprehend that the intestine had been too far altered to recover its powers.

On the succeeding day he was still alive, but his pulse was feeble, his countenance sunken, his body covered with a cold sweat, and his abdomen very much distended. He died on the following morning.

My house pupil, Mr. Jones, examined the body, and found the intestines highly inflamed; and he brought away the portion which had been strangulated, as well as the crural arch and the adjacent parts, of which I have given a Plate. The intestine which had been strangulated remained in the same state as at the time of the operation.

CASE VIII.

Hernia mistaken for an Abscess.

Mr. Bethune, Surgeon, of Woodford Bridge, informed me he was witness to the case of a person who had a tumour in the left groin attended with an interrupted state of the bowels, to which a poultice was applied, under the idea of its being in the progress to suppuration. After the symptoms had continued three days the tumour was opened by a small incision, and air immediately escaped from the wound. A discharge of feculent matter succeeded, accompanied with symptoms of inflamed intestine. When glysters were injected a part of them escaped at the wound in the groin, and the patient died in ten days after the opening had been made. It was probable that the sygmoid flexure of the colon had been contained within this hernia.

In the four following cases mortification had taken place in the intestine prior to the operation.

CASE IX.

A man, aged fifty-three, was admitted into Guy's Hospital at four o'clock in the afternoon of May 24, 1804, with a strangulated crural hernia, which had been in that state since the twenty-first; and previous to his admission poultices had been applied to it, under the idea of its being a suppurating bubo. Some attempts had been made to reduce it, but without effect, and at seven in the same evening I performed the operation. The swelling at this time was very obscure, but it bore some resemblance to a suppurating bubo, for the skin over it was inflamed.

When the skin was cut through, which was done by a crucial incision, the fascia was exposed lying over the swelling, and upon this was a quantity of grumous blood very offensive to the smell, and a bloody serum mixed with drops of animal oil. When the fascia was divided, and the sac exposed, it appeared soft and pulpy, and I easily made a small opening into it with my finger nail, which I afterwards enlarged with a knife on a director.

No fluid was found in the sac, but omentum, and intestine had both descended. The former was of a brownish red colour, as if tinged with blood; the intestine, in most parts, was of a coffee colour, but with several black spots, which were evidently mortified. A very offensive smell issued both from the omentum and intestine.

Having examined these parts, I passed a director between the fascia and the sac, and attempted to divide the stricture without opening the sac; but as I still found a stricture at the mouth of the hernial sac, I carried a probe-pointed bistoury within this, and divided the orifice of the sac directly inwards along the linea ileo pectinea.

As the intestine was mortified, I passed a needle and ligature through the mesentery, and fixed it to the mouth of the hernial sac, then made a large opening into it, and discharged the fæces. I also left the omentum within the sac, and covered the whole with a poultice. The man appearing in a dying state, he was immediately carried to bed, and in about an hour afterwards I found him in a cold perspiration. As no fæces had passed from the wound in the course of two hours, I dilated the stricture at the orifice of the sac somewhat more freely, and then the fæces rushed down into the mortified intestine and were discharged by the opening in it.

On the next day he still vomited, and his extremities were cold, but his mind was composed, and he was insensible of his danger; his pulse was small, but scarcely quicker than natural; he had no hiccough, nor any pain. At four o'clock in the afternoon he vomited violently, and suddenly expired.

DISSECTION.

The intestines were all inflamed and glued together within the cavity of the abdomen, and were greatly distended with air and fæces. There was no appearance of mortification in any other part of the intestine than that which had descended into the hernial sac; nor was any other disease found, excepting ossification at the beginning of the aorta.

CASE X.

On December 24, 1806, I was requested by Mr. SMITH, at Chertsey, in Surry, to visit Mrs. WEBB of that place, who had a crural hernia on the left side, and of whose situation Mr. SMITH gave me the following account. On Tuesday the 16th of December, she complained of much pain about the region of the uterus, attended with bearing down, suppression of urine, pain in the back, and a quick pulse. She mentioned that she had been subject to a bearing down pain (her own expression) before, but that this was more violent than ever.

Mr. S. gave her some Castor oil, which was soon rejected, and then a solution of Magnesia Vitriolata, which, although longer retained, was also eventually rejected.

Wednesday—She had vomited during the night, and now, for the first time, complained of a swelling in the groin, which Mr. S. found to be an hernia; after administering a glyster, he made an attempt to reduce it, but in vain. She was thought to vomit fæculent matter during this afternoon.

Thursday—Mr. WHITE requested his friends Mr. IVES and Messrs. TOTHILL, of Staines, to assist him in consultation, as the case was becoming extremely dangerous; and they continued to visit the patient daily until I saw her. During this period, bleeding, the warm bath, opium, glysters, and cathartics were tried, but without avail. Ice, and the solution of Ammonia Muriata were also used; and on Tuesday the 23d, the tobacco smoke was thrown up.

Wednesday the 24th, I met Mr. SMITH, and the gentlemen above mentioned, at the patient's house. The tumour was slightly inflamed, and very tender to the touch. The abdomen but little distended, and not very sore upon pressure; her pulse, however, was quick and very feeble; her countenance anxious; her frame weak and languid, and she had occasional hiccough. It was immediately agreed that the operation gave the only chance of saving her life, although that hope was small.

In performing the operation two incisions were made through the integuments, three inches long, and in the form of the letter T reversed. By the second incision the superficial fascia, which was much thickened, was divided, and the fascia covering the sac was exposed. A small opening being made in this, a director was introduced behind it, and it was divided by the curved bistoury to the crural arch.

The sac was next opened by a very small cut, and afterwards dilated in a similar manner to the fascia.

The omentum was first exposed, which was of a dark colour, and had a feculent smell; behind this, and involved in the posterior part of the omentum, was found a portion of intestine seven inches long, perfectly gangrenous, but there was no opening in it, so that the feculent smell which was observed in the sac, and its contents, was the effect of transudation after the death of the parts. The finger was now passed to the orifice of the hernial sac, and the stricture was found not at the opening in the crural sheath, but much higher up, and could be distinctly felt, formed on the inner side by the interior insertion of the external oblique muscle and the fascia behind it, on the anterior by the posterior edge of the crural arch, and externally by the process of fascia on the inner side of the crural vein.

I passed the probe-pointed bistoury into the sac, and cut the posterior edge of the crural arch upwards, and slightly inwards; and then made an opening into the mortified portion of intestine to discharge the fæces, and left the part to slough.

During the operation her pulse became very feeble, and she was very languid. I saw her about half an hour after she was put to bed, and then she appeared to be sinking; and Mr. SMITH wrote to me the following day, to say, that in an hour after I left her, she complained of much pain in her abdomen; was covered with a cold perspiration; her pulse was extremely feeble; she was sensible of her approaching dissolution; said that she should not live more than an hour, and in about that time she died.

It ought to be remarked that the circumstances usually considered as denoting the presence of mortification, did not occur in this patient, for there never was any sudden change of symptoms, any abatement of pain, or considerable alteration in the state of the pulse. The only circumstance which induced me to expect to find a mortified intestine, was the inflammation and tenderness of the skin over the tumour, and the duration of the symptoms of strangulation.

CASE XI.

.... CLARK, aged fifty, was attacked with symptoms of strangulated hernia on the 1st of November 1806, which she supposed were produced by carrying a great weight upon her head. On the 6th in the evening, my friend Mr. SAUNDERS, Surgeon, knowing my wish to see every example of hernia that I could, informed me of the case, and I found a crural hernia in the right side. She vomited frequently; was completely constipated, and had fits of pain at the interval of a few minutes; but the abdomen, though tense, was not sore upon pressure, and this induced me to hope that the operation might still preserve her life. I staid with her more than an hour, strongly urging her to consent to its being performed, but she refused to submit to it at that time, as she thought herself somewhat better.

On Saturday the 8th, I was sent for to perform the operation, as she was then very anxious to have it done. At this time she had the following symptoms: Obstinate constipation, for she has had no stool for eight days; frequent vomiting of a yellowish fluid, free of fæculent smell; abdomen distended, and rather painful when pressed; the tumour red, hard, and exquisitely painful to the touch; her pulse 130, and strong; her tongue furred and dry; great thirst; countenance sunken and distressed.

The operation was performed at one o'clock, in presence of Dr. FARRE and Mr. SAUNDERS.

The first incision, which was in the form of the reversed T, exposed the superficial fascia very much thickened, and this being turned aside, the fascia propria of the sac was exposed, and being opened, the hernial sac was laid bare. The appearance of the sac was very unusual, it looked like a bladder which had been long macerated in water, and doubts were expressed if it were not intestine. When it was struck with the finger it fluctuated, but upon feeling through the fluid the intestine could be perceived at the upper part of the sac forming a hard tumour there, and involved in a quantity of fluid. A strong fæculent smell issued from the external surface of the sac, and we therefore concluded the intestine was mortified, and that fæces had escaped into the sac. An incision was made through the hernial sac with very great caution, and a quantity of liquid fæces immediately escaped from it, and at the upper part of the sac close to the crural sheath the intestine was found mortified, and occupying not more than one-third of the cavity of the sac, and having a large circular opening in it, with thickened and inverted edges, which were of the colour of venous blood. I introduced my bistoury upon the finger into the hernial sac, and cut the orifice of the crural sheath, but still I was unable to draw down the intestine, and passing my finger further within the sac, I felt the posterior edge of the crural arch and fascia behind it forming a strong stricture, which I divided upwards and inwards, and thus liberated the intestine, for then a large quantity of fæculent matter issued from the opening in it.

The portion of intestine which had been strangulated, and which was about two inches and a half in length, was then cut away and the ends of the intestines joined by three sutures, so as to leave a small opening for the discharge of fæces, and the ligature which passed through the back part of the intestine next the mysentery was confined to the mouth of the hernial sac.

The edges of the wound were brought together by sutures, excepting that a small opening was left for the escape of the fæces.

During the operation she vomited frequently, but only once after it was concluded; her pulse were then 108 and languid. Thirty drops of Tincture of Opium were ordered her after the operation.

Evening, the vomiting had ceased; abdomen less tense and painful; pulse about 112; tongue dry and furred; countenance distressed; eyes frequently rolled upwards; extremities warm; she had not slept, although she had taken a grain of opium in addition to the thirty drops.

November 9th, the vomiting had not returned; abdomen soft; but she complained of slight pain in the stomach; the wound discharged freely, and the fluid was similar to that which she had previously vomited; but she had no evacuation per anum, and whatever she drank in a few minutes escaped at the wound; her pulse 130, and she denied her having slept.

November 10, every symptom as above, with increasing debility; tongue very brown; skin hot; complained much of want of rest, and an opiate was given her. The nourishment she took, consisting of tea, broth, and porter, was speedily discharged at the groin.

November 11, she remained very much in the same state, excepting that the debility every hour increased, and she died in the morning of the 12th, sensible to the last, and complaining of pain in the abdomen.

EXAMINATION.

The abdomen was flaccid, the integuments over the artificial anus were of a livid colour, but not mortified.

The stomach was pale and contracted. The small intestines between the stomach and the protruded intestine were inflamed, the minute vessels being all turgid with blood.

The ilium was the protruded intestine, and it was its upper part which had descended; below the protruded part to the cecum, the intestine was pale and contracted.

The large intestines were not inflamed; there was no effusion of fluid into the cavity of the peritoneum, nor any adhesion of the intestine within the abdomen; but the protruded intestine was firmly glued to the inner side of the sac.

On the opposite side I found a small crural hernia, of which I have given a Plate.

For the account of the symptoms after the operation, I am indebted to my friend Dr. Farre, whose judgment, accuracy, and perseverance, are required only to be better known to raise him to the highest rank in his profession.

CASE XII.

Emma Dollett, of Haggerstone, aged sixty-eight, was attacked on Sunday, July 26, 1806, with symptoms of strangulated hernia, which continued until the next Thursday, when she sent for Mr. Weston, Surgeon, in Shoreditch. Mr. Heriot (Mr. Weston's assistant) visited her, and found a crural hernia on the right side, which he made some efforts to reduce. Mr. Weston, who saw her three hours afterwards, repeated the attempts to reduce it; but, although the tumour lessened, it did not entirely disappear. At nine o'clock in the same evening, I was sent for, and found a crural hernia on the right side, the skin over it much inflamed, and it pitted under the application of my finger. The tumour diminished under the pressure I made, but did not disappear. She had considerable pain in the abdomen, vomited frequently, and had a slight hiccough; her pulse was small and frequent, but she thought the symptoms less violent than in the morning. However, as the tumour remained, the symptoms continued, and the state of the skin indicated the greatest mischief in the intestine, I thought it right to advise the operation, to which she readily consented. A crucial incision was made through the skin, and the cellular membrane beneath it was found very much thickened and condensed. A fascia which distinctly involved the hernial sac was cut open, after which the sac was divided, and a quantity of omentum (about half an ounce) was found, which had a strong feculent smell; and, when I pressed upon it, a liquid feculent matter issued from the inner corner of the sac, though, on farther examination, no portion of intestine could be found from which this discharge could have issued.

I next dilated the stricture, and thought whilst doing this that I could perceive a small portion of intestine within the orifice of the hernial sac, and securing it between my finger and thumb, I carefully dilated the orifice of the sac.

I then drew forwards the substance which I held, and found it to be a portion of intestine, about the size of the end of my finger, and about three quarters of an inch long, of a very dark colour, and it had two small holes in it, one which would almost admit the blunt end of my probe, and the other only the point. Both these holes were circular and passed through the coats of the intestine, so that feculent matter escaped through them when I pressed upon the portion of bowels adjoining to them. It now became an object of consideration to determine what should be done with this perforated portion of intestine. It might either be sewed to the sac, and left in that situation, so as to allow of the escape of the fæces, or it might be returned into the cavity of the abdomen, or a portion of it might be cut away, and the ends united; I preferred the latter mode, therefore spreading the portion of strangulated intestine in my hand, with a pair of scissars, I cut off the sphacelated piece, and then made three sutures upon the intestine to bring its edges together. The divided edges bled freely; but this was checked when the ligature were drawn together. The intestine was then pushed as near as possible to the mouth of the hernial sac, and the threads left hanging from the wound; the protruded omentum was cut off, and the edges of the wound were brought together every where, except in the center, so that if feculent matter did escape from the intestine it might pass through the wound, and be prevented from being effused into the cavity of the abdomen.

Immediately after the operation, she was seized with violent shivering and sense of coldness, but when she got into bed she soon became warm, and her pulse, which was small during the operation, became fuller after it, and she said her pain wass less.

Friday, August 1, she had passed a good night, having slept several hours; her belly is still tense, but much less sore when pressed. The intestine appears florid. She has had no feculent discharge from the wound, nor any stool: she has vomited once since the operation, and the eructations still continue; her pulse is 96, and she has little constitutional irritation.

Saturday, August 2, I received the following account from Mr. Weston:—A large quantity of liquid fæces have passed from the wound; the abdomen has become flaccid; she passed a good night, and her pulse is only 92.

Saturday 3, Mr. WESTON wrote that he had seen our patient this morning, and found the parts looking well, the belly soft, fæces discharging at the wound, mixed with a quantity of gelatinous matter, having the appearance of coagulable lymph effused under inflammation. The pulse 84; the tongue cleaner, and all the appearances very favourable.

Monday 4, I saw her; she has passed a good night; her belly is quite reduced from the state of tension; she has no vomiting; her pulse is 84, but rather feeble; her stools are not feculent, but of a green colour, and mixed with the mucus of the intestine; when she drinks, the fluid passes from the artificial anus in an hour. Some veal she also took passed off in an hour very little changed.

The intestine appears florid, but it seems to have a tendency to protrude, and I ordered a dossil of lint to be pressed upon it, and to be occasionally removed for the evacuation of the fæces.

Wednesday 6, she was entirely free from constitutional irritation, and much invigorated by having taken some wine. The intestine appears florid, and has a quantity of mucus hanging from it. The artificial anus appears to be established, and the opening into the intestine is sufficiently large to admit the finger.

From this time to the 23d of September, I had occasionally reports respecting her from Mr. WESTON, and sometimes saw her myself, but nothing occurred worthy of notice, excepting that the skin surrounding the wound was often inflamed by the discharge from the intestine, and required the application of a lotion of acetite of lead, with tincture of opium, and sometimes a saturnine ointment, an aperture being left in the lint for the discharge of the fæces.

On the 23d of Sept. I was sent for on account of the discharge of the fæces having stopped. I found the wound very much contracted, and the hole into the intestine so small, that it would not admit a bougie. She had been eating some rabbit and roasted apple before the discharge of fæces had ceased. I advised that a poultice should be placed on the wound, and nothing farther done, supposing some portion of the apple, undissolved, had stopped the aperture of the intestine. She vomited, and the belly became distended. After having remained in that state forty-eight hours, a large discharge of fæces took place from the wound: but she became very feeble, and never entirely recovered her former strength. She died on the 9th of October.

I opened the body, and found the abdomen free from inflammation. The lower part of the ilium formed the artificial anus. The colon and the large intestines had become of very small size, and contained only a little mucus. The orifices of the intestine were both very small, but more especially the lower, that which was continued to the large intestine.

These four cases strongly point out the danger of delay, and so strongly am I impressed with this belief, that if I were myself the subject of strangulated crural hernia, I should only try the effect of tobacco glysters, and if they did not succeed, would have the operation performed in twelve hours from the accession of the symptoms.

The two following cases are related to shew the danger of the operation of dividing the stricture directly inwards, or towards the symphisis pubis, in the way which has been recommended by GIMBERNAT.

CASE XIII.

Mrs. PHILLIPS, aged fifty years, was seized on Wednesday, February 16, 1804, with symptoms of strangulation, in a hernia, to which she had been subject for twelve years, during which time it had been occasionally smaller or larger, but never completely reduced. On the day above mentioned it suddenly increased, during a violent exertion, became very painful, and produced much uneasiness in the bowels, with frequent vomiting. On the 24th, Mr. ROBERT KENT was called to her, who advised her going to St. Thomas's Hospital, and she was accordingly admitted on the 25th.

The tumour was on the left side, its long axis, passing in the direction of the crural arch, or POUPART's ligament, anterior to which it was situated. It bore so strong a resemblance to an incipient inguinal hernia, as to deceive several of the most intelligent pupils; but on examining her, and drawing the tumour downwards,

I found the crural arch passing above the sac, and the tuberosity of the pubis on its inner side, which made the true nature of the case sufficiently obvious.

The symptoms were not so urgent as might have been expected from the duration of the disease, for the tumour was not inflamed, the abdomen but slightly tense and painful, and the countenance did not shew any remarkable sign of anxiety. Her pulse, however, was quick and *thready*. After an unsuccessful trial of the taxis, and a tobacco glyster, I proceeded to perform the operation.

An incision was made in the long axis of the tumour, (transversely, therefore, to the neck of the sac), and the fascia which it exposed was next divided to bring the sac in view. This was next opened, and a little clear serum escaped. A director being introduced, the opening into the sac was extended up into its neck, which shewed both intestine and omentum strangulated; the former, discoloured as much as is usual in these circumstances, but not to any remarkable degree. The intestine being drawn towards the spine of the ilium, which was obliged to be done to reach the stricture, a director was passed up into the mouth of the sac on its inner side opposite the pubis, and a common probed bistoury being slid upon this, the stricture was divided inwards along the margin of the pubis. The intestine was then easily returnable; but, as the last portion of it was entering the abdomen, a small quantity of feculent matter escaped from the orifice of the sac, but too late to prevent the return of the intestine, which, had I observed this circumstance sooner, I should have done, and made a small suture upon it. The omentum was then returned, and the wound dressed. I saw her an hour and a half afterwards, when she complained of violent pain in the abdomen, and was extremely restless. I removed the dressings, and saw fæces discharged from the wound, on which I ordered a poultice only to be applied. The pain and restlessness continued till her death, which happened within four hours and a half after the operation.

On examining the body I found the fæces effused into the cavity of the abdomen, the intestines universally inflamed, the portion of gut which had been strangulated, but little altered in colour, but with a hole in it opposite the stricture.

Whether in this case the intestine gave way at the strictured part by drawing it aside, or was injured by the knife, it is impossible to determine, but I was resolved never again to cut inwards, on account of the danger of tearing, as well as of cutting the intestine.

CASE XIV.

A woman, aged forty-five, who had long been troubled with crural hernia on the right side, was seized with symptoms of strangulated hernia. They had begun at eight o'clock in the evening, and (as she stated) were brought on by suddenly rising from her chair.

On the whole of the following day she vomited frequently, had great pain in the tumour, and her pulse was small and frequent.

Eight ounces of blood were taken from the arm, and attempts were made to reduce the hernia by the taxis, but without success. She was ordered into a warm bath, and the attempts at reduction were repeated, but in vain. A tobacco glyster was thrown up, but it also failed.

At noon on the following day the operation was performed. The intestine, which was discoloured, was found adhering to the sac; but these adhesions were separated without much difficulty, and the stricture at the mouth of the sac was divided inwards, or towards the symphysis pubis; but several incisions were required before the aperture was large enough to allow of the return of the hernia.*

As the intestine was about to be pushed back into the abdomen, its contents were seen to escape from a considerable opening in it. It was therefore confined to the mouth of the sac; and dressings being applied, she was put to bed. I saw her soon after the operation, when she was in most violent pain, and she died at seven o'clock in the same evening.

* I was not present at this operation, but was informed of the particulars by two very intelligent persons who witnessed it.

DISSECTION.

Having obtained leave to inspect the body, I found fæces extravasated in the cavity of the abdomen. The intestines were much inflamed, and, as usual, red lines appeared on them, passing longitudinally on the points at which they adhered. The portion of intestine which had descended into the hernial sac was discoloured, and it was much inflamed above that part; and two openings were found in the portion which had been placed at the mouth of the hernial sac. One of these openings had been confined within the sac, but the other had escaped observation, and had been returned into the cavity of the abdomen; and it was from this that the fæces had been extravasated, which so speedily brought on a fatal termination. See Plate relative to the operation.

OF UMBILICAL HERNIA.

CHAPTER I.

Of the Symptoms and Causes of Umbilical Hernia.

IF I had followed the order of frequency of occurrence in my description of the several species of hernia, I should not have hesitated to place the Umbilical next in order to the Inguinal; but as the parts connected with Crural Hernia are not only contiguous to, but really form a part of those concerned in the Inguinal, I have chosen to describe the Crural Hernia immediately after it, that the subject may more readily be understood. Next in frequency to the inguinal.

The umbilical hernia passes through a hole at the navel, which is formed in the fœtal state for the passage of the umbilical cord. This hole is situated near the center of the linea alba, and it naturally becomes closed after the funis is tied; but it is never entirely filled by tendon, but only by a condensed cellular membrane, containing the remains of the umbilical vein and arteries. When this part is dissected, the peritoneum is found behind it covered above by the remains of the umbilical vein, and below by the ligament of the bladder and the two umbilical arteries, and the peritoneum will be found to adhere with more firmness here than it does to the rest of the linea alba. Umbilical ring and hole.

A hole which will admit a common sized quill exists at this part of the tendon, but is naturally filled up by a condensed cellular membrane. The skin of the umbilicus is reflected inwards, to adhere to the external part of this hole, and it is this reflection which gives the peculiar form of the navel.

If the umbilical hole was situated at the lower part of the abdomen no person could escape hernia, and placed as it is, protrusions very frequently take place at different periods of life through this aperture, (which continues for life) and the disease takes the name of *Exomphalos*, or Umbilical Hernia. The peritoneum, however, is as complete here as at any other part of the abdomen, which I mention particularly, because some have erroneously supposed, that the umbilical cord passed through a hole in the peritoneum behind the umbilicus, and consequently that when the intestine protruded, during infancy, the umbilical hernia was not covered with peritoneum. But though in the adult the umbilical hernia is sometimes found without a sac, and always when the hernia is large with a sac extremely thin, yet this is not the cause of that variety; and it should be remembered, that the remains of the umbilical arteries and vein are no where situated *within* the peritoneum, but *before* it; for the umbilical arteries passing from the internal iliac arteries by the side of the bladder, are continued to the navel between the peritoneum and abdominal muscles; and the umbilical vein, after entering the navel, is also continued between the peritoneum and abdominal muscles to form the round ligament of the liver. The only natural deficiency of tendon is at the navel, where an opening is formed for the passage of the blood-vessels, in the same manner as openings are left at the abdominal rings for the passage of the spermatic cords. Peritoneum complete behind the hole.

It has been asserted, that the umbilical hernia does not pass through the umbilical hole, but by an aperture on its side or near it, but from the dissections which I have made, I believe that it very generally passes through this aperture; and I suppose that the contrary opinion has been founded upon the circumstance of the swelling being rarely just at the center of the navel, for as there is a strong adhesion of the skin to the center of the opening, the cicatrix rather gives way upon either side than directly at the center.

Umbilical hernia begins in the form of a small tumour, about the size of the tip of the finger, at the navel, which can be returned by very slight pressure into the cavity of the abdomen; but by directing the patient to cough, it immediately reappears. As it increases in bulk it begins to gravitate, so that the ante- First appearance.

Pendulous. rior extremity of the bend is generally below the level of the umbilical opening. If the person is thin, it becomes very pendulous and distinctly circumscribed, and is then usually of a pyriform shape. If nothing is done to check its growth, it grows to an enormous size, extending downwards towards the pubis. The disease in this state produces a great deal of suffering, and often endangers life if the hernia is intestinal.

Effects of. Almost every thing that is eaten too produces flatulency, pain in the protruded part, and sickness; and even slight pressure to return it, gives the same uneasy sensations when the intestine is passing back through the abdominal opening. If no bandage is habitually worn to confine the hernia, the patient feels so much weakness and sinking at the pit of the stomach as to be often incapable of any exertion. The bowels also are generally irregular, and if the tumour becomes inflamed, it swells to a great size, and vomiting and constipation ensue. These symptoms are much more frequently happening in this than in the other species of hernia, but at the same time they are generally more easily removed.

I have never seen the umbilical hernia in the adult but that it contained omentum, and the intestine is also often found, and most frequently the colon.

Diagnosis of the intestinal. The symptoms of uneasiness and sickness above mentioned belong to this hernia when it is intestinal, and this may readily be distinguished from the omental by its great elasticity, by its uniform feel, and by the ease with which the motion of the air and fæces within the hernia may be felt, which produces that guggling noise which in other kinds of hernia is generally only to be perceived at the time of their reduction.

Diagnosis of the omental. An umbilical omental hernia produces a tumour, irregular upon its surface, and in which the lobules of fat that compose it, when the hernia is large, may be felt through the skin if it is thin. The feel is also doughy, and the person experiences but little pain, and scarcely any of that uneasy sensation of sinking and irregularity of bowels that distinguish the intestinal hernia. Still, however, a swelling of this kind requires attention, as its increase is sometimes very rapid, the intestine is very apt to protrude where omentum has once passed, and the omentum itself sometimes becomes strangulated.

Diagnosis when both are contained. When omentum and intestine are both contained in the sac two tumours are formed in it, which may sometimes be readily distinguished from each other: one of them, which consists of omentum, forms the upper and anterior part of the tumour; the other, which contains the intestine, forms the lower. But if the quantity of omentum is very large, the intestine is so much involved in it that it cannot be very distinctly felt.

Umbilical hernia in infants. The umbilical hernia is very frequent in the young subject, and forms a tumour like the inflated finger of a glove, with a slight obliquity downwards. It very generally contains intestine, which may be easily returned, unless the orifice is very small, in which case the cries of the child shew that some pain is given. Irregular bowels and costiveness, succeeded by griping and long continued purging, are attendant on this disease.

Fascia. A fascia may be distinctly traced over the tumour when the hernia is small, but when it becomes of large size, the skin, sac, and fascia become so united at the anterior part of the swelling, that it is difficult to separate them there, although the fascia may still be distinctly observed on the sides of the tumour.

Varieties. There are some varieties in the umbilical hernia which require to be mentioned. First, with respect to *Figure.* figure, in a thin subject it is generally pyriform, as I have already stated, but in fat persons it forms a broad and flat swelling, which extends as much upwards as downwards. Sometimes, in consequence of there being a large quantity of fat which separates the skin at a great distance from the abdominal muscles, the hernia projects as far as the skin of the navel, and then extends upwards and downwards, so as to form a tumour which is scarcely apparent on a superficial examination. But when the hernia assumes this extended and flattened form in thin persons (which is sometimes the case), it can be embraced by the hand, and its dimensions readily ascertained. I have also seen this umbilical hernia divided into a number of different cells.

Sac. Besides this variety in the figure of the hernia, there is a great difference in the state of the sac. When this is small, it is as complete as in other herniæ; but I have an example in my possession of the sac having been either absorbed or burst, by which openings have been formed and portions of omentum protruded through them, producing small herniæ through the sac of the large one. Mr. CLIFF has made me an excellent drawing of this hernia, from which a Plate is given in this work. In this instance two small omental herniæ are seen protruded through the hernial sac, and on the opposite side an opening may be observed through which either omentum or intestine might have passed.

In the subject of the Plate to which I have alluded, the anterior part of the sac was entirely absorbed, so that the omentum was brought in contact with the skin, to which it firmly adhered, and the skin had been the subject of repeated ulcerations in consequence of the magnitude and weight of the tumour, and of the daily exertions which the woman was obliged to make for her maintenance. Since then it is demonstrable, that either by absorption or laceration a portion of the sac may be lost, this will fully account for the apparent absence of the sac altogether, without having recourse to the supposition, that the peritoneum was originally wanting opposite the umbilicus, and, excepting in this instance, and in one which I once saw in the possession of Dr. MARSHALL, teacher of Anatomy in London, I have known no example of this hernia being without a sac. The reasons which have led to a belief of its being generally so, are two:—first, from a mistaken idea of the structure of the part, by supposing that the peritoneum was naturally deficient behind the umbilicus; and secondly, because the sac is thin and generally adheres firmly to the skin at the anterior part of the tumour. *Sac absorbed or lacerated.*

Another and very curious variety, which is in the collection of preparations at St. Thomas's Hospital, was taken from the body of a woman who had been a patient of Mr. CLINE's in that hospital, by Mr. SMITH. In performing the operation for umbilical hernia, after returning the intestine from the hernial sac, on putting the finger into the abdomen an opening could be felt about half an inch from that by which the finger passed, which led into another tumour by the side of the former. This patient recovered from the operation, but was admitted about twelve months afterwards with the hernia again strangulated. The operation was repeated, and the patient recovered, but she died after five months of another disease, which gave me an opportunity of making a dissection of the two sacs, of which figures are given in the Plate of Umbilical Herniæ; and this case, described by Mr. SMITH, is particularly detailed hereafter. *Two sacs.*

I have also several times seen, with Mr. AGAR, Surgeon, in Whitechapel, a lady who has two hernial tumours at the umbilicus, one very large, and the other small, a little to the left side of the former. See Cases.

Of the Causes of Umbilical Hernia.

Pregnancy is the most common cause of this complaint. When the gravid uterus rises above the brim of the pelvis it pushes the bowels upwards, and contracts the space which they usually occupy. The origin of this complaint therefore, is generally at this period, or if it had existed before, it is then aggravated. Women often also ascribe this disease to laborious parturition. Another very frequent cause of this complaint is, an extraordinary degree of obesity, which by enlarging the omentum and mesentery renders the abdomen less capable of retaining its contents. When women who have had many children become corpulent, the abdominal muscles being loose and pendulous, render them peculiarly liable to this disease. From these circumstances it will be seen that women are more subject to this disease than men. *Pregnancy. Obesity.*

We often see during ascites the umbilicus projecting, the skin thin, and a fluid evidently contained within it, and sometimes the water has been discharged by puncturing it with a lancet. I believe, however, that generally this is rather the consequence than the cause of hernia. Mr. WARNER, formerly Surgeon of Guy's Hospital, and author of several surgical tracts and cases, gives an account of a hernia being produced by puncturing the navel in dropsy, which is a valid objection against tapping the abdomen either at the navel or above it, both because it may lay the foundation of hernia, and because it is possible that a portion of intestine may adhere to the umbilicus, which would be wounded by the puncture. *Ascites.*

Children, however, are most frequently the subjects of this complaint, and in them it appears very soon after birth, as the opening for the passage of the umbilical cord into the abdomen is at that time large, and will readily allow of the escape of the intestine. This complaint is more frequent in some families than in others, and I am disposed to attribute it to the size of the funis, as I know an instance of three children in the same family who have this disease, and in whom at birth the funis was larger than usual. *Large Funis.*

Children are sometimes born with a deficiency of the abdominal muscles at the umbilical aperture, which gives rise to a large protrusion, a little on one side of which is the funis, and the covering is so thin that the intestines may be seen through it. The edges of the skin surrounding the tumour are of a red colour, and somewhat thickened and retracted. On this subject I have had the honour of receiving a very valuable communication from Dr. HAMILTON, Professor of Midwifery in the University of Edinburgh. See Cases. *Abdominal muscles deficient.*

Fleshy tumour at the navel.

A small tumour sometimes projects from the navel of children, which Surgeons have mistaken for hernia. It hangs in the hollow of the navel, is of a florid red colour, and is attached by a small neck.

The first case of this kind which I saw was brought to me from the neighbourhood of Sittingbourne in Kent. The child was seven years old, and during the four first years of its life it had a discharge from the navel, and the funis which had sloughed further from the navel than usual, had never healed. A small red and fungous tumour then appeared which bled frequently, and at other times discharged a bloody serum, and was painful when irritated by exercise. On examining this substance, I found it arose from the circumstance of the funis being so long, as to project beyond the skin of the navel, which prevented cicatrization. I made a ligature around it, which gave the child scarcely any pain, and on the following day I removed it with scissars.

I have seen another case of a similar kind.

CHAPTER II.

Of the Reducible and Irreducible Umbilical Hernia.

WHEN the attempt is made to return the intestine into the cavity of the abdomen, particular attention must be paid to relax the abdominal muscles. For this purpose the shoulders must be elevated, the pelvis raised, and the thighs brought at right angles with the body. This position gives the greatest possible room for the return of the intestine. Position for reduction.

In making the reduction the Surgeon grasps the tumour in his hands and directs it upwards, as the opening which leads from the swelling into the abdomen is not directly in the center of the tumour, but a little above it, and he then kneads the neck of the tumour with the finger and thumb of the other hand; but if the swelling is small and projects only from the abdominal muscles to the navel without spreading on each side, a direct pressure may be made upon the surface of the tumour with the thumbs, so as to force it into the cavity of the abdomen. The most difficult species of umbilical hernia to reduce, is that which lies between the skin and abdominal muscles imbedded in fat, and scarcely projecting the integuments; for this tumour cannot easily be grasped in the hands, and all that can be done is to bring its sides together as closely as possible by a general pressure over the contiguous part of the abdomen. Taxis.

When the hernia is returned, some kind of bandage must be applied, and the one that I prefer for a hernia of small size is a spring truss, made exactly on the same principle as the truss for inguinal hernia. A small circular pad is made to press upon the navel, and the steel spring reaches from this point round to the back a little further than the spine, and the circle is completed by a strap which buckles upon the pad. In taking measure for this truss, nothing more is necessary than to take the girt of the abdomen at the level of the navel. This simple bandage I have found to answer all the purpose of the most complicated, and it has the additional advantage of taking up so little room as to be easily concealed. Truss.

If the navel is very deep, owing to great corpulency, I generally order an ivory ball, from half an inch to an inch and an half in diameter, (according to the size of the tumour) to be cut in half, and this to be first put into the navel and kept in its situation, by applying the pad of the truss over it. The more common method of making pressure, when the navel is very hollow, is to unite a small cushion to the pad, which is to fill the hollow; but as the common exertions of the body will cause a slight motion in the pad, the cushion slips out of the navel, and the hernia is liable to pass down by its side. Whereas, if the ivory ball is introduced in the way mentioned, a slight variation in the position of the truss will not displace the ball. Ball.

Very large herniæ, especially if they are accompanied by a pendulous belly, require a truss which exerts a more extended pressure on the abdomen. For this purpose very broad thin pads are applied, which both keep back the hernia and give a support to the abdomen, which is very comfortable to the patient's feelings. Large hernia.

A truss of this kind is represented in the Plate of Umbilical Hernia, and together with it is a very ingenious one for the same purpose, invented by Mr. MORRISON, of Leeds, in which the pad is supported by a spring extending from the arm of the truss, and which he considers as an improvement upon that which is delineated in Mr. HEY's Work. When the umbilical hernia is small, it may sometimes be kept up, and finally cured by the following method:—A small circular piece of adhesive plaster is laid on the navel, (after reduction) over which are placed successive circles of plaster, gradually increasing in diameter, so as to form a solid cone, with the apex inwards, till the navel is quite filled, after which a large piece of plaster is fixed over the whole. A medical man who had a hernia after ascites, informed me that he had cured himself by this method of treatment. Adhesive plasters.

Infantile hernia.

With regard to the umbilical hernia of children, if they are not very young, a truss like that for the adult may be employed; but if they are quite infants, the plan which I have found the most effectual is the following:—a small section of an ivory ball is laid on the navel; over this is to be applied a piece of adhesive plaster of the size of the palm of the hand, and a linen belt over the whole round the abdomen. As soon as the child begins to walk two thigh straps are to be added to the bottom of the belt to prevent it from slipping. If this application be carefully persisted in for a length of time, the cure of this disease is very sure to be effected.

Tying the tumour.

It has been recommended by some foreign Surgeons in the umbilical hernia of children, to press the intestine carefully into the cavity of the abdomen, and then to make a ligature round the root of the hernia, and to leave both the integuments and sac to slough. But although this operation may be with safety performed, yet it is not entirely destitute of danger, both from inflammation of the sac and injury to the intestine, and it is so very painful and violent that, in my opinion, it ought not to be performed. Besides, even after the operation, it is necessary to have recourse to the same pressure to prevent a relapse, which is employed to produce a cure.

Fœtal hernia.

In those cases in which from an original deficiency of the linea alba around the umbilical aperture a hernia forms in the funis of the child, it is right, after reducing the intestine, to place a small piece of linen upon the navel, to bring the sides of the aperture together by pieces of adhesive plaster, to place a pad of linen over the part, and a belt which is to go around the abdomen, over the whole.

Of the Irreducible Umbilical Hernia.

Causes of.

The same causes which render inguinal hernia irreducible generally operate here. Of these the most frequent is adhesion of the omentum; and sometimes of the intestine. An extraordinary growth of the omentum, the mesentery, and the appendices epiploïcæ, will render the hernia irreducible even without adhesion. Sometimes, too, this may be brought about by the hernial sac giving way at some part, and allowing the omentum to pass through the opening, where it remains confined, as I have already explained.

Size enormous.

The irreducible umbilical hernia sometimes grows to an enormous size in women whose bellies are pendulous from bearing a great number of children. In three such instances, I have seen the hernia extending so low from the navel as entirely to cover the pudendum. One example which Dr. POLE, of Bristol, took from the body of a patient of his measured ten inches in length, and eight in breadth at the upper part, and seven at the lower. In such cases, however, the umbilicus cannot remain at its usual distance from the pubes, but from the constant weight of the hernia the opening is brought considerably lower. I have given a Case of this description from the authority of Mr. DUNDAS, of Richmond, Serjeant Surgeon to his Majesty.

Ulceration of.

A tumour of such uncommon magnitude produces so much inconvenience as almost to unfit the sufferer for any exertion. This happens partly from the excessive weight of the tumour, and partly from ulceration of the integuments, which frequently occurs, and which is extremely difficult to heal, and often impracticable without confining the patient to a recumbent posture. Specimens of ulcerated integuments will be seen in the first of the two Plates which illustrate umbilical hernia.

Danger of.

This state of enormous tumefaction also exposes the person to considerable hazard from blows or falls, which endanger the bursting of the intestine; an accident that is certainly and speedily fatal.

Suppuration of.

Suppuration now and then takes place in the omentum of an irreducible umbilical hernia. An account of a case of this kind is given in my former work, p. 27, of a woman who had three herniæ, one of which was umbilical, and in the sac, which contained the omentum, was found about half an ounce of pus.

Hollow truss.

When the hernia is evidently become irreducible a hollow truss should be applied to prevent its increase. For this purpose it should be made in the form of the inner part of a saucer, but with its edges a little rounded to prevent any painful pressure on the abdomen, and with a spring attached to each side. Thus constructed it may be worn with as little inconvenience as a common truss. The material of the pad may be tin covered with leather. A lady I saw, to whom expence was no object, had it made of silver, which is the best material, as this metal will not, like tin, be rusted by the perspiration with which the leather is always damp.

Large herniæ supported by a belt.

When the irreducible hernia has grown very large no truss can be worn, and in this uncomfortable situation all that can be done is to carry a broad belt under the tumour, which being crossed round the shoulders, will take off a part of the weight with which the sufferer is encumbered.

CHAPTER III.

Of the strangulated Umbilical Hernia.

The symptoms of strangulation are generally less urgent in this than in the inguinal or crural hernia, but as they do not, in other respects, materially differ from those which have been mentioned in the descriptions of those herniæ, it will be unnecessary to repeat them in this place. There is one circumstance of danger however which is peculiar to the umbilical hernia, which is that when the skin has become very thin over the tumour, the pressure simply of the protruded parts, under strangulation, will sometimes very early destroy the life of that portion of integument by stopping the circulation through it. It first turns green, the cuticle separates from it, and that portion of skin becomes dry and of a brown colour, and in both the instances in which this circumstance came under my observation the patients died. These cases will be detailed at large in a subsequent chapter. *Symptoms.*

The time in which strangulated umbilical hernia proves fatal varies considerably. The earliest period from the accession of the symptoms at which I have known death to happen was seventeen hours and an half. In general when death is late, the hernia consists chiefly of omentum, and sometimes (though very rarely) entirely so. *Time in which it proves fatal.*

The most frequent cause of strangulation is indiscretion, both in the quantity and quality of food, so that persons subject to this complaint should eat rather sparingly at any one time, and should avoid every thing that tends to flatulency. This last circumstance seems to be confirmed by the observation which has been made, that cases of strangulated hernia are more common in the season when green vegetables are most abundant. Meat of an indigestible kind is to be equally avoided, as it passes through the greater part of the intestinal canal undissolved, as I have observed in cases of artificial anus, when a large quantity of ham, or fat, had been taken. *Cause of.*

The seat of strangulation is in the edge of the tendon forming the linea alba, which forms the umbilical aperture, and which always becomes extremely thickened, so that in the operation I have felt it resisting the knife like cartilage. The sac also is thicker in this part than elsewhere, and sometimes prevents the return of the protruded parts. *Seat of.*

Strangulation, however, may also arise from a hole in the sac itself through which a part of the hernia will protrude, as will be seen in the case of Mrs. Marshall.

With regard to the treatment of strangulated umbilical hernia, the first object is to attempt the reduction by the taxis, for which purpose the patient is to be placed in the relaxed position already described, and a gentle and uniform pressure is to be kept up for half an hour or more. *Treatment.*

When the simple taxis had previously failed, I have known instances in which it has succeeded, after having given large doses of Calomel, (ten grains, for example, for an adult) combined with a grain of opium, followed up with Magnesia Vitriolata and Infusion of Roses, and if the skin is inflamed, drawing away some blood by leeches. The remedy, however, on which I place the greatest reliance, and which I have found more successful here than in any other species of hernia is the tobacco glyster, employed with the same precautions as have been detailed at large in the first part of this work. I attended a lady with Mr. Toulmin, of Hackney, who laboured under severe symptoms of strangulation from umbilical hernia, in which the tumour was very tense, and where all previous attempts at reduction by the hand had failed. In twenty minutes after the tobacco enema had been thrown up, faintness came on, the tumour became quite flaccid, and with slight pressure the hernia returned into the cavity of the abdomen. I saw a patient of Mr. Hammond's, at Southgate, thus quickly relieved after a strangulation of forty-eight hours continuance, and a person who came to my house informed me, that she had been repeatedly relieved by this glyster of the symptoms of strangulation. If the symptoms of strangulation do not yield to the tobacco glyster and continue urgent, the effect of cold may be tried, either by inclosing ice in a bladder and letting it remain on the part, or (what has been also found successful) by dashing cold water repeatedly on the naked belly; but if the vomiting is frequent much time must not be spent in these attempts. *Medicine.* *Tobacco glyster.* *Cold.*

If the patient is plethoric blood should be taken from the arm; but as the subjects of this disease are generally women of relaxed fibre, I have seldom found venesection advisable.

Omental hernia. In strangulated omental hernia, after all attempts at reduction had failed by the taxis, I have seen the omentum gradually reduced by bleeding from the arm, applying leeches, and afterwards a bladder containing ice and water. See Cases.

Two sacs. As there are sometimes two hernial sacs involved in the same tumour, care should be taken that no deception arises from reducing the larger alone, whilst the other remains strangulated. In a case of this kind that occurred to me, with Mr. AGAR, in Whitechapel, I found that on compressing the larger swelling, the air and fluid in the intestine could be felt returning into the abdomen with a guggling noise, after which a smaller tumour was felt on the left side of the larger, the contents of which were strangulated, and which remained irreducible till the tobacco glyster had been employed.

Of the Operation for Umbilical Hernia.

Small hernia. If this hernia is not of considerable size, and if the parts do not adhere, the operation is very simple: an incision is made from the upper to the lower part of the tumour, which must be performed with caution to avoid wounding the intestine, as it is not always covered by a sac, and when it is, the sac is extremely thin. The sac (if any) is then to be divided by a small opening, a quantity of fluid escapes, and the contents of the hernia are exposed, of which, if both omentum and intestine are present, the omentum first appears, and on turning it aside the intestine is found behind, and in some degree involved in it. When the opening is sufficiently dilated by the director, the finger is to be gently introduced at the upper part of the intestine between it and the omentum, and directed to the orifice of the umbilicus, which is thus easily found. The omentum being then drawn aside, a probe-pointed bistoury is to be carried upon the finger, and the linea alba divided towards the sternum to an extent proportioned to the size of the parts which have descended, so as to allow of their return without using more than gentle force. In most instances from half an inch to an inch of dilatation will be sufficient.

Dilatation upwards.

The intestines are first to be returned if in a state to admit of it, after which the omentum is to be either cut away or returned according to the state in which it is found, and the integuments brought together by suture.

The operation which I have just described is easily performed, and is that which is generally employed; but it is one which exposes the patient to the risk of peritoneal inflammation, in consequence of a direct opening being left through the integuments into the cavity of the abdomen. I have, therefore, in two instances performed the following operation. As the opening into the abdomen is placed towards the upper part of the tumour, I began the incision a little below it, that is, at the middle of the swelling, and extended it to its lowest part. I then made a second incision at the upper part of the first, and at right angles with it, so that the double incision was in the form of the letter T, the top of which crossed the middle of the tumour. The integuments being thus divided, the angles of the incision were turned down, which exposed a considerable portion of the hernial sac. This being then carefully opened, the finger was passed below the intestine to the orifice of the sac at the umbilicus, and the probe-pointed bistoury being introduced upon it, I directed it into the opening at the navel, and divided the linea alba *downwards* to the requisite degree, instead of *upwards*, as in the former operation.

Dilatation downwards.

When the omentum and intestine are returned, the portion of integument and sac which is left at the upper part undivided, falls over the opening at the umbilicus, covers it and unites to its edge, and thus lessens the risk of peritoneal inflammation by more readily closing the wound.

Large herniæ, Sac unopened. I have mentioned in the former part of this work the advantage which is derived in large herniæ, from dividing the stricture, when in the surrounding tendon only, without opening the hernial sac itself. Mrs. AARON's case hereafter detailed was of that kind. It was very large, and had been irreducible for many years. A portion of intestine descended into it, and it became strangulated. I was called to her, and advised the operation, as many hours had already elapsed since the symptoms commenced, and several unsuccessful attempts had been made to return it. I made a very small incision opposite the neck of the tumour, exposed the fascia which covered it, passed my probe-pointed bistoury between the fascia and the sac, and divided the former to the edge of the umbilical ring, then putting my finger to the edge of the linea alba, I passed my knife through the umbilical hole behind the linea alba and made a small division of it upwards, then, with drawing the knife, I pressed upon the tumour and it immediately returned. This operation did not take more than four miuutes in its performance; it is attended with no more danger than the taxis; and, if insufficient, the operation may be afterwards performed in the common way by extending the same incision.

In the case of Mrs. HERBERT, patient of Mr. HUNTER's, in Tower Street, where the hernia was intestinal, and had been long irreducible; I made the incision upon the orifice of the sac, opened it and passed in a probe-pointed bistoury, and dilated the stricture upwards, then pressing upon the intestine, I discharged its contents into the intestine within the abdomen, left it in the sac, and brought the edges of the wound together with very little exposure of the protruded parts, and with relief to all the symptoms of strangulation. See Cases. *Large hernia. Stricture at the mouth of the sac.*

In dilating the mouth of the hernial sac and the linea alba, whether the stricture be divided above or below, it requires great care not to wound the intestine, as it is not unfrequent to find it adhering to the peritoneum within the abdomen close to the mouth of the hernial sac; an example of which is seen in one of the Plates, taken from a subject dissected by Mr. FORBES, of Camberwell. The intestine in this case adheres so generally to the orifice of the hernial sac, that unless the finger precedes the knife, and the dilatation is performed very gradually, the intestine must be wounded. Much difficulty also attends the returning the intestine into the abdomen under these circumstances, and if the adhesions are very firm it is best to leave the intestine in the sac, and to bring the edges of the skin together over it, closing it with great care: in short to perform the operation as it was done in the case of Mrs. HERBERT. *Intestine adhering to the mouth of the sac.*

The colon is the intestine usually found in the umbilical hernia, and the appendices epiploïcæ of this intestine undergo more alteration in fat subjects than the intestine itself. In the case of Mrs. PICKERING, I was under the necessity of removing several of them which had become of a very dark colour, before I could safely return the intestine into the cavity of the abdomen; for if they had been left adhering to the intestine, it was probable from their altered state, that they would have sloughed within the abdomen, which must have destroyed the patient. *Appendices epiploïcæ.*

The intestine often adheres to the inner side of the sac. If these adhesions are recent they may be readily and safely torn through by the finger: if they are long, they may be divided with the knife; but when short and firm, the sac must be cut away at the adhering part, which may be safely done in this case, as no vessels of any consequence can be injured by the incision, as happens in inguinal hernia. *Intestine adhering to the sac.*

With respect to the omentum, if the sac contains a very large quantity of it, or if in consequence of long continued protrusion it adheres extensively and has become very hard, it should be removed by the knife, taking care to secure the small vessels by ligature if they bleed, and the portion of divided omentum is to be left to form a plug to fill up the orifice of the hernial sac. In one of the subjoined Cases the omentum was left to slough, by which a troublesome sore was produced, and a considerable discharge was kept up for a great length of time. In the case of Mrs. PONDER, it will be seen that in consequence of its general adhesion, I left the omentum within the sac, and brought the integument closely together over it, which united without difficulty. *Omentum removed. Sloughs left.*

In dividing the orifice of the hernial sac and the linea alba there is no risk of cutting through any vessel of sufficient consequence to endanger life; for it is refining upon anatomy to mention the umbilical vein or arteries in this operation, as the two latter are mere cords, and the former, even if it were open and divided, would be readily closed by a dossil of lint. The danger in this operation, therefore, is that of wounding the intestine, and not the blood-vessels. *Vessels.*

After the parts are returned, great care should be taken to close the wound by sutures; this is required in all operations for hernia, but especially in the umbilical, where the passage into the abdomen is nearly direct, and the danger of peritoneal inflammation very considerable. *Sutures.*

CASES OF UMBILICAL HERNIA.

I am indebted to Mr. AGAR, Surgeon, in Whitechapel, for the following account.

CASE I.

Mrs. ...., about sixteen years ago, whilst getting over a stile, felt something crack above the navel, being then in the fifth month of pregnancy. An umbilical hernia was the consequence, which, in the succeeding years, increased very considerably, without however producing any particular indisposition: it was during this period confined with an elastic truss in the day, which at night was usually laid aside. Of late, however, a smaller tumour has been formed near to the left side of the larger, and it is this which has occasioned the following symptoms.

On January 9, 1805, the patient was seized about eleven at night with a violent pain about the navel, and the other symptoms of strangulated hernia. Ten grains of Calomel, with one of Opium, were immediately given, without however affording relief; and at six in the morning two opening pills were taken, but soon returned by vomiting, and a cathartic clyster was almost instantly rejected. The symptoms continuing, about six in the evening, by the advice of Mr. ASTLEY COOPER, the Calomel and Opium were repeated; and half an hour afterwards a clyster of half a drachm of Tobacco, infused in half a pint of water, was administered, which produced the usual depressing effects, and in a few minutes procured relief, so that nothing farther was required but keeping the bowels open, by giving of Rochelle salts occasionally.

On the 19th, the symptoms returned, and early on the following morning rapidly increased, when Mr. COOPER recommended the Calomel and Opium pills, and Tobacco clyster to be repeated; by which plan immediate relief was obtained.

April 20, 1806, the patient was attacked with heartburn, which was soon followed by pain and vomiting; but the pain was not now incessant, as it had been on the former occasions, experiencing sometimes intervals of a quarter of an hour. Two days previous to this she had taken two opening pills, to which she had occasionally had recourse for twenty years past, without any unpleasant consequence, and generally with the desired effect; but in this instance they operated very violently. Mr. COOPER recommended a repetition of the Calomel and Opium pills, the application of leeches, with fomentation to the part affected, and the use of Rochelle salts occasionally, which effectually removed the complaint.

On the night of December 2, the patient in a violent fit of coughing felt something pass through the part, which soon produced pain and sickness. The Calomel pills with Opium were given, and the protrusion in some degree returned; but she had some sleep from twelve till towards six in the morning, when the cough brought on a return of the rupture, with more violent vomiting than the patient had ever experienced before. About eight, Mr. COOPER arriving, advised the Calomel pills with Opium to be repeated, and a Tobacco clyster administered, which instantly returned; and, as the symptoms increased, in about an hour a second clyster was tried, which soon procured the desired relief. Since that time the Rochelle salts have been occasionally taken; but the patient experienced more debility than after any former attack. The Calomel also in this instance produced a troublesome salivation.

This was a case of double umbilical hernia. The larger contained both omentum and intestine, for the lobules of fat in the former could be readily felt, and the guggling noise in the latter be easily heard. The larger I could partially return after a few moments pressure; but upon the smaller I could make no impression until the Calomel and Opium had been given, and a Tobacco glyster administered.

CASE II.

Mrs. B........., a patient of Messrs. Jourdan and Castle, Bermondsey Street, was seized on the 20th of January last, with pain at the navel, which continued on the 21st, when, of her own accord, she took an opening medicine, which succeeded in procuring some stools. The pain, however, still continuing at the navel, and being attended with sickness and pain in the stomach, on the 22d she sent for Mr. Jourdan.

He found a tumour at the navel, about the size of a pullet's egg, which was very tender to the touch, and resisted every attempt to return it into the abdomen. He took away blood from the arm, applied leeches to the swelling, which relieved her with respect to the pain she had suffered, but still she vomited once on this day.

On the 23d, as her bowels were constipated, Mr. Jourdan ordered her some opening medicine, which procured several evacuations.

24th, I was sent for; the tumour was still of the same size, very tender to the touch, and very hard, entirely free from elasticity, rather knotted on its surface, did not project the integument, but was embedded in the fat between the muscles and the skin. It had the feel of omental hernia. She said, that upon the whole, she was in less pain since Mr. Jourdan bled her and applied the leeches. I ordered ice, inclosed in a bladder, to be applied to the tumour, and the purgative medicine to be continued.

25th, She has had stools; the part is not so sore to the touch, but the tumour is very hard. Upon the whole she thinks herself better.

27th, I was informed that she was better, and that she continued the ice and purgative medicine.

28th, I saw her, and the swelling was much reduced. Its tenderness has ceased; her bowels are regular.

February 3d, the tumour is almost entirely reduced, and she is doing well.

CASE III.

Mrs. Marshall, aged forty-eight, who resided in Prescot Street, Goodman's Fields, and who had a very large irreducible umbilical hernia, at six o'clock in the afternoon of the 21st of August, 1806, was seized with symptoms of strangulation. She sent for Mr. White, Surgeon, in the New Road, who reached her house by seven o'clock, and, after giving her a purgative medicine, came for me. It was ten o'clock at night before I saw her; the tumour was then very hard and large, and before I made any attempt to reduce it, I ordered a drachm of tobacco to be infused in a pint of water, and half to be injected. When this had been done a quarter of an hour, I made an attempt to reduce part of the swelling, but it was unsuccessful. The other half of the tobacco enema was then thrown up, and at the same time five grains of Calomel, and two of Opium were given; after which another attempt was made to reduce the hernia, but unsuccessfully. Indeed, the swelling was so tender to the touch, her cries were so violent at each attempt, and she made such resistance to every trial, that it was impossible to persevere sufficiently to give a chance of success.

She passed the night in dreadful agony, disturbing not only the persons in the house, but the neighbours with her cries, and scarcely five minutes elapsed without her vomiting; in short, I never observed in any person the symptoms so violent.

August 22, I called upon her at half past seven in the morning, and found mortification had began in the skin over the tumour, where the umbilicus had been originally placed; the skin there seemed to be particularly thin, it had changed to a green colour, but the cuticle had not separated. All the other symptoms were the same, except that her cries were not so loud and piercing, for she seemed already beginning to sink. Under these circumstances there appeared no chance of saving her life by an operation; a very slight mention of which excited the utmost horror in her mind. I therefore merely ordered fomentations to the part, and Opium internally.

Mr. White informed me, she continued in great pain after I quitted her in the morning; she vomited frequently, and was occasionally delirious; that about eleven o'clock, she brought up, with a slight effort, a large quantity of coffee-coloured fluid; that she afterwards became extremely feeble, and at half past eleven o'clock she expired.

Dr. Babington had been sent for, but she died before he reached the house. She lived only seventeen hours and a half after the strangulation began.

DISSECTION.

Upon opening the tumour, it was found to contain a very large portion of colon, and opposite the umbilicus, where the mortification in the skin had appeared, there was a little pouch protruding from the general cavity of the sac, in which a separate portion of the colon had been strangulated, and had there undergone a much greater change of colour than that in the larger portion of the bag.

Several small pouches were found in the side of the sac at different parts, and the whole tumour bore much resemblance to the shape of a melon.

The intestine adhered generally to the inner side of the sac; the quantity which had descended was so large, and the time which it required in the dead body to return it into the cavity of the abdomen was such, that I am perfectly satisfied that the operation could not have been performed at any time with hopes of success, if the hernial sac had been opened in the usual manner.

CASE IV.

The following Case I was favoured with by Mr. Dundas, of Richmond, Serjeant Surgeon to his Majesty.

DEAR SIR, Richmond, October 25, 1805.

I was sent for on Tuesday to a woman, about sixty, and very fat, who had an umbilical hernia for near thirty years, of a monstrous size, and which had been in a state of strangulation for three days. After much perseverance, I succeeded in returning the whole into the abdomen, and the opening through the umbilicus was so wide, that I could push my four fingers and thumb into it.

The poor woman was for twelve hours apparently better, the vomiting ceased, and she had a stool; but, like our patient last year at Teddington, her pulse continued very quick, her weakness increased, and her pain diminished.

In the course of the evening, notwithstanding my attempts to retain it, the hernia returned as large as ever, and she died yesterday morning.

I meant to have removed the integuments and the sac as well as the umbilicus, but both were so completely sphacelated, it was impracticable; almost all the bowels contained in the sac (as much as would fill a hat) were mortified.

I removed the umbilicus, which is so wide, that one would think it would have been impossible for it to have occasioned a strangulation of the bowels; but the quantity protruded made it produce the same effect as a narrower passage would have done.

I have sent the umbilicus to you in its rude state, as you may, perhaps, not dislike to see its extraordinary appearance.

I apprehend mortification of the bowels had taken place before I reduced them; perhaps that was the case with Mrs. D.* I remain, Sir, with great regard,

Your obedient humble Servant,

DAVID DUNDAS.

CASE V.

Mary Harris, aged sixty years, who lived at N° 3, Bryant Street, Webb Square, Shoreditch, had an umbilical hernia for twenty years, the origin of which she attributed to parturition. The hernia became of very large size, and four years before her death the skin ulcerated; the sores were difficult to cure, but did not remain healed for any length of time.

Symptoms of strangulation began in this hernia on July the 21st, 1805, soon after a hearty dinner of beans and bacon. She had a continued inclination to go to stool, but could not evacuate; and then began to vomit every thing she swallowed. She complained of excessive pain in the stomach, and in the hernia.

---

* Mr. Dundas here refers to the case of a lady at Teddington, in whom I partially returned an umbilical hernia, but without relief to the symptoms.

Mr. WESTON was called to her. Calomel and Cathartic Extract, Magnesia Vitriolata, and infusion of Senna were given without advantage; glysters were also injected, and fomentations applied to the abdomen, without diminishing the urgency of the symptoms.

At ten o'clock at night of the 23d, in getting out of bed, she fell forwards upon the floor; her husband ran up stairs to help her, but she complained of violent pain, and refused to be removed from the place on which she was lying; she was, therefore, covered with the bed clothes and suffered to remain upon the spot, and after a few minutes she died.

INSPECTION.

Upon opening the abdomen, the intestines appeared but slightly inflamed, and there was no effusion into this cavity, but the bowels were extremely inflated.

Cutting open the tumour, the intestine was found burst in two places, so that the fæces had escaped into the hernial sac, and in one part the inner coat of the intestine was burst without any rupture of the external peritoneal covering.

The hernial sac was absorbed at the place at which the ulcers in the integuments had existed, and to this part the omentum adhered with a degree of firmness, which made it impossible to separate it. The hernial sac had given way in two different places on the left side, and in one on the right, and through each of these holes the omentum had passed, so as to form two small herniæ between the sac and the skin.

The strangulation still remained complete at the umbilical ring. See Plate.

CASE VI.

Mr. PIDCOCK, Surgeon, of Watford, favoured me with the following account.

Watford, Monday, May 1, 1797.

Mrs. PICKERING, aged sixty-four, of a fat corpulent make, had been afflicted with an umbilical hernia for many years, which had been reduced four or five times in the week by herself on going to rest. About five years ago it was slightly strangulated, when the tumour was not one-third so large as at this time. This was reduced by the great assiduity and attention of a Surgeon in town.

On Saturday evening last, about ten o'clock, after having spent the evening in a cheerful party, on going to bed a descent of the contents of the hernia suddenly took place, attended with severe pain and vomiting. At one in the morning Mr. STRUT attended, and administered some opening pills. On the Sunday morning early I saw her, when the tumour was irregular and very hard, the vomiting violent, and she suffered a severe pain in the abdomen, and part affected. The pills had not been retained upon the stomach. I administered a glyster, and made attempts to reduce the protruded parts, but without success, and the pain continued violent, and the vomiting incessant. I ordered a draught, with ten drops of Tinct. Opii, to be taken every two hours, which seemed to produce a remission of the pain, and the tumour became more soft. About three o'clock, P. M. I kept the part constantly wet with cloths dipped in a solution of Sal Ammon. in vinegar and water for an hour, and then made a long continued attempt to reduce it without any success. Previous to this I had taken away about twelve ounces of blood, and the pulse was still small and feeble. The sickness having continued without intermission during the day, at night I ordered a glyster, with one drachm of tobacco, infused in a pint of boiling water, to be thrown up, which, however, was forced away a few minutes after being administered. A few pills of Calomel and Opium were given, but could not be retained in the stomach.

In this state she remained during the night without sleep, with the tumour soft, the pulse feeble, great thirst, no hiccough, nor tumour of the abdomen, great sickness and no stool.

Early on Monday morning, when I saw her, I found that she had passed a very restless night, that the sickness was continual, the pulse small and feeble, the tumour and abdomen still painful, and she had had no stool. I again repeated the tobacco glyster as last night, which was immediately rejected, and made a slight attempt to reduce the hernia, but to no purpose.

Seeing no prospect of returning the hernia, and that nothing but an operation could save her life, which, if done immediately, might turn out favourably, since there had been no great degree of inflammation, or any symptoms of gangrene, we thought it best immediately to propose it to the patient, to which she consented, and Mr. ASTLEY COOPER was immediately sent for from London, and the operation performed as soon as he arrived.

OPERATION.

Mr. C. made a crucial incision through the integuments, and having exposed the hernial sac, which was very thin, he made a small opening into it, and the omentum protruded at the aperture. The opening being dilated, a large quantity of water escaped from the sac, and the intestine was exposed by drawing the omentum upwards. The intestine, which was of a dark colour, was the colon, as appeared, from its membranous bands, and appendices epiploïcæ, the latter of which were of a dark venous colour.

The stricture was next divided by passing the finger to the umbilical ring, and by dilating it upwards, or towards the sternum.

A considerable quantity of water then issued from the abdomen, whence it appeared that she had laboured under ascites; when this was discharged the intestine was particularly examined, and it was not so much discoloured but that it might be safely returned into the abdomen; the appendices epiploïcæ were thought to be too much altered to recover their natural state, and several of those bodies were cut away, and the intestine was then returned. The omentum was also returned into the abdomen, where it rested opposite the mouth of the hernial sac.

May 2, (the morning after the operation.) A glyster given last night staid for some time, but brought away no stool. Has passed a restless night, and complains of pain in the part and abdomen; but there is no tension nor swelling; she was inclined to vomit during the night; the pulse is small and quick; thirst not so great; a quantity of water has discharged by the wound, but the dressings remain unmoved.

The following medicine was given:—℞. Ol. Ricini ʒi—Infus. Sennæ, S. ʒij—Vitelli Ovi unius—Aq. Menth. Pip. ʒij—Spt. Vol. Aromat. ʒifs. M. ft. Mistura cujus capiat cochl. ij. secundis horis donec alvus solutus fuerit.

On taking the second dose, a large and copious evacuation took place, from which she felt herself much relieved, and during the afternoon was easier, and much inclined to sleep.

Evening.—Has rested well during the afternoon; the pain is less, and the vomiting is something abated; the pulse is quick and feeble; the thirst considerable; has no pain in her head. She omitted the mixture, after having had two copious stools. Sumat h. s. Haust. Anod. cum T. Opii gtt xxx.

May 3, Wednesday morning.—Has had no sleep during the night; the vomiting decreases; has had two stools; the urine is high-coloured, and deposits a lateritious sediment; the tongue is dry; the skin moist and cool; the pulse small, but not particularly frequent; the matter vomited up is principally bile; there is no tension, nor hardness of the abdomen, and no inclination to eat. The wound, which was dressed with a simple ointment, looks extremely well, without tumefaction, redness, or inflammation; and upon the whole she feels herself much better. In the afternoon, she conceived that a portion of the gut had fallen into the sac; but, on examination, I found no return of the parts. The vomiting continues slightly.

Haust. Salin. ʒifs—Conf. Aromat. ʒi.—Pulv. Rhub. gr. 10. M. ft. haustus—4^{tis} horis sumendus.

Evening.—Has slept near two hours this afternoon; the parts and other particulars remain as yesterday and this morning. Her sickness is not violent, and has ceased since taking the draught; the pain is less; the pulse better and stronger. She has drank a little beer, and taken some nourishment.

May 4th, Thursday.—Has slept more this night than the preceding one; the sickness continues with a discharge of a greenish colour; has had two stools in the night; the abdomen remains soft and less painful; there is no soreness to the touch; the pulse continues soft and regular.

Cont. Haust. Salin. 4^{tis} horis.

Evening.—Has had a stool in the day; has continued a little sick, but by no means so frequently; has little or no pain in the abdomen; the pulse is as before; has had a little desire for food, which she retains.

May 5th, Friday.—Had a very indifferent night; was restless and sick, and very rarely retained what food she took; had a stool in the night; and a watery discharge flowed from the wound, which emitted a fœtid smell; the pain and soreness in the abdomen are much the same. I removed the sutures, and fomented with Anodyne fomentation. Her spirits are very low; the pulse feeble, but regular; the appearance of the wound healthy; a part of the omentum or appendices epiploïcæ sloughed away; she drinks a little beer; had a stool during the day.

Sumat Haust. Cardiac. h. s.

May 6th, Saturday.—Has slept much better during the night; the sickness has entirely left her; she is free from any febrile symptoms; the pulse rather quick; appetite better; little thirst; tongue moist; no pain in the abdomen, nor tension. She feels a smarting in the wound, which is very slightly inflamed. There is a suppuration, with a sloughing of that part of the omentum that was left at the wound. Retains both medicine and food on the stomach.

Persistat in usu Fotus, & Haust. Cardiac.

May 7th, Sunday.—Has not had so good a night; has been restless, and the wound has discharged a watery matter, and is slightly inflamed; removed a part of the omentum that was about to slough off, fomented, and dressed with digestive and dry lint. Had a natural stool; no fever; the pulse regular.

Evening.—Has had a little return of the sickness; is very low and faint. The part gives out a very fœtid discharge, but neither the pain nor local inflammation are increased.

Adde Tinct. Opii g^{ttas} xxv. haustui, h. s. sumendo.

May 9th, Tuesday.—Slept but very indifferently at night; her strength and her appetite increased; she is free from any unpleasant symptoms; the pulse regular; has two or three natural stools every day; no sickness, nor pain nor tension in the abdomen. The wound appears remarkably well; the remaining part of the omentum came away with the dressings; but there is another sphacelated part on the point of separating, which looks very much like the sac of the hernia. A good discharge of pus appears, and the part is much contracted and diminished in size. Upon the whole she is in a very favourable way.

Foment and poultice night and morning. Dress with dry lint.

R. Decoct. Cinchonæ, Mixt. Camph. aa ʒi. Tinct. Stomach. ʒij. M. ft. Haust. bis in die sumendus.

R. Ext. Opii g^r ifs. Conf. Aromat. ʒfs. M. ft.—Bolus. h. s. sumendus.

Saturday 13th.—The part which on Tuesday was sloughing off, bearing the appearance of the sac, has come away from that time in portions, and yesterday the whole was removed, and is very evidently the hernial sac. The wound discharged very good pus, and the whole of it is very much contracted. She sleeps better, but as yet very indifferently; has continued perfectly free from fever. Vomiting very rarely occurs. Has one or two regular motions every day, without the assistance of purgatives. There is no swelling, fulness, nor tension of the abdomen; and she is, in every respect, in a more favourable state.

Fomentation and poultice night and morning. Application—Dry lint.

Monday 15th.—Has had a very restless night, and a constant sickness and vomiting of a bilious matter, and a very large fœtid discharge of a sanious nature, with a quantity of water from the cavity of the abdomen; the pulse low and feeble; no appetite; much thirst; the wound looks flaccid and unhealthy.

R. Haust. Salin. ʒi. Conf. Arom. ʒi. Rhub. gr. ij. Tinct. Gentian. C. ʒij. M. 4^{tis} horis—Dry lint, and a spirituous embrocation were applied.

Tuesday 16th.—The sickness much less; the discharge still considerable and very fœtid; her pulse is stronger, and the thirst has abated; in other respects well and very cheerful. This watery discharge must have been retained in the abdomen for some time, and its evacuation arises from some change in the patient's position in lying and sitting; but I am at a loss to what to attribute the extreme fœtor, except to the discharge from the wound having gravitated into the cavity of the abdomen. The wound itself looks very favourably to day.

Thursday 25th.—From the day of the last minutes the discharge has been fœtid: on some days very little or not any; on others more copious. The wound is filling up with granulations, and the discharge (as simply connected with the wound) very good. The sickness continues at times, but is rarely very distressing; her bowels perform their office regularly; her appetite on the whole is tolerable. She sleeps the greatest part of the night. Her complaints now are a dry parching heat in the mouth and tongue; restlessness, and great dejection of spirits, and a wandering pain about the abdomen. She makes as much water as usual; has no fever, and the most distressing symptom is, a frequent vomiting of a bilious matter.

From the time of making the above minutes, that is from the 25th of May, to August 16th, the time when

Mr. Cooper saw her a second time, the wound was continually diminishing in size; the discharge decreased, and the former distressing symptoms were then very slight.

The discharge had during this time varied very much; on some days it was in great quantity, and very watery, in others less in quantity, but more purulent. Whenever the discharge decreased suddenly, she felt pain and distention in the epigastric region, and sometimes vomited a watery matter; but on the return of the discharge these symptoms disappeared.

Whenever she walked much, took more than ordinary exercise, or accidentally pressed upon the wound, it became painful and inflamed, but on the application of a poultice these symptoms subsided. Her appetite for food, and general debility, with indifferent nights, continued much the same, until about a fortnight ago, since which she has increased in strength very rapidly. She now sleeps extremely well, and relishes her food and drink as much as before her confinement.

She moves about at this time with the assistance of a small stick, and now and then expresses herself, as feeling better in health and freer from indisposition than she has been many years.

The wound is scarcely the size of a small horse bean, but at the upper part of the original wound, a small sinus continues to discharge in a trifling degree, and a probe will pass by it towards the cavity of the abdomen several inches. She is now left to dress herself, with no other application than a simple plaster of white Cerate.

She occasionally takes a few opening pills, and they have been the only medicine of this kind she has required since the second week of the operation. Her appetite is good; she sleeps well; is not in any degree troubled with sickness, flatulency, colic, or nausea, dryness of the tongue or fauces. No anasarcous appearance appears, except a slight puffiness in the ancles. Her spirits are good, and she walks about with ease, and is in all respects wonderfully recovered.

November 20th, 1797.—She is now perfectly well, the wound is completely closed, and does not afford the most trifling discharge. She is remarkably lively and cheerful. Her bowels regular; one or two small distentions appear in some part of the parietes of the abdomen, but nothing of consequence.

CASE VII.

Mrs. Culf, of Tottenham High Cross, had long laboured under a large umbilical hernia, which became strangulated at three in the morning of the 17th of September, 1801, and the symptoms continued undiminished till seven in the morning of the 18th, when Mr. Holmes, of Tottenham, her Surgeon, requested me to see her. I found her vomiting violently; incapable of having a stool, and with frequent eructations, and excessive pain across the middle of the abdomen, which came on by paroxysms, at the interval of about ten minutes, and the belly was very much swollen. The tumour, which could be distinctly felt to be in part omentum, and partly intestine, was not equally tense with the abdomen, which I attributed to the large quantity of omentum which had descended.

As there was no hope of preserving her life, but by an operation, (and, indeed, from her extraordinary bulk, even this was attended with much danger,) I instantly proposed it, to which she very readily consented.

The first incision was made across the middle of the tumour, and the second at right angles with it at its lower part; and after dividing the hernial sac in the same direction, eight inches of the great arch of the colon, and a large portion of omentum became exposed. I removed the stricture by cutting the linea alba towards the pubis, for which purpose an incision of an inch in extent was required. The intestine was then easily returned into the abdomen, but the omentum I left in the hernial sac, and having brought the edges of the wound together over it, I laid an adhesive plaster upon the part. She became easy immediately after the operation, and when I left her, was disposed to sleep.

19th.—She was hot and restless the whole of yesterday, and had a restless night; she has had no sickness, but has passed a great number of very liquid stools; her menses, which were discharging the day preceding the accession of the symptoms, still continue; her pulse is 140 and fluttering; the abdomen swollen and tense. I bled her to the amount of six ounces; ordered the navel to be fomented and poulticed, as there appeared a disposition to gangrene about the edges of the wound.

20th.—She was better, being less restless, continuing to have stools, and to menstruate; the belly was less tense, and the gangrenous appearance had somewhat subsided, but her pulse was still 120, and weak; I therefore ordered her to take nourishment.

21st.—I found her low, but her pulse was not so quick; the menstrual discharge continues, and she has had one stool; the tumour, however, is tense, and one of its edges is sloughy.

24th.—Her health continued to improve until to day, when I found her complaining of pain in her head and giddiness. She was also hot, and her pulse was quick. I opened the wound a little, the edges of which were slightly gangrenous; and I found the omentum which I had left in the sac in a sloughy state. I ordered bark, wine and water, and a nourishing diet.

26th.—She is much improved in health; but the omentum continues to slough. A poultice is the only application, and which she says is productive of great ease.

29th.—Her health is improving, but the omentum continues to slough, and keeps up a great discharge.

As she resided five miles from town, I did not see her afterwards but at distant intervals; the omentum did not entirely separate until the end of the month of April, and she was not perfectly cured until the middle of May.

In the following Case I divided the stricture without attempting to return the protruded parts.

CASE VIII.

Mrs. HERBERT, aged forty-four years, a patient of Mr. HUNTER's, in Tower Street, sent to him at half past two o'clock in the morning of the 18th of May, 1804, having had no stool for three days, and having been seized with violent pain at the navel, and across the upper part of the cavity of the abdomen.

She had long been subject to an irreducible umbilical hernia, which now appeared full, and somewhat painful to the touch, and she had strong eructations, frequent vomiting, and violent pain in the abdomen; her pulse was quick and hard. Calomel and Colocynth, Oleum Ricini, and other medicines of that class had been given without effect. On Saturday the 19th, I was sent for, as she still continued in the same state. I saw her at nine o'clock in the morning, and met Dr. ELLIOTT and Mr. HUNTER.

The tumour was now tense and painful to the touch; but, after considerable and long continued pressure, I thought it became somewhat softer. I ordered a Tobacco Enema, and ice broken and put into a bladder, to be applied to the swelling. The medicines which were ordered her, were Calomel and Colocynth, united with Opium.

At one o'clock on the same day, I saw her, when she was in less pain, her pulse less quick and hard, but she had no stool. At eleven o'clock at night I was sent for, on account of her suffering more pain; her pulse was quicker; she had frequent eructations, and occasional vomiting, and still had no stool; the tumour was tender to the touch, and the abdomen sore upon pressure.

As it was clear, therefore, that the inflammation was extending into the abdomen, and that it would soon be too late to expect success from the operation, I immediately performed it.

I made a small incision upon the upper part of the tumour, opposite the umbilicus, and cut through a quantity of fat which lay between the skin and the hernial sac: then the sac appeared, which was opened by a very small incision, and intestine was seen adhering within it. No fluid was found in the hernial sac, although the adhesion of the intestine was by no means general. I passed my finger along the surface of the intestine to the mouth of the sac, and found I could insinuate it into the cavity of the abdomen, though with difficulty, without dilating the orifice.

Upon my finger I carried a probe-pointed bistoury within the orifice of the hernia, and dilated it upwards, till the finger could readily pass by the side of the intestines into the abdomen, so that they were left quite free from pressure; but as I found the intestine adhering to the internal surface of the sac, in such a manner that it would require a large opening to be made, and a long continued dissection to divide the adhesions, I thought it better to leave the intestine adhering, and to bring the edges of the wound in contact. I therefore sewed up the small wound I had made, and covered it with adhesive plaster.

Her pulse became extremely quick during the operation, and continued so till I left her, at a quarter before one in the morning; the eructations also continued, but still she expressed herself more free from pain.

Sunday, ten o'clock in the morning. She had a stool in three quarters of an hour after I left her, and has had several since; the pain and soreness of the abdomen have disappeared; the pulse, however, is 120 in a minute, and the tumour is inflamed; the eructations continue. I ordered a poultice to be applied.

Sunday evening, at ten o'clock I met Dr. LETTSOM; her pulse was then nearly natural; she was perfectly easy, and had many stools; the eructations had ceased. She was ordered saline medicine, with an absorbent earth, as she complained of heartburn.

Monday 21st.—The abdomen was free from pain, the pulse soft, and nearly natural; but she has stools in great numbers; and I therefore ordered her opium. The tumour being inflamed a poultice was ordered to be continued on it.

Tuesday 22d.—She took last night Opium, with Magnesia Vitriolata, on account of her having vomited. She passed a good night, and feels much better this morning. Her pulse is less quick than it was last night; the tumour is relaxed, but the skin over it is slightly inflamed, and shews a tendency to slough at the edge; the tongue is a little furred, and the skin somewhat moist. A poultice of stale beer grounds was ordered.

Wednesday 23d.—As she had little constitutional irritation, she was ordered more nourishment, and allowed to drink a small quantity of ale.

Thursday 24.—The ale purged her, and she was obliged to take opium to check it.

Friday 25.—The skin was hot; her pulse full and quick; and she vomited last night. Opium was given, which immediately checked the vomiting, and improved her feelings.

Saturday 26.—She was purged frequently; the threads seemed separating, and I removed them all, excepting one. The edges of the skin now appear healthy.

Monday 28.—I took away the remaining thread.

Tuesday 29.—The wound appears to be healing quickly under the application of a poultice.

On June 15.—She was perfectly well.

CASE IX.

Mrs. ...., a patient of Mr. ANDERSON, in Walbrook, who had an umbilical hernia, which was in part irreducible, had symptoms of strangulation on the 1st of September, 1802, which continued until the 4th, when it became necessary to operate.

I made an incision at the lower part of the tumour, following the same course as in the former cases, and exposed a portion of omentum, which was very much hardened, adhering strongly to the inner part of the sac, and forming membranous bands across it.

At the upper part of the sac I felt a fold of intestine passing through the opening at the umbilicus, which opening was sufficiently large to allow, by the yielding of the omentum, a passage for my finger into the abdomen. Still, however, as some force would have been necessary to return the intestine into the abdomen, I thought it proper to divide the stricture, which I did with a probe-pointed bistoury upwards, and found it of a cartilaginous hardness. I then easily returned the intestine, but the omentum was left within the hernial sac without separating its adhesions. The integuments were brought together by sutures.

She had stools soon after the operation, but the inflammation in the abdomen proceeded, and she soon became delirious. She died sixteen hours after the operation.

CASE X.

Mrs. ...., aged fifty-two, a patient of Mr. JOURDAN's, in Bermondsey Street, was on March 27, 1803, seized with symptoms of strangulated hernia.

On the 28th, I first saw her, and found a hernia at the navel, about the size of a small orange, and projecting upwards towards the sternum, instead of descending in its usual manner towards the pubis.

Her symptoms were, frequent vomiting, pain across the middle of the abdomen, which was tense, but not tender when handled; her bowels were constipated; her pulse 100, and she was extremely restless; the tumour was slightly inflamed, and a portion of skin, about the extent of half a crown, at the lower part of the tumour was mortified. Any pressure of the tumour with the hand excited a disposition to vomit.

I ordered her a glyster, containing half a drachm of Tobacco in infusion, which immediately as it was thrown up produced a disposition to evacuate, but the glyster only came away; her pulse immediately after the injection rose to 120.

On the 29th.—Her general symptoms were the same as before; the vomiting, and constipation continued, but the mortification had increased in extent; however, as the symptoms were not such as to lead me to believe that mortification had yet extended to the intestine, I resolved to cut through the skin at the part already mortified, and to return the intestine into the abdomen; I therefore made an incision through the dead part of the skin only, and found intestine within the hernial sac, which I returned into the cavity of the abdomen.

The pain in the abdomen, which she had previously suffered, became increased by this operation, and the vomiting was equally urgent; her bowels continued constipated, and she had no alvine evacuation. She died the following night, and I could not obtain permission to inspect the body.

CASE XI.

Mrs. Bond, a patient of Messrs. Johnson, John Street, Minories, who had for many years been subject to an umbilical hernia, and which had been often strangulated, was, after a violent cough, again seized on Saturday, June 28, with the symptoms of strangulation. Various trials were made by Messrs. Johnson to reduce it; the Tobacco glyster was repeated six times on Monday the 30th, in the quantity of a scruple of Tobacco, in infusion, but each time without effect; and on Tuesday, July 1, at eleven o'clock in the morning, having previously made a trial to reduce the hernia, which proved unsuccessful, I performed the operation.

My first incision was made at the linea alba, at the upper part of the tumour, and having exposed an aponeurosis which covered the sac, I put a curved bistoury between the aponeurosis and the sac, and cut the linea alba upwards, at the part at which it embraced the sac. Still, however, the intestine could not be reduced, and I therefore opened the sac at its upper part, when a small quantity of fluid escaped, and the omentum was found adhering and thickened. The adhesions of the omentum being then separated, the strangulated portion of intestine was exposed, which was of a deep red colour. Passing my finger upon its upper portion, and a curved bistoury upon my finger, I opened the mouth of the sac upwards. Next, I examined the intestine, and finding that though it was much altered, it soon, in a great degree, recovered its natural appearance, I returned it into the cavity of the abdomen, and brought the edges of the wound together, correctly, by means of sutures.

In pushing back the intestine, I felt a large tumour within the abdomen, which seemed to be a solid mass, reaching from the pelvis above the umbilicus; and on enquiry, respecting her general health, I was informed that it had been gradually declining, and that from extreme obesity she had, without any obvious cause, gradually become thin.

Evening.—I found that from the time of the operation, the pain of which she had previously complained had ceased, but that the vomiting had continued without abatement, and that the flatus had not passed the protruded portion of intestine, for she had almost incessant eructation. She had no stool; her pulse was scarcely perceptible at the wrist; she was extremely restless; her countenance was anxious; her body was covered with a cold sweat. She was ordered thirty drops of Tinct. of Opium, which quieted her a little.

Wednesday, July 2.—I was informed that she died during the night.

DISSECTION.

Thursday, July 3.—At one o'clock, accompanied by Messrs. Charles and George Johnson, I opened the body.

On cutting open the hernial sac, we found in it a portion of the intestine, which had descended since the operation; the omentum adhered to the mouth of the hernial sac. The intestines within the cavity of the abdomen were generally inflamed, and the omentum was reddened by inflammation, a great number of blood-vessels being visible upon it, which are not seen when it is in a healthy state.

The lower part of the abdomen was occupied by the tumour, which was felt during the operation. I found it proceeded from the uterus, which had a great number of external polypi upon it; one of which was so large as to project as high as the navel. I removed the uterus that I might make a preparation of the disease, and weighing the tumours the same afternoon, I found their weight to be six pounds and three quarters.

This case serves to shew that any considerable disease which would not of itself prove immediately mortal will prevent the success of an operation, the result of which might be otherwise favourable.

CASE XII.

On the 23d of January last, I was requested by Mr. Wilson, Assistant Apothecary of Guy's Hospital, to visit with him Mrs. Ponder, of Maze Pond, aged seventy years and five days, who had, as he informed me, symptoms of strangulated hernia, and a tumour at the navel as large as a swan's egg. Mr. Wilson had ordered a Tobacco enema, and made use of the taxis, but it did not seem that any impression could be made upon the swelling.

I found the tumour of the size he described, situated a little on the right side of the cicatrix of the navel, although projecting through the umbilical ring; it was hard and somewhat irregular to the touch, and I could make no alteration in its bulk after a long continued attempt to return it. As she vomited frequently and violently, and nothing would pass through the bowels, I requested her consent to the operation, and it was immediately performed.

As soon as the integuments were divided by a very superficial incision, the hernial sac was exposed, and on opening it a small quantity of clear serum escaped, and the omentum appeared. The incision was then extended from the upper to the lower part of the tumour, and the parts completely exposed. The omentum being next unfolded, a portion of intestine was seen of a claret colour, and all the vessels on it very turgid with blood. I carried my finger behind the omentum, and between it and the intestine, and felt the stricture at the umbilical aperture, which was completely lined by the adhering omentum.

A probe-pointed bistoury was directed by my finger into the orifice of the sac at the umbilicus, between the omentum and intestine, and keeping the blade close to the posterior part of the linea alba, so as to prevent the intestine slipping before it, I divided the stricture (through the omentum,) upwards, to the extent of about three quarters of an inch.

The intestine was then returned with slight pressure.

As the omentum adhered very generally to the inner side of the sac, and its vessels appeared unusually large, and the subject, from age, extremely feeble, I did not choose either to return or remove it, but I brought the edges of the skin very closely together by sutures, and left it in the hernial sac, covering the wound with adhesive plaster.

Almost immediately as the operation was concluded, she had a stool.

24th.—She informed me that she had eleven evacuations in the afternoon and night, and she appears this morning free from pain, and cheerful; the pulse is good; the belly soft, and the eructations with which she had been much troubled before the operation, had ceased.

25th.—Tongue a little furred; pulse rather quicker than natural; has had two stools; the part was very sore, but her abdomen is flaccid and free from pain.

26th.—I found her sitting in her chair, in which she had fainted. I insisted upon her immediately going to bed. Fortunately the sutures had not given way.

27th.—Mr. Wilson and myself visited her together, and we found her free from every bad symptom.

30th.—She seems low, and a painful tumour is capable of being felt in the beginning of the arch of the colon on the right side. Mr. Wilson gave her Calomel.

Feb. 2d.—Tumour disappeared after the evacuation. She is very cheerful, and the abdomen is quite soft.

4th.—I dressed the wound, which appears healthy.

8th.—The wound was again dressed; it is now but small, and is healing fast.

In the following Case the operation was performed without opening the hernial sac.

CASE XIII.

February 5, 1807.—I was called by Mr. SHANNON to see Mrs. AARON, a patient of his, aged fifty-two years, who had symptoms of strangulated hernia. She had long had an irreducible omental exempholos, of the form of a melon, for which a hollow truss had been worn; the pad of which was formed of pewter, and covered with leather. For a month prior to this period she had a very violent cough, with difficulty of breathing, and in a fit of coughing on January the 31st, felt the tumour become tense, with violent pain in the abdomen, constipation of the bowels and sickness. On February the 2d, however, she had several motions, but on the 3d, was in much greater pain and vomited frequently, which continued on the 4th and 5th.

As the symptoms had remained so long, and I could make no impression on the swelling by the taxis, I proposed the operation, to which she immediately consented, and it was performed at one o'clock, P. M. in the following manner.

I directed Mr. SHANNON to draw down the tumour towards the pubis, and then I made an incision two inches long through the skin only, opposite the upper part of the neck of the hernial sac. This incision exposed a fascia, into which I next made an opening large enough to admit a director, which was carried to the aperture at the umbilicus and cut upon.

I then passed my finger between the mouth of the sac and the linea alba, where it forms the umbilical aperture, and having carried a probe-pointed bistoury upon the finger behind the linea alba, I cut it to about the extent of three-fourths of an inch.

Pressure was then made upon the tumour, and a portion of intestine immediately returned into the cavity of the abdomen. A piece of adhesive plaster was applied upon the wound. The sac was thus left unopened, and the stricture having been seated in the tendon and not in the mouth of the sac, this simple and easy operation was sufficient to enable me to return the hernia.

Evening.—She had two stools immediately after the operation, and in the afternoon six others. The vomiting had ceased, and the tumour is quite flaccid.

February 6th.—At three o'clock in the morning she was attacked with pain and heat in the abdomen, and sickness, immediately after a violent fit of coughing, and she continued vomiting until nine o'clock, when Mr. SHANNON came for me. I found the tumour tense as before the operation, and upon pressing it the intestine returned with a guggling noise, and I was much gratified I had not opened the sac, as her death, if I had, would have almost certainly ensued from this return of the protrusion. I ordered fourteen ounces of blood to be taken away, and applied the truss upon the tumour.

Evening.—She had three stools in the morning after the reduction of the intestine.

Feb. 7th.—Complained of abdominal pain this morning at two o'clock, and Mr. SHANNON again bled her, and ordered her a cathartic, from which there were four evacuations. She had taken off her truss, which I replaced, with positive orders that it might not be again removed.

Feb. 8th.—She has had evacuations, and is perfectly free from pain. Broths, and other liquid nourishment were allowed.

Feb. 10th.—Her cough is troublesome, but all the symptoms arising from the hernia have ceased. The wound discharges healthy pus.

Feb. 12th.—I pronounced her out of danger from the operation.

Feb. 15th.—She has been sitting up for the three last days. Her cough is the only remaining complaint; the wound requires no further application.

I am obliged to Mr. SMITH, Surgeon, for the history of the following Case.

CASE XIV.

MARY CROSS, admitted February 6, 1801, under the care of Mr. CLINE, on account of a strangulated umbilical hernia. It was found necessary to perform an operation, which was accordingly done, and it proved successful; but she remained in the hospital for other complaints till the 28th of May.

In February 1802, her hernia again became strangulated, and she was taken to the hospital. From the urgency of the symptoms, Mr. Cline thought it necessary to have recourse to the operation immediately, as the usual means had been tried before her admission; and this time it also proved successful. But other complaints again detained her in the hospital till her death, the 27th July, more than five months after the operation. Her complaints after both operations were pain in the abdomen and right leg and thigh, the latter was œdematous. In addition to which, since the last operation, she had a bad cough, and great pain in her loins.

I obtained leave to inspect the body. The hernia formed two tumours, and Mr. Cline at the time of the operation could feel a membranous band between them. I took out the hernia entire, and in the tumour that was most inferior I found a small portion of the ilium and part of the cæcum. In the other tumour there was a portion of colon, and which adhered to the sac. This last tumour I was told had formerly suppurated, and the fæces were discharged from it, and the part afterwards healed; which I think probable, as the skin was extremely thin and appeared like a cicatrix.

When I opened the abdomen I found a mass of disease on the loins, which appeared to be the glands enlarged to a great size; some of them were hard and as large as a goose's egg, others were very soft, and contained a curd-like matter. These glands were more enlarged on the right side than on the left, which probably was the cause of the swelling of the right leg and thigh. In the left kidney there were some small calculi, and in the right there was a large rough stone, about an inch and a half long and half an inch broad, with a process that lay in the ureter, and also about four ounces of a white fluid. The process of stone that lay in the ureter prevented the fluid passing into the bladder. The liver had a great number of tubercles, and the spleen was somewhat enlarged. The lungs adhered to the pleura costalis in every part. The pericardium had no cavity, for it adhered rather firmly to the whole surface of the heart.

She gave me the following account a few days after the first operation: the hernia was produced about four years and a half ago by coughing, but it never was of much inconvenience till about two years ago, when she was attacked with symptoms of strangulation, from which she got better in a day or two, but they returned again in about a month with greater violence. She continued in great pain, the tumour increasing in size, for three weeks, when it burst and discharged a quantity of greenish fœtid fluid by four apertures, and then the pain was somewhat relieved. Poultices were applied to the part, which continued discharging the same kind of fluid in great quantity for seven or eight weeks, after which it gradually ceased, and the apertures continued for eleven weeks longer before they healed. She said that her food was found in the poultices for the first seven or eight weeks.

CASE XV.

To Dr. Barclay, Teacher of Anatomy, in Edinburgh.

MY DEAR SIR,

It affords me great pleasure to have it in my power to communicate any information either to your good self, or to my old Fellow-Student Mr. Astley Cooper.

The case to which he alludes occurred about the 14th of July, 1804. It was the smallest congenite umbilical hernia, or what we call ventral tumour, I had ever met with, for its size did not exceed that of a large hen's egg. And the deficiency of abdominal parietes could have been covered by a half crown piece. The edges of the teguments of the abdomen surrounding the base of the tumour were, as I have always observed in such cases, thickened and somewhat retracted, and of a deep pink colour. The tumour itself was not nearly so transparent as I have usually found it, but the navel string terminated as it ordinarily does in similar cases, that is a little to one side, and not on the apex.

On examining accurately the appearances, it occurred to me that the protruded contents might be reduced, and that the edges of the defective parts might me brought together. I therefore immediately sent for my friend Mr. James Anderson, Surgeon, and requested his assistance in the operation.

After a little difficulty the contents of the sac were reduced, a ligature was then tied firmly round its base, after which the sac was cautiously opened. It proved to be the sheath of the umbilical chord. With two silver pins and some adhesive straps the edges of the separated parietes abdominis were brought closely together. The sac was allowed to drop off, and in a few days the cure was complete.

The infant lived and throve well for nearly eight months, when it became affected with some internal disorder, which the mother called " Bowel hyve," and died after a week's illness. But the woman declared to me a few days ago, that it had never seemed to suffer (after the cure) from the former disease.

The result of this case led me to fear that I had often lost the opportunity of saving life, for I had hitherto always considered such cases as strictly desperate. But I have since found that sometimes there is such a deficiency of the parietes abdominis as to render it impossible to reduce the protruded viscera. Sometimes the expansion of the sheath of the cord adheres to the peritoneum; and in some cases besides this, there is a firm adhesion of the peritoneum to the external surface of the liver. This I found in a case last Spring, where I had advised an operation merely as a dernier resource.

On the whole I have seen on an average for seventeen years past two cases of this congenite malconformation annually.

I remain, Dear Sir, with best compliments to Mr. COOPER,

Your's most sincerely,

JAMES HAMILTON, JUN.

Nicholson's Square,
Oct. 3, 1806.

OF THE VENTRAL HERNIA.

The Ventral Hernia differs from the umbilical only in its seat. Every hernia protruding through the anterior or lateral parts of the abdomen, except at the umbilicus or the abdominal rings, has the name of ventral.

<small>Unfrequent.</small> This disease is not very frequent, for though my situation at the hospitals gives me the opportunity of seeing a great number of herniæ, yet neither my notes, or my memory, furnish me with more than twenty examples of this disease in as many years.

<small>Seat.</small> In most of the cases that I have seen, it has been seated in the linea alba, and in the greater number, about half way between the umbilicus and the ensiform cartilage. I have also met with it in the linea semilunaris in three examples, in all of which they have been placed below the level of the umbilicus. One of these was in a young lady not more than twenty-two years of age, which was irreducible; another in a corpulent gentleman, advanced in years, patient of Mr. Maiden's, at Stratford; and the third in a young woman, whose case will be hereafter given, on whom the operation was performed.

<small>Symptoms.</small> The symptoms attending this complaint are generally the same as those which accompany the umbilical hernia, except that when the hernia is situated at the upper part of the linea alba it usually contains the stomach, which gives rise to some peculiar symptoms; for a part of the food by passing into the tumour occasions an increase of it after eating, and the patient is subject to a sinking sensation at the scrobiculus cordis, great flatulency, and depression of spirits. An eminent literary character once consulted me respecting a small tumour of this kind. I applied a truss, which readily prevented the parts from protruding, on which he expressed his wish that I could as easily remove the flatulency, indigestion, and sinking at the stomach which he constantly felt. I told him it was probable the application of the truss might remove all these symptoms, and when I met him in the country a short time afterwards, he informed me that the truss perfectly answered the purpose intended, and that he believed I was right in my opinion as to the cause of his symptoms of indigestion.

<small>Causes.</small>
<small>Natural apertures.</small> There are four different causes of this disease so far as I have been able to observe; the first and most common is, that apertures are left in the linea alba and linea semilunaris, and between the fibres of the muscles, for the passage of small blood-vessels, and these holes are sometimes larger than is sufficient to allow the vessels to pass, and protrusions of the viscera readily occur through them.

<small>Malformation.</small> A second cause is, that the formation of the linea alba is sometimes defective in children. I have a cast in my possession, taken from a child who was brought to Guy's Hospital as an out patient, who had three herniæ in the linea alba, arising from such a malformation. I once saw a tumour about four inches long, and one and a half broad, reaching from the navel, to where the umbilical vein passes to the liver, produced by the absence of that portion of the linea alba, but without any corresponding defect in the skin. This species is readily distinguished from the other, by the great size of the opening through which the hernia passes.

<small>Muscles torn.</small> A third cause is, a laceration of some of the fibres of the abdominal muscles under violent exertions, which allows the peritoneum to pass between them. I never, however, ascertained this by dissection, but am disposed to believe it, from the sudden appearance of the disease after a sensation of laceration.

<small>Wounds.</small> The fourth cause of ventral hernia, is a wound through the parietes of the abdomen, in which the skin after-

wards heals, but the muscles never unite. An example of this has been communicated to me by my friend Mr. James Wardroper, of Edinburgh, and will be found at the end of this chapter. Sometimes in these wounds a protrusion of the intestine occurs, which is lacerated by the injury, and an artificial anus remains during life. Of this an example was lately to be seen in St. Thomas's Hospital, sent there by Mr. James of Hoddesdon. The subject of it was a woman who had been gored by an ox, and the horn tore the intestine as well as the parietes, the intestine became protruded and inverted, and the fæces were discharged through the opening.

The dissection of the ventral hernia offers the following observations. In examining the small one, (of which I have given a Plate,) which was situated a little above the navel when I cut through the skin, a loose fascia was exposed, which was the aponeurosis of the external oblique muscle, and to the inner side of this was glued another, which proceeded from the edge of the aperture in the linea alba, and which seemed to be a fascia formed to fill up the opening in the tendon. Under these fasciæ there was a considerable quantity of fat, which being dissected away, exposed the hernial sac, which was of a dark blue colour. Between the fascia and the sac a small blood-vessel was observed, which passed through the same opening with the hernia. *Dissection of.*

In the large ventral hernia, of which I have given two views, I found only one fascia covering the sac, in other respects it resembled the former. In both, the umbilical vein had been pushed into the sac, and adhered to its anterior part.

Of the Reducible Ventral Hernia.

When this hernia is situated in the linea alba, and can be returned into the cavity of the abdomen, it requires the same small truss as that which I have recommended for the incipient umbilical hernia. If, however, it arises from any extensive deficiency of this tendinous line it is necessary that the form of the pad should be varied so as to cover a greater extent of surface than the tumour, in which case the pad should be from four to five inches long, and two inches broad. *Reducible.*

If the hernia is placed at the lower part of the linea semilunaris, it is proper to apply a truss similar in its general form to that which is made use of in the inguinal hernia, but the pad in this case is to be turned upwards, instead of taking its usual direction. The truss is to be applied round the pelvis, and the pad is to be turned towards the linea semilunaris so as to cover the orifice of the hernial sac. *Truss peculiar.*

The Irreducible Ventral Hernia requires the pad of the truss to be made hollow. The general form of the truss resembles that used in the umbilical. It was in an irreducible ventral hernia at the lower part of the linea semilunaris that I applied the inguinal truss, with the direction of the pad reversed, which I have described above, and as the hernia appeared to be omental, I had the pad made hollow to gently compress the tumour. The patient wore the truss with ease, but as she lived at a distance in the country, I have not had an opportunity of learning whether the tumour has been absorbed. *Irreducible*

Of the Strangulated Ventral Hernia.

As the ventral hernia, like the umbilical, is pendulous, the Surgeon, in employing the taxis to reduce this hernia, ought, after grasping the tumour, to direct his pressure upwards, as the orifice of the sac is placed in that direction. *Strangulated taxis.*

The same general means which have been directed in the strangulated umbilical hernia are to be here employed; and it may be observed that in this hernia, as well as the umbilical, medical treatment alone will more frequently succeed in reducing this hernia than either the inguinal or crural. I have been twice called to a patient of Mr. Maiden's, of Stratford, who had a ventral hernia in the linea semilunaris, and laboured under symptoms of strangulation; he appeared to be more relieved by purgative medicine, by glysters, leeches, and fomentations, than by the use of the taxis, which it was difficult to employ on account of the size of the tumour, and its being embedded in adeps. *Medical treatment.*

In performing the operation for this species of hernia, the sac should be opened by a similar incision to that we have recommended in the umbilical hernia, that is to say, in the form of the letter T, which leaves a valve of *Operation.*

skin to cover the opening, after which the mouth of the sac is to be opened, and the linea semilunaris dilated at its inferior part; but if the tumour is placed at the lower part of that line, the sac is to be dilated upwards or downwards according to the situation of the epigastric artery, which crosses the linea semilunaris at its lower part.

Large hernia.   But if this hernia is very large, it will be right to make a small opening through the skin to the tendon which surrounds the sac, and to divide the tendon without opening the sac, in the way which has been stated in treating of the Umbilical Hernia. I shall conclude this account of ventral hernia with the following cases.

CASE.

DEAR SIR,   Edinburgh, 25th October, 1806.

The case about which you enquire was as follows.

A strong healthy man of twenty-four years of age, twelve years ago, when sliding down a rope, a piece of wood fixed to it, forcibly penetrated the abdominal parietes. It entered about half way between the anterior spinous process of the ilium and pubis, passed in the direction of the tendinous fibres of the external oblique muscle, and again appeared exteriorly about four inches above the first wound. The intestines immediately came out at both wounds; they were reduced, and in about two months the wounds were healed.

Ever after the accident he observed a swelling at the place where the parietes were wounded, which has gradually been enlarging. When I saw him the tumour was about six inches in length, four in breadth, and of a rounded form. It was a soft elastic mass, and could by moderate pressure be made to entirely disappear, but when the pressure was removed, in a few minutes it regained its former bulk; the motions of the intestines could be seen as they filled the bag, and they rushed in with a gurgling noise. The coats of the tumour were very thin, and the external skin was marked with cicatrix. There was a very considerable loss of substance of the abdominal parietes, and the opening between the sac and cavity of the abdomen was very large. He was employed as a shoemaker for eleven years after the accident, and he afterwards found so little inconvenience from the swelling that he returned to sea.

I am yours, &c.

JAMES WARDROPER.

CASE.

On Sunday the 23d of March 1806, I was sent for by Mr. Holt, of Tottenham, to see Mrs. W........., of Tanners End, who had a ventral hernia, which had become strangulated on Sunday, the preceding day.

On Monday morning at one o'clock, I met Mr. Holt there, and found a hernia about as large as my fist, situated in the linea semilunaris, about an inch and a half below the level of the umbilicus. After a long continued attempt I succeeded in reducing it, and her truss was applied, which was not only originally badly constructed, but was nearly worn out by continued use. Some opening medicines were ordered her, and she was desired to keep her bed.

I was surprised at being sent for to her on the afternoon of the same day, on account of the hernia having again descended, and upon inquiry found that, soon after we quitted her, she had got out of bed, and sat for some time near the fire, and that the truss had allowed the hernia to redescend. Mr. Holt had attempted to reduce it, and I repeated the attempts without success, and it was, therefore, agreed that the operation should be performed, as she had already very urgent symptoms, and the abdomen was becoming tender to the touch.

The operation was well performed by Mr. Holt. He made an incision across the middle of the tumour, which was covered with a large quantity of adeps; the sac being opened, exposed omentum only, which adhered very generally to the inner side of the sac. The opening of the sac was with difficulty found, on account of the adhesions of the omentum, but a probe-pointed bistoury was with care insinuated into it, and the stricture divided. The omentum was returned into the cavity of the abdomen, the integuments were brought together, and the wound carefully closed.

After the operation she had several stools, and great hopes were reasonably entertained of her recovery; but on Tuesday, she had no evacuation from the bowels, had frequent eructations, and repeated vomitings, which, together with increasing soreness of the abdomen, clearly shewed that peritoneal inflammation had come on.

Mr. Holt bled her largely, and she had glysters administered.

On Wednesday, I found her vomiting frequently, her abdomen extremely tense, and tender to the touch, and she had frequent hiccough.

On Thursday morning she died.

Her body was not examined, but it was sufficiently obvious that she died of peritoneal inflammation.

OF THE PUDENDAL HERNIA.

Situation.
This hernia is situated in the middle of the external labium pudendi, a little above a line drawn from the orifice of the vagina outwards.

Size.
The size of those which I have seen, has been that of a pigeon's egg, and the figure of each was pyriform.

Figure.
They were elastic to the touch, conveying the impression to my mind that they contained intestine only.

Intestinal.
Like other herniæ they descended in the erect, and ascended in the recumbent posture, dilated when the person coughed, became occasionally tense and painful, and produced frequent interruptions in the functions of the bowels, but the patients were generally easily able to return them into the cavity of the abdomen.

Diagnosis.
This hernia is very readily distinguished from the common inguinal, which also passes into the labium pudendi, because the species of hernia I am now describing has no communication with the abdominal ring, and the upper part of the labium is entirely free from swelling, whilst the tumour in this case occupies nearly the center of the labium, and extends on the inner side of the branch of the ischium into the cavity of the pelvis.

This tumour is felt as a ball in the labium, and if the finger is passed into the vagina, it is found to extend upwards into the cavity of the pelvis between the ischium and the vagina, till it ceases to be felt at the os uteri.

The lower extremity of this swelling occupies the doubling of the external labium; its middle part is situated between the ischium and the vagina, and its orifice into the cavity of the pelvis is placed near to the os uteri.

Differs from the lateral vaginal.
This hernia differs but little from the lateral vaginal in its commencement, but at its lower part, instead of pressing the vagina forward, in form of a hernial tumour, it passes beyond the vagina, and appears in the labium pudendi.

Mistaken for the hernia foraminis ovalis.
I am inclined to believe that this disease has been mistaken for the hernia foraminis ovalis, and that it has been observed by other medical men, who examining it in the living subject when it was not in a strangulated state, have been led into a mistake with regard to its real nature. I once asked Dr. Lowder. Lecturer on Midwifery, if he had seen any example of the hernia foraminis ovalis, he said that he had, and that it had extended inwards so far from the foramen ovale as to reach the middle of the external labium, whence it could be easily pressed into the cavity of the pelvis. Upon farther inquiry, I found, that he conceived it had passed through the foramen ovale, and afterwards turning inwards at a right angle with its neck extended to the middle of the external labium pudendi. But when we attentively consider this subject, we shall find it scarcely possible that the hernia foraminis ovalis, which is small in size, and embedded in the triceps muscle, should pass through the gracilis first, and afterwards the fascia of the thigh, and extend itself so far as to distend the labium, and produce an appearance like that I have here described. At all events, the cases which I have seen were not of that description.

Liable to be confounded with the diseases of the lacuneæ.
This swelling is liable to be confounded with a disease, which does not unfrequently occur on the inner side of the labium, in the form of a tumour that distends the labium;* it is elastic to the touch, and often becomes of con-

---

* I was called by Mr. Benjamin Atkinson, Nicholas's Lane, to a patient of his, who had one of these tumours situated on the inner part of the labium, near the os externum vaginæ. It appeared through the nymphæ of a light blue colour, tense and elastic, and had an obscure sense of fluctuation; it did not dilate in coughing, and pressure made no difference in it. I advised its being opened, to which she would not consent.

A woman in St. Martin's Le Grand, came to me last Summer with a tumour of this kind. I called at her house, and passed a small seton through it, and a glary fluid was discharged; a considerable degree of inflammation arose from the part, and constitutional irritation supervened; I withdrew the thread after ten days, when the suppuration was completed, and she got well.

Dr. Haighton desired I might meet him to see a patient of his, who had a similar tumour larger than a pigeon's egg on the inner side the left labium. I made an incision into it, and introduced lint into the cavity. She got well in three weeks with little constitutional irritation.

siderable magnitude. It arises from an obstruction of the lacunæ, situated near the orifice of the meatus urinarius and vagina, in consequence of which an accumulation of fluid takes place, which either proceeds to the production of a large tumour, containing a fluid like the white of an egg, or sometimes occasions inflammation terminating in abscess. These swellings, though they resemble each other somewhat in their seat, are found by attentive inspection to differ so much as to be capable of being distinguished from each other.

The tumour which I have just mentioned does not dilate on coughing; fluctuates; cannot be traced entirely into the cavity of the pelvis by the side of the vagina, and the pubis ischium can be felt behind it; it does not descend in the erect, or disappear in the recumbent posture.

To the following Case I was called by Dr. Best, of York, who at the time this occurred was attending the Carey Street Dispensary.

CASE I.

Dr. Best called on me the evening of the 18th of May, 1802, to request me to see Sophia Hall, aged twenty-two years, who laboured under symptoms of strangulated hernia. He informed me he had made a slight attempt to return the hernia about an hour before, but it was unsuccessful; its size was about that of a pigeon's egg, and it was situated in the left labium; it had frequently descended during the last six months, and she was able to reduce it herself with little effort and little pain.

The hernia had at this time been down three weeks, and upon the whole of the 16th and 17th, (that is the two preceding days,) it had given her great pain when it was touched, but still more when she coughed.

As she had been ill from a peculiar nervous attack, Dr. Best thought that she was probably prevented by this cause from attempting to return it herself, as she had been in the habit of doing. When I examined the swelling, I was surprised to find it situated below the middle of the labium, and the upper part of the labium, the abdominal ring, and the parts about it, quite free from tumefaction. Examining her per vaginam, I found a tumour extending by its side nearly as far as the os uteri. I desired her to cough, and found it immediately dilated. I then grasped the swelling, and pressing on it with some little force, which gave her a great deal of pain, in about three minutes it went up with a guggling noise, and she became easy. The labium then felt flaccid as if a tumour had been taken from it, and when the finger was placed upon this flaccid and hollow portion of skin, it could be forced back into a circular orifice on the inner side of the branch of the ischium, and between it and the vagina. The only method she has since used to keep the hernia up, is to wear a common female bandage between the thighs, and fixed around the abdomen.. The last time Dr. Best heard of her was in the August following, at which time she was in perfect health.*

The following is Dr. Best's Letter.

* DEAR SIR, York, May 19, 1806.

The young woman to whose case you allude, and whom you was so kind as to visit on my account, was twenty-two years of age. How long she had been subject to hernia, or how it first commenced, I am unable to inform you. I remember, however, her saying, that it had frequently come down during the last five or six months, and that she had always before been able to reduce it herself without either difficulty or pain. At the time you saw her, which was on the evening of the 18th of May, 1802, the hernia had been down nearly three weeks, and the whole of that and the preceding day, had given her much pain both when she coughed, and when it was touched. The illness and extreme debility, under which she laboured, had, I suppose, prevented her from reducing the tumour in the first instance, as she had always done on former occasions.

About an hour before you saw her, I examined the tumour, and made some ineffectual attempts to reduce it. To the best of my recollection, it was somewhat less than a pigeon's egg, of a smaller diameter, but more oblong form.

At the time you reduced it, she was laid in a supine posture. You sat on the bedside on her left hand, with your face towards the upper part of the bed. The time you employed in reducing the tumour could not be more than two or three minutes, perhaps not so much, but she complained of the process giving her very severe pain. The only method she used to prevent a return of the tumour was, passing a bandage under the perineum, connected at both its ends with another bandage, which surrounds her waist. For six or seven weeks previous to your seeing her, she had been afflicted with an irregular, severe, nervous disorder, an account of which I left in your possession. She was then convalescent, fat, and was perfectly well in about a month afterwards. The last time I heard of her, was in the August following, when she was in perfect health, and did not complain of any return of the hernia. She resided at the time we saw her with a married sister, N° 4, Axe Court, Hackney Road. Her sister's name was Kemp, her own Sophia Hall. I remain, &c. &c.

CHARLES BEST.

CASE II.

A young woman whose age was twenty-two years, called at my house, complaining of a tumour of a similar kind with the above, in the right labium pudendi. Its size was somewhat less than that of the former case; it descended in the erect, and returned into the abdomen in the recumbent posture, it dilated upon coughing, and became much distended during the evacuation of the fæces. She supposed it had been occasioned by having been thrown out of a One-horse Chair, by which accident she received a blow on the lower part of her belly, and soon afterwards she observed the swelling.

I ordered her to wear a small pessary of sponge in the vagina, and I have not since seen her.

When this species of hernia is in the reducible state, it may be prevented from becoming larger, and occasioning inconvenience, either by wearing a common female bandage, or, what would answer the purpose better, by the application of the truss employed for the relief of the prolapsus ani; its distance from the vagina is too considerable for it to be readily prevented descending by the use of the pessary, unless the instrument were of very large size, yet it can only be by such an instrument that a prospect of a cure can be reasonably entertained, as no other can close the orifice of the sac.

In the irreducible state, it cannot be otherwise relieved, than by the constant support of a bandage, which would tend to prevent its growth.

When this hernia becomes strangulated, the mode of attempting its reduction consists in the Surgeon placing himself upon the diseased side of the patient, and then embracing the tumour with his fingers, he is to press it with gentle and regular force, against the inner side of the branch of the ischium, and from the yielding nature of the parts through which this hernia descends, I am inclined to believe that these efforts will very generally be attended with success. If they were unsuccessful, the warm bath, bleeding, and the Tobacco glyster ought to be tried, and then the attempt at reduction should be repeated.

If the hernia cannot be reduced, and the symptoms of strangulation continue, an operation ought to be performed, which, although difficult, is certainly far from impracticable. An incision should be made into the labium, to expose the lower part of the tumour, and the hernial sac being carefully opened, and the intestine exposed, a concealed bistoury should be passed up the sac, and directed by the finger previously introduced into the vagina, the division of the mouth of the sac ought to be made directly inward towards the vagina. The bladder should be emptied previous to the operation, and even before the first attempts at reduction are made.

OF THE VAGINAL HERNIA.

Those who are in the habit of practising Midwifery must necessarily see this disease more frequently than I have had an opportunity of doing; only two examples of it have occurred under my observation.

<small>Case.</small> The first was in a young woman, aged twenty years, who had never had children, and whose case I was informed by Mr. Stocker, Apothecary, of Guy's Hospital, was worth examination, on account of a tumour which projected into the vagina. She was ordered to place herself in the recumbent posture, with her shoulders a little elevated, and an examination being made per vaginam, I felt a swelling a little above the os externum vaginæ, the size of which was that of a small billiard ball. It was situated at the posterior part of the vagina, but rather to the left side; it was elastic, and not at all painful to the touch. When I compressed it, it readily passed away, but upon directing her to cough it was reproduced. When I ordered her to place herself on her knees the swelling became very tense and much larger than before, and when she coughed it dilated as any other hernia, only more forcibly.

<small>Symptoms.</small> Having placed herself again in the recumbent posture, I pressed the swelling entirely away by keeping the fingers about half a minute on the posterior part of the vagina, and then carrying the fingers higher up in the vagina above the seat of the tumour near to the os uteri, and having pushed the vagina towards the rectum, I directed her to cough, and the tumour was not reproduced. Still pressing at the same part, I desired her to rise, and so long as the pressure was supported the hernia did not return, but almost immediately as the fingers were removed the tumour became as large as before.

The inconvenience she suffered was, that she was incapable of taking much exercise, and could not engage in those laborious exertions which were required for her support, as she was in indigent circumstances; for she found whenever she exerted herself much a sense of bearing down as if something would burst its way through the part. She was ordered to wear a pessary; but when I last heard of her she had not followed this advice, and she continued to suffer the same inconvenience from the tumour.

<small>Seat.</small> This hernia protrudes into the space that is left between the uterus and rectum, which allows the intestines to descend between them. This space is bounded below by the peritoneum, which is reflected from the vagina to the fore part of the rectum, and between this reflection and the perineum is situated a loose cellular membrane. The pressure of the intestine then upon the portion of peritoneum forces it downwards to the perineum, and being unable to pass further in that direction, it is pushed towards the vagina, and projects its posterior part forwards. This hernia has been sometimes found placed more laterally, producing a tumour on the side of the vagina instead of its posterior part.

If this tumour then were dissected, the vagina would be found covering it anteriorly; behind this is placed the peritoneum, and then the intestine would be seen in the peritoneal sac between the vagina and the rectum. I wish it, however, to be understood that I have had no opportunity of examining this disease in the dead body, and that I am here describing it, from what is known of the structure of the parts, and not from actual dissection.

<small>Reason why it is not more frequent.</small> It appeared astonishing to me when I first considered this subject, that the disease did not occur more frequently, for the small intestines always descend into the pelvis, and the reflection of the peritoneum is too feeble to be able to support any considerable pressure. But I believe the reason of its being comparatively rare, is, that the oblique position of the pelvis is unfavourable to its production. In the erect, as well as in the sitting posture, the intestines fall rather upon the symphisis pubis, and the bladder, than on the posterior part of the pelvis, and when thus gravitating into the anterior part of the pelvis they push the uterus

against the rectum, and close the space which would be otherwise existing between them. But for the oblique position of the pelvis this must be a very frequent disease, for upon passing my fingers in the dead body from behind the uterus within the cavity of the pelvis in women who have died a few weeks after delivery, I have found that I could thrust the reflection of peritoneum between the uterus and rectum readily down to the perineum.

Intestinal. It appears in the case which I have related, as well as in those which I have been permitted by my friend Dr. John Sims hereafter to describe, that these herniæ contained intestine, and that will very generally happen, because although the omentum is sufficiently long to reach into this part of the pelvis, yet it is generally situated between the intestines and the anterior parietes abdominis.

Hernia of the anterior part of the vagina. The other case of vaginal hernia which I have seen, was that of a girl, a patient of mine in Guy's Hospital, who was admitted for what was supposed to be a prolapsus uteri. Her age was seventeen. When I examined her, a tumour was found situated just under the meatus urinarius, forcing the anterior part of the vagina through the os externum. In passing my finger to ascertain the state of the os uteri, when I pressed upon this swelling her urine was immediately discharged, and the tumour became flaccid. This induced me to make a more particular examination, and I then found the following circumstances. There appeared a tumour just under the meatus urinarius, of a florid red colour, projecting the anterior part of the vagina beyond the os externum vaginæ. The tumour was broader than it was deep, being about two inches in breadth, and one and an half in depth. I pressed upon it, and the urine immediately flowed from the meatus urinarius. I directed her to discharge her urine, and the swelling became quite flaccid, but on the following day when the urine had reaccumulated, the tumour was as large as before. Dr. Haighton, who examined her, found the same appearances. She continued some weeks in the Hospital, but I could suggest no relief for her complaint.

Dr. Sims's case. Dr. John Sims had a lady under his care with a hernia of a similar kind; it projected the anterior part of the vagina, was situated under the meatus urinarius, and when compressed the urine was discharged by the meatus, and the swelling became flaccid. This disease probably arises from a relaxed state of the portion of peritoneum which is reflected from the bladder to the uterus, which allows the bladder to yield to the superincumbent weight of the intestines.

Case of vaginal hernia of large size. To the same gentleman I am also indebted for the following cases of herniæ at the posterior part of the vagina. He was called to Mrs. P............, a lady under thirty years of age, who had a tumour at the posterior part of the vagina, which passed down between it and the rectum, and thrust the vagina forwards. The nature of this case had been dubious to those who had previously attended, but the Doctor became acquainted with its real nature, from finding that he could distinguish solid fæces within the tumour. He directed a glyster to be thrown up, and the swelling became soft, and then yielded to the pressure which he made upon it. Notwithstanding the swelling was very large, she continued to have children, but she suffered great inconvenience from a sense of bearing down whenever she used exercise, so that she is on that account prevented from taking it, and all the persons the Doctor has seen in this disease suffered extremely from the same symptom.

When this hernia is in the reducible state a pessary is obliged to be worn to prevent its descent.

Treatment illustrated by a case. A lady, aged about thirty-five years, consulted Dr. Sims for a hernia at the posterior part of the vagina, which rendered it difficult for her to use any exercise, and entirely incapacitated her from doing so if she did not wear a pessary. Pieces of sponge were at first used for the purpose of preventing the descent of the hernia, but they were found to be inadequate to the purpose, and she is under the necessity of wearing a globe pessary, which succeeds extremely well, at least in removing the uneasiness and sense of weight in the part, of which she had previously complained.

OF THE PERINEAL HERNIA.

This hernia descends in men between the bladder and the rectum, and in women between the rectum and the vagina. Seat.

It protrudes as far as the skin of the perineum, but does not project it so as to form an external tumour; its existence in the male can be only ascertained during life, by an examination by the rectum; but in the female, it may be felt both by the rectum and by the vagina. No external tumour.

The Plate which I have given of this disease, was taken from the body of a male subject brought for dissection to St. Thomas's Hospital; the preparation is now in the possession of Mr. CUTCLIFFE, Surgeon, at Barnstaple, in Devonshire, to whom the subject belonged. This drawing was made whilst the parts were in the recent state, and it differs from the preparation in half the bladder being represented as being removed, as it would have prevented the hernia from being seen.

The peritoneum, which is naturally reflected from the posterior part of the bladder to the anterior part of the rectum, was pushed down to the perineum by this hernia, but the skin did not appear to have yielded so as to have formed any external swelling. Dissection of.

The lower extremity of the hernial sac was placed before the anus.

The prostate gland was situated immediately anterior to the fundus of the sac.

The fundus of the vesicula seminalis was placed upon the lateral part of the sac, its apex was situated before it.

The bladder covered about one inch and three quarters of the anterior part of the hernia.

The mouth of the sac was two inches and an half from the anus.

As to the symptoms which this disease had produced, I had no opportunity of ascertaining them, for this person being accidentally brought for dissection, his previous history could not be traced. Symptoms.

Its existence might certainly have been ascertained by passing the finger up the rectum, but in the reducible or irreducible state nothing could have been done but to afford him temporary relief, by emptying the tumour when it pressed very heavily upon the rectum. If this hernia were strangulated, pressure might be made upon it from the rectum, and the intestine be possibly reduced, but I have no experience of this having been practised. Treatment.

Mr. BROMFIELD gives the following curious case of this disease in his Chirurgical Observations, p. 264. Mr. Bromfield's case.

"A lad between six and seven years of age, was put under my care to be cut for the stone. The staff, in the attempt to introduce it into the bladder, met with resistance from a stone, which seemed to be lodged in the membranous part of the urethra, or a little lower down in the neck of the bladder: I made my incision as usual through the integuments and muscles, to get at the groove of the staff; I then pressed the blade of my knife into the sulcus at the extremity of the staff, being able to divide only the membranous part of the urethra, and a very small portion, if any, of the prostate gland: by the examination of the parts with my fingers, I then found that this hard body was a process continued from the body of the stone contained in the bladder; I therefore took the double gorgeret, without the cutting blade affixed, intending only to push back the stone, and to dilate the neck of the bladder, which I did, by getting the beak of the gorgeret into the sulcus of the staff, and pressing it against the point of the stone, following its course with the instrument as the stone retired: but the direction that the gorgeret took, alarmed me, as it ascended under the ossa pubis with great obliquity: I then concluded that the instrument had taken a wrong route, as I could not in this case have the advantage of the groove of the staff farther than the extremity of the membranous part of the urethra; but on withdrawing the upper half of the gorgeret, I introduced the fore finger of my right hand into the bladder by the under part of the instrument, which remained in the bladder, and was now no more than the common gorgeret; by which I was soon convinced that it was in the bladder, whose situation was raised much higher in the pelvis than usual: I then introduced my forceps, and while I was searching for the stone, *a thin diaphanous vesicle like an hydatid appeared, rather below my forceps, which on the child's screaming, soon burst and discharged a clear water, as if forced from a syringe; the next scream brought down a large quantity of the lesser intestines.* I need not say, that this was sufficient to embarrass a much better operator than myself; however, I proceeded in the operation with great tranquillity, being conscious that this very extraordinary event was not owing to any error in the operation: but the difficulty was to keep the intestines out of the cheeks of the forceps, when I should again attempt to lay hold of the stone; the extraction of which would be very difficult to effect, from the unusual situation of the bladder in this subject. The lower part of the gorgeret remaining in the bladder, the forceps were again easily introduced, which being done, with the fingers of my right hand I pressed back the intestines, and with my left supported the forceps. I then got an assistant to keep up the intestines while I laid hold of the stone; but, during the extraction, the intestines were pushed out again by the child's screaming: nevertheless, as I had the stone secure in the forceps, I proceeded to extract it, which I did very easily. Before I introduced the common gorgeret, for the introduction of the forceps the next time, I got up the intestines again, and desired my assistant to keep them up till I got hold of a second stone, which I likewise extracted; and repeated the same process on account of another piece of stone, which from its shape appeared to be that which had got into the neck of the bladder. As soon as I was convinced by the examination with my finger that the bladder was totally freed from any pieces of stone, I again returned the intestines into the pelvis, and brought the child's thighs close together; a piece of dry lint was applied on the wound, and a pledget of digestive over it; he was then sent to bed with no hope of his surviving till the next day: but, contrary to expectation, the child had a very good night, and was perfectly well in a little more than a fortnight, without one alarming symptom during the process of cure: neither did the intestines ever once descend through the ruptured peritonæum, after they had been returned when the operation was finished."

Mr. B. proceeds to explain his ideas of the nature of this case.

" After the incision of the integuments and muscles was made, as usual, there soon appeared in the wound something like an hydatid, which proved afterwards to be that part of the peritonæum which is extended from the left side of the bladder and intestinum rectum to its attachment on the inside of the left os innominatum; by which attachment that part of the peritonæum, when in a natural state, does the office of a ligament, thereby preventing the lesser intestines from falling down too low in the pelvis; therefore, in this case, this expansion of the peritonæum must have been forced out of its usual situation.

" Suffering daily more and more extension, it will at length permit the intestines to fall down to the very bottom of the pelvis, between the bladder and rectum: therefore, when in the case above related the resistance of the integuments and muscles was taken off by the operation, the peritonæum was forced out, and at first was filled only with lymph, which gave it the appearance of an hydatid; but its thinness not being able to resist any longer the force of the adominal muscles pressing the viscera downward, it burst, and the intestines soon followed through the aperture. If this is allowed, we can easily account for the oblique course that the gorgeret took when first introduced, as the intestines had raised up the fundus of the bladder against the back part of the ossa pubis, so that my forceps could not be conveyed into the bladder, but almost in a perpendicular direction; and I was obliged to press with my hand on the lower part of the abdomen, just above the pubes, to bring the bladder and its contents sufficiently low, for my laying hold of the last stone with my forceps."

Female.

In the female the existence of this disease may be ascertained by examination, either by the vagina, or by the rectum, as the tumour is placed between the two canals.

Dr. Marcet's case.

Dr. MARCET, Physician to Guy's Hospital, read a paper at the Medical and Chirurgical Society of London, during the last Spring, containing an account of the dissection of a patient of his who had been six weeks in Guy's Hospital, and who laboured under vomiting and constipation for the greater part of that time, and when her body was examined after death, it was found that the uterus was retroverted without pregnancy, and the fundus uteri being turned into the space between the vagina and the rectum, had pressed upon the latter with so much force as to prevent the passage of the fæces. The preparation of this disease is preserved in the collection of morbid parts in Guy's Hospital.

Dr. JOHN SIMS informed me, that he had been consulted by a lady who had been married several years, but had never borne children, and being desired to examine her, he found a swelling at the posterior part of the vagina, pushing the os uteri forwards. After long continued, but slight pressure, he succeeded in returning the tumour into the cavity of the pelvis, and the os uteri then resumed its natural situation. She soon after conceived, and has never since complained of those cholicky sensations under which she had laboured previous to the tumour being reduced. She has had, however, but one child, although this circumstance occurred four years ago. *Dr. Sims's case.*

Dr. HAIGHTON, Lecturer on Midwifery at Guy's Hospital, informed me that he had seen an example of a tumour of this kind descending between the vagina and rectum. When pressed upon from the vagina, it protruded the rectum, if compressed from the rectum it forced the vagina through the os externum. *Dr. Haighton's case.*

Whilst the perineal hernia is capable of being reduced, it may be prevented from descending by the pressure of a pessary, which must be of large size.

Both this hernia and the vaginal may sometimes become dangerous during gestation, as the following case will prove.

Dr. SMELLIE was called to a woman, who about five weeks before she fell in labour had a tumour of this kind, which she had been previously able to reduce, increase to such a degree that she could not reduce it. The Doctor found her in great agony; the tumour was livid, and all round the edge of a fiery red colour. She lay on her side, and when turned upon her back to examine the tumour, it broke in the middle where the skin was thin, and there issued about a spoonful of pus mixed with blood, and next a thin fluid of a greyish colour, to the quantity of half a pint. She exclaimed that the intestine was gone up, and that she was free from pain. She recovered, went to her full time, and was delivered by Mr. TOMKINS, and some months after her delivery called upon Dr. S., when he found the hernia had kept up, and the part appeared firm, though a little ichor continued to ooze from a small orifice. In about five months after this the rupture reappeared, and she being again pregnant, it was several times reduced by one of his pupils, by whom she was likewise safely delivered. See SMELLIE's cases on Midwifery, 8vo. p. 132, Case V. Also Cases IV, and VI, of a somewhat similar disease. *Dr. Smellie's case.*

OF THE THYROIDEAL HERNIA;

OR,

HERNIA FORAMINIS OVALIS.

Thyroid foramen.
A CONSIDERABLE opening is left in the anterior and upper part of the Obturator or Thyroid Foramen of the pelvis for the passage of a nerve, an artery, and a vein.

This aperture is sometimes so incompletely filled by the vessels and nerve as to permit the descent of a portion of omentum or intestine, and the peritoneum lining the cavity of the pelvis is pushed down before it.

Example of a male hernia.
The only example which I have seen of this disease, is in the collection of preparations at St. Thomas's Hospital, and in this case the hernial sac was so small that I doubted the propriety of including it amongst my Plates. But when I considered that the danger of a hernia is proportioned rather to the smallness of its size than to its great magnitude, and that this small sac explains equally well with the largest the situation of the disease; and, moreover, when I considered that it is probable that this hernia seldom becomes of great size, I thought it right to introduce it.

This hernia existed in a male subject, and was accidentally observed in making a preparation of an inguinal hernia on the same side.

It descended through the aperture in the ligament of the foramen thyroideum, above the two obturatores muscles.

Seat of.
The pubis was placed immediately before the neck of the sac.

Three-fourths of it was surrounded by the ligament of the foramen.

The fundus of the sac was placed under the heads of the pectineus and adductor brevis muscles.

The size of the hernial sac within the thigh was that only of a nutmeg.

The obturator or thyroid artery and nerve were situated behind the neck of the sac, and a little to its inner side.

Case of.
In a paper of Mr. GARENGEOT's, in the Memoirs of the Royal Academy of Surgery at Paris, the following account is given from M. DUVERNEY. " He found in the pelvis of a woman that he dissected two portions of intestine, which had forced the peritoneum through the superior part of the two oval or thyroideal foramina, and had formed two tumours, each of the size of an egg, between the anterior ends of the triceps muscles of each side; and as these intestinal tumours were not yet sufficiently advanced to produce a projection of the fat and skin which covered them, no tumour was perceived from without." p. 714, Vol. I.

Several cases of this disease are given in the same paper.

Reducible.
It requires that this tumour should be of large size before it can be detected by external examination; but it sometimes becomes of considerable magnitude. The author of the Memoir above mentioned, gives a case to which he was called, of a woman who after a fall, felt an extremely violent pain at the upper part of the right thigh, near the labium pudendi, attended with vomiting, which continued three days. When Mr. G. examined her, he found a tumour on the inner and upper part of the right thigh, about a finger's breadth from the pudendum, and five or six inches in length. Raising the pelvis and knees, and rubbing the tumour with his hand from below upwards, the intestine was returned, and the tumour disappeared, the patient feeling at the same instant a guggling sensation in the abdomen. The symptoms all ceased, and she had an evacuation in half a quarter of an hour afterwards. Memoirs of the Royal Academy of Surgery, Vol. I. p. 709.

When this hernia is reducible the truss which would best answer the purpose of preventing the descent of the tumour, is that which I have described for the large crural hernia, only that the extremity of the pad must be much thicker, to make a deeper impression upon the thigh. Truss.

With respect to its strangulated state, if the means which are recommended in other herniæ, viz. the taxis, warm bath, bleeding, and the Tobacco glyster have failed, the operation of cutting the ligament which embraces the sac, is the only hope of preserving life. This operation must be extremely difficult, and so far as I am informed, it has never been performed. The only attempt, I believe, of that kind which has been made, is one mentioned in the Memoir already alluded to by M. MALAVAL, who being called to a girl who had a hernia of the foramen ovale, attempted to reduce it, and succeeded in returning the intestine, but could not reduce the omentum. He advised her to apply to M. ARNAUD, and the following operation was performed. The intestine was first reduced, after which an incision was made through the skin and fat to the hernial sac, which was opened, and a portion of omentum found of the size of a nut, which was cut away, as well as a portion of the sac, and the remaining part was pushed between the heads of the triceps muscle. This operation, he adds, succeeded; but it must be at once seen it was entirely unnecessary, for as the parts were not strangulated, a truss would have answered the purpose effected by this operation. Operation.

If the operation for this hernia, when strangulated, is ever performed, the division of the ligament of the foramen and the mouth of the sac should be made inwards, on account of the situation of the obturator artery.

OF THE CYSTIC HERNIA;

OR,

HERNIA OF THE BLADDER.

I introduce this subject merely to give my reasons for not at present proceeding to describe the disease. Although I have seen it in the living body, I have never had an opportunity of dissecting any one who had this complaint, and there are several circumstances in its anatomy which are by no means clear in the descriptions of it which I have read. If an opportunity presents itself of my dissecting this disease, I will give a description of it in the form of an Appendix to this work, and shall only here add, that I have seen the complaint twice in the living subject, forming inguinal herniæ. In the first case it was rendered very obvious, by its being distended when the bladder was full, and disappearing as the urine was discharged. In the second, that of a gentleman I have visited for another complaint, the tumour descends into the scrotum, and in order to empty the protruded part of the bladder, he is obliged to raise the scrotum to a level with the abdominal ring, and then the urine passes off, and the tumour becomes very flaccid, but does not entirely disappear.

OF THE ISCHIATIC HERNIA.

A rare disease. This is either a very rare disease, or, from its producing but little, if any, external tumour, it has generally escaped observation; but I am inclined rather to believe the former, because, from the manner in which the lower extremity is dissected, in the subjects brought into our dissecting-rooms, the muscles, nerves, and blood-vessels of the pelvis being generally traced, it could scarcely have escaped detection, if it happened frequently.

I am indebted to my friend, Dr. Jones, of the island of Barbadoes, (who is well known to the public by his excellent treatise on the processes employed by nature in suppressing hemorrhage from divided and punctured arteries,) for having an opportunity of dissecting the only case of this disease, which has occurred within my knowledge: and as the Docter watched daily the symptoms under which the patient laboured, an opportunity is given of comparing the symptoms with the appearances on dissection.

Dr. JONES informed me, that he had been inspecting the body of a man who had died of ischiatic hernia, and that he had found a small portion of intestine strangulated. After considerable difficulties the Doctor and myself opened the body a second time, and I removed the portion of the pelvis, in which the hernia was situated, and which will be seen in Plate XII. and XIII. of this work. I shall first give Dr. JONES's account of this case during his attendance, and then describe the appearances upon dissection

CASE.

"On the 18th of April, 1800, I was requested to attend a young man about 27 years of age, who had been attacked a few hours before with nausea, retching, and violent pain in the epigastric region. His pulse was rather smaller and slower than natural, and his skin covered with perspiration. His employment was that of warehousekeeper to a respectable mercantile house in the city: he was not conscious of any cause to which he could attribute his symptoms, but said, that he had once before been attacked in a similar manner, though by no means so severely; and on that occasion, as soon as the disordered state of his stomach was relieved by Tinct. Opii, a dose of Ol. Ricini. had effected his cure. He had taken fifteen drops Tinct. Opii about an hour previous to my seeing him; but as it had not afforded him any relief, and the symptoms continued very urgent, I ordered a grain of Opium made into a pill, with one drop of Ol. Menthæ pip. to be immediately given him; and as soon as his stomach appeared more quiet, to take the following medicine:

℞ Calomel pp^t .... g^r v.
Pulv. Scammon. ... g^r viii.
Sapon Opt. .... g^r vi.
Syr. simp. q. s. ut f. pil. N° 3.

"On seeing him at eight o'clock in the evening, I was informed that the opium had procured him ease for a short time, and had in some measure quieted and composed his stomach, though not sufficiently to enable him to retain the Cathartic pills, which, with the Opium, were therefore repeated that night, during which he slept but little, had occasional returns of retching, but no purgative effect was produced. The day following (the 19th) I found him troubled with frequent eructations, which he said inconvenienced him much, and requested I would give him something to remove them, as he now conceived flatus to be the cause of his pain. The following draught was therefore ordered to be taken immediately, and repeated, if found useful and agreeable to the stomach.

Sp^t Ammon. Comp. ...... ʒj.
Lavendul. .... ʒj.
Aq. Menth. sativ. .... ʒj. m. f. Haustus.

"At nine in the evening he told me he had taken three of the draughts, and he imagined they had been of service to him; for though he had not been perfectly free from nausea and retching, yet he had been more composed and easy than usual. The eructation had quite gone off, and the pain, which had left his stomach, was now situated just below the umbilicus, and was not increased by slight pressure being made on it.

"I enquired of him if ever he had a rupture; he said he had not. No evacuation per anum having been yet procured, I ordered a laxative glyster with Ol. Ricini to be injected, and repeated, should the first prove ineffectual, after waiting a certain time; and that he should take another draught, with the addition of twenty drops of Tinct. Opii. Two enemas were administered, but each was immediately returned, without any discharge of fæces: he slept however rather better than on the former night. On the 20th, the pain below the umbilicus continued, but was not worse; he also complained of a sense of weight and fulness about the stomach. I again enquired of him if he was sure he had no rupture; he replied that he had not; however, as I felt myself very much embarrassed to account for the obstinacy of his symptoms, and knowing that a protrusion may have taken place, sufficient to have occasioned them, but so small as to have escaped his notice, I requested he would allow me to examine him, to which he readily consented, and I cautiously examined the abdominal ring, and Poupart's ligament, on each side, and every part of the parietes of the abdomen, but found them perfectly free from hernia. As he did not complain of pain about the parts at which hernia is perceived, when it occurs at the foramen ovale, or ischiatic notch, I did not conceive it necessary to examine them.

"My attempt to procure evacuations by Calomel and Scammony having twice proved ineffectual, I determined to try an infusion of Senna, which, without any other addition than a few prunes, he had been accustomed to take as a cathartic, and which I therefore should have prescribed for him at first, had not the extreme irritability of his stomach induced me to suppose, from its being more bulky and nauseous than the pills, it was less likely to be retained. In the course of this day he took nearly xij. ℥ s. of a strong infusion of Senna with prunes, taking small quantities at intervals; but neither did much of this remain on his stomach, although cataplasms of mustard were occasionally applied to the epigastric region, nor was any purgative effect produced. As he continued to complain of the sense of weight and fulness about his stomach, attended with constant nausea, and retching, more indeed than he did of the pain below the navel: and as the ordinary means had failed to give relief, I thought it might be advisable to encourage the disposition to vomit, and thus completely to empty the stomach; with this view he took 12 g^{rs} pulv. Ipecac. which however was probably immediately returned, as it produced no alteration either in his state or sensations. After this he took a composing draught, and I requested that some one else might be called to him. The next day, however (the 21st), when I went to see him, he said he found himself better, and had therefore considered it unnecessary to call in another person: he had passed a better night than usual, and imputed his apparent amendment to his having perspired very profusely: his pulse (except during some periods of languor, which had occasionally come on within the last twenty-four hours) continued as at first, rather small, and slower than natural, and he remained during the whole day more composed than he had hitherto been, but was not perfectly free from retching, and complained more of the pain below the umbilicus: six leeches were therefore applied to the part, by which a copious discharge of blood was obtained. In the evening two laxative enemas were thrown up, and were followed by two small evacuations of fæces, after which he took a composing draught, nevertheless he got but little sleep; and on the 22d, finding he still complained of the pain (but not of its being worse), for he could bear gentle pressure on his abdomen, and it was not at all tense, a large blister was applied to the part, and the infusion of Senna repeated, but without effect. In the evening, he complained very much of pain, which he imputed to the blister; the Senna having proved ineffectual, the glysters were repeated, but not with much success, a very small quantity only of fæces being discharged. After three had been injected, the composing draught was repeated, but did not produce him a good night; and on the 23d I again desired some further advice might be had for him, but he told his friends he felt easier, and prevailed on them not to send for any other physician. In the course of the day he again took the draughts, in consequence of the recurrence of the eructation.

" On visiting him the next day, the 24th, I found him sitting up in bed: he informed me he had that morning taken some toast, and drank two cups of tea, which he had never before done during the whole of his illness: he said he found himself so well, that he had been inclined to go to business, but wished to consult me first. I advised him by no means to think of that for a few days. On feeling his pulse I found it so perfectly good, that it alone would not have given me an idea either of that he had been, or was at that time, even indisposed: however, as he was much reduced, I ordered for him an infusion of Serpentaria with Tinct. Cort. Peruv. of which he took only two small doses. In the evening I heard from him, and was informed he continued as well as when I saw him in the morning, complaining only of weakness and soreness from the blister. He slept but little during the night, and between three and four o'clock in the morning of the 25th he got out of bed, and went below from his chamber, which was on a floor four stories high, but soon returned, said he felt very unwell, and from that time gradually sunk, till seven o'clock in the evening, when he died."

DISSECTION.

Having obtained permission to examine the body, on opening the abdomen it was found that the ilium had descended on the right side of the rectum into the pelvis, and that a fold of it was protruded into a small sac, which passed out of the pelvis at the Ischiatic notch. In order to get at the part more conveniently, a ligature was made on the ilium, just at the place where it entered the pelvis, and round all the intestines above the pelvis: this gave a fair and ample opportunity of perfectly satisfying ourselves with regard to the nature of the case: after which the intestine was gradually withdrawn from the sac, in which it was rather firmly confined; and on examining the surface of that part which had been contained in the sac, it was found to have adhered at two points by coagulated lymph. The strictured part of the intestine, and about three inches of it on each side, were very black; the intestines from the hernia towards the stomach were very much distended with air, and had here and there a livid spot on them: there was also a dark coloured spot on the stomach, just above the pylorus. The colon, as far as its sigmoid flexure, was so rigidly contracted, as not even to admit the passage of air through it, but was of its natural colour, and the inflammation had scarcely extended to the cæcum.

Upon a careful dissection of the parts, after they had been brought to my house, we found a small orifice in the side of the pelvis, anterior to, but a little above the sciatic nerve, and on the forepart of the pyriformis muscle. When the finger was passed into this opening, it entered a bag situated under the gluteus maximus muscle, and this was the hernial sac in which the portion of intestine had been strangulated. The cellular membrane, which connects the sciatic nerve to the surrounding parts of the ischiatic notch, had yielded to the pressure of the peritoneum and viscera. The orifice of the hernial sac was placed anterior to the internal iliac artery and vein below the obturator artery, and above the obturator vein; its neck was situated anteriorly to the sciatic nerve, and its fundus, which was on the outer part of the pelvis, was covered by the gluteus maximus. Anterior to, but a little below the fundus of the sac was situated the sciatic nerve, behind it the gluteal artery. Above, it was placed near to the bone, and below, appeared the muscles and ligaments of the pelvis. *Anatomy of this hernia.*

If this hernia should in any case be obvious to the feel, and should be found reducible, a spring truss might be easily constructed to keep it within the pelvis. If it has become strangulated, and an operation is ventured to be performed, the safest direction in which the orifice of the sac can be dilated, will be directly forwards. *Treatment.*

OF THE PHRENIC HERNIA.

Three causes. Protrusions of the abdominal viscera through the diaphragm arise from three different causes.

First, natural apertures. First, from this muscle, like the other parietes of the abdomen, being naturally formed with apertures for the blood-vessels and nerves. The aorta, the vena cava inferior, and the intercostal nerves have openings formed for their passage; and the œsophagus passes through its muscular part by a considerable aperture.

Second, malconstruction. Secondly, a species of hernia is produced by a defect in the structure of this muscle, in consequence of which unnatural openings are formed, and a direct passage is given for the abdominal viscera into the cavity of the chest.

Third, wounds or lacerations. And thirdly, wounds or lacerations of the muscle sometimes occur, which remain open during the continuance of life, and allow of the protrusion of the abdominal viscera.

Symptoms; more of hernia and asthma. From which ever of these causes the disease arises, its symptoms are particularly distressing, as in addition to the common symptoms of other hernia, viz. an interrupted state of the bowels, vomiting, constipation, and extreme abdominal pain, the patient suffers from the pressure upon the lungs great difficulty of breathing, and a very severe cough.

Sacs: some have them, others not. Some of these herniæ are included in sacs, others are not; those which arise from gradual protrusion at the natural apertures have sacs, formed by the peritoneum and pleura; but of those which I shall describe, arising from malconstruction, some are contained in sacs, and others not, whilst those which arise from laceration are always without sacs.

First kind. **Rare.** With respect to that species of phrenic hernia, in which the viscera protrude through one of the natural apertures of the diaphragm, I have seen no example of it, and I believe it to be a rare occurrence. This probably arises from the bowels having to pass contrary to gravity, for if such an opening as that which is formed for the passage of the œsophagus, existed at the lower part of the abdomen, protrusions would almost constantly occur, which is also confirmed by its being a more frequent occurrence in quadrupeds than in man; the position of their bodies being more favourable for its production.

Examples in Mortgagni. However, examples may be found in Mortgagni of this disease. One is described, in which a part of the colon, and a still larger portion of omentum and pancreas were thrust through the passage which transmits the intercostal nerve.

Another case is mentioned in the same work, in which the person had a vehement cardialgia come on in the morning at break of day, attended with very frequent vomiting of an incredible quantity of blackish matter, and with straining to vomit, so that the young man died on the following night; and within the thorax was found, together with the omentum and intestine, the duodenum, with the jejunum, and a part of the ilium, so distended with that matter and with flatus, as to compress into a very narrow compass the heart and lungs, having been admitted into that cavity by the same foramen through which the gula (œsophagus) is brought down, this foramen being greatly dilated and deprived of its tone. (See Mortgagni, Epist. LIV. Art. 13.)

Second cause, malconstruction. The second species of Phrenic hernia, which arises from a malconstruction of the diaphragm, is a more frequent disease.

Children born with it. It is not unusual to find in a child dying almost immediately after birth, a very large opening in this muscle, which permits the passage of the more moveable viscera into the cavity of the chest.

Cases at St. Thomas's Hospital. There are two preparations in the collection at St. Thomas's Hospital of this disease. One of these has an opening so large as to permit the passage of the small intestines into the cavity of the chest, and in the other, although the muscle is less defective, a considerable part of the stomach was protruded. In each preparation the malformation appears in the left muscular part of the diaphragm, whence the viscera protruded into the left cavity of the chest. (See Plate.)

Two cases of this kind are also related by Dr. George Macauley, in the Medical Observations and Enquiries, Vol. I. p. 25. In the first case, the child was a full grown boy, remarkably fat and fleshy; the child when first born, started and shuddered, so that the nurse apprehended his going into fits; he breathed also with difficulty, and it was some time before he could cry, and when he did, there was something particular in the note. The child seemed to revive a little in about half an hour, and breathe more freely, but soon relapsed, and died before he was an hour and a half old. Upon dissection, when the sternum was raised, the stomach, and greatest part of the intestines, with the spleen, and part of the pancreas were found in the left cavity of the thorax, having been protruded through a discontinuation, or rather an aperture of the diaphragm, about an inch from the natural passage of the œsophagus.

From the extraordinary bulk of the parts contained in the left side of the thorax, the mediustinum, the heart, the œsophagus, and the descending aorta, were forced a considerable way towards the right side, and the left lobes of the lungs were not larger than a small nutmeg, and about two-thirds less than the right, though neither of them were diseased. The viscera being replaced in their natural situation in the abdomen, there was found a large chasm or hole in the diaphragm on the left side, through which the parts might freely pass into the thorax. From its appearance, as well as from that of the other parts, it seems extremely probable that in this case, there was an original malconformation of the diaphragm, by which means the abdominal viscera had very easily slipped into the thorax, because there was not the least mark of rupture, or inflammation about the edges of this opening, and became the diminished size of the left lobes of the lungs of the heart, and the mediustinum, and their inclination towards the right side seemed to be produced by a gradual enlargement of the protruded abdominal viscera, increasing with the growth of the fœtus.

In the second case, the child was a female; it first breathed with great difficulty, cried once feebly, sighed for about three quarters of an hour, and expired.

This case is the reverse of the former, as the abdominal viscera had passed into the right side of the thorax. In both the displacement of the abdominal viscera seemed to be owing to an original malconstruction of the diaphragm, and not the effect of rupture or violence.

As the lungs perform no very essential part of the fœtal economy, whilst children so constructed remain in utero, the imperfect state of the diaphragm does not interfere with the functions necessary to that state of existence, and therefore these infants are perfectly formed in other respects; but when respiration begins, the great size of the opening of the diaphragm will allow the abdominal viscera to be forced into the chest in such quantity as to compress the lungs and destroy life.

When this unnatural opening of the diaphragm is small, the consequences are not so immediately fatal. It produces at first some inconvenience, which increases in the progress of life, and at length destroys, as in other hernia, by a strangulation of protruded parts.

I shall take the liberty of extracting two cases, which I published in the year 1798, in the Medical Records and Researches, in which an opportunity was given of combining the appearances upon dissection, with a short history of the symptoms which the complaint produced during life.

This disease was discovered in a subject brought to St. Thomas's Hospital for dissection, where a preparation made from it is still preserved.

CASE.

Sarah Homan, aged twenty-eight, had from her childhood been afflicted with oppression in breathing. As she advanced in years, the least hurry in exercise or exertion of strength produced pain in her left side, a frequent cough, and very laborious respiration.

These symptoms were unaccompanied with any other marks of disease; and as her appetite was good, she grew fat, and, to common observation, appeared healthy. The family with whom she lived suspected her of indolence, and her complaints being considered as a pretext for the non-performance of her duty, she was forced to undertake employments of the most laborious kind.

This treatment she supported with patience, though often ready to sink under its consequences. After any great exertion, she was frequently attacked with pain in the upper part of the abdomen, with vomiting, and a sensation, as she expressed it, of something dragging to the right side; which sensation she always referred to the region of the stomach.

The cessation of these symptoms used to be sudden, as their accession; after suffering severely for a short time, all pain and sickness ceased, and allowed her to resume her usual employments.

As her age increased she became more liable to a repetition of these attacks; and as they were also of longer continuance than in the early part of life, she was at length rendered incapable of labouring for her support.

Some days previous to her death she was seized with the usual symptoms of strangulated hernia, viz. frequent vomitings, costiveness and pain; the pain was confined to the upper part of the abdomen, which was tense and sore when pressed.

As these symptoms were unaccompanied with any local swelling which indicated the existence of hernia, they were supposed to be produced by an inflammation of the intestines; but there were other symptoms that could not be attributed to this cause, which occasioned much obscurity with respect to the true nature of the complaint, and seemed to indicate a disease in the thorax. She was unable to lie on her right side, had a constant pain in the left, a cough, and difficulty of breathing, attended with the same dragging sensation of which she had formerly complained.

The signs of inflamed intestines, with the addition of a troublesome hiccough, continued without any abatement for three days, when she expressed herself better in these respects; but the morbid symptom in the thorax remained as violent as at first, and in the fourth day from their commencement she expired.

DISSECTION.

When the abdomen was opened, there appeared a very unusual disposition of the viscera.

The stomach and the left lobe of the liver were thrust from their natural situation towards the right side.

On tracing the various convolutions of the small intestines, they were found to retain their usual situation; but lines of inflammation extended along such of their surfaces as lay in contact. This appearance the adhesive inflammation assumes in its early stage, and it is highly probable that if the approach of death had been less rapid, these surfaces of the intestines would have been glued together by the effusion of coagulated lymph.

When the large intestines were examined the great arch of the colon, instead of being stretched from one kidney to the other, was discovered to have been pushed into the left cavity of the chest, through an aperture in the diaphragm.

The cæcum and beginning of the colon were much distended with air, and appeared, therefore, larger than natural; but the colon on the left side, as it descended toward the rectum, was smaller than it is commonly found.

A small part only of the omentum could be discovered in the cavity of the abdomen, a considerable portion of it having been protruded into the chest through the same opening by which the arch of the colon had passed.

The displacement of the stomach and left lobe of the liver, had arisen from the altered position of the colon and omentum, which, in their preternatural course towards tne diaphragm, occupied the situation of each of these parts.

When the chest was examined, the left lung did not appear of more than one-third of its natural size; it was placed at the upper part of the left cavity of the thorax, and was united to the pleura costalis by recent adhesions.

The protruded omentum and colon were found at the lower part of the left cavity of the chest, between the lung and the diaphragm, floating in a pint of blood coloured serum. The colon in colour was darker than usual, in texture softer, distended with fæculent matter mixed with a brownish mucus. The portion of the intestine contained within the chest measured eleven inches.

The omentum was also slightly altered in its colour, being rather darker than natural; but in other respects this viscus was not changed: it adhered firmly to the edge of the aperture, and more than half of its substance was contained within the chest.

The opening through which these viscera had protruded was placed in the muscular part of the diaphragm, three inches from the œsophagus: it was of a circular figure, and two inches in diameter; its edge was smooth, but thicker than the other parts of the muscle.

The peritoneum terminated abruptly at the edge of this aperture, so that the protruding parts were not contained in a sac, as in cases of common hernia, but floated loosely, and without covering, in the cavity of the chest, of which they occupied so large a space, as to occasion considerable pressure on the left lung, and to produce the diminution I have before remarked. The right side of the chest, and the right lung, were free from disease, and the heart was in a sound state. See Plate.

When the size of the opening, and the importance of the diaphragm, as an agent in respiration, are considered, it seems singular that this disease had not proved fatal at an earlier age; but it is probable that the aperture was originally small, and had been gradually enlarged by the protrusion of the abdominal viscera.

Before it became thus dilated, it was probably closed in common inspiration by pressure from some abdominal viscus, most likely by the omentum, as this part adhered firmly to its edge. But under the deeper inspirations consequent upon extraordinaty exertions, the abdominal viscera, instead of simply covering the orifice, were forced into it, and then becoming compressed by its edge, slight symptoms of strangulation succeeded; hence the sickness, pain, and the dragging sensation of which she so frequently complained. The situation of the aperture however favoured the descent, and consequently, the return of the protruded parts into the abdomen; the symptoms, therefore, though they so frequently recurred, remained only for a short time, and then suddenly disappeared.

By these frequent protrusions the opening became gradually enlarged, whence she was rendered more liable to subsequent attacks of pain and sickness, because the viscera entered the chest with greater ease and in larger quantities. At length a large proportion of the omentum and intestines was forced through the opening; their bulk prevented their return, and the pressure of the edge of the opening occasioned inflammation in the protruded intestine, and all the common symptoms of strangulated hernia; and by pressure on the lungs, produced oppression in breathing, pain in the left side, and a difficulty in lying on the right.

Dr. CLARKE has lately published in the Transactions of the Society for the Improvement of medical and surgical Knowledge a case of a similar kind; and Dr. MUNRO, Junior, has related one in his Treatise on Crural Hernia.

It will be difficult in the living subject to decide on the nature of this disease; yet the judgment may be directed in some degree by the combination of symptoms of strangulated hernia with those of an oppression on the chest; that is to say, by vomiting, costiveness, hiccough, pain and tension of the abdomen; together with cough, oppressed breathing, and inability to lie on one side.

Little could be done for the relief of such patients, even if the disease was certainly known, except by strongly recommending that quiet, which indeed their own feelings will prompt them to adopt. But hard must be their lot, if they are placed under the circumstances of this young woman, obliged to labour under unfeeling employers, who suspect the sufferings she described to arise from a disposition to indolence.

If the deficiency in the diaphragm is unaccompanied by a defective state of the peritoneum and pleura, these membranes form a double covering to the protruded parts, as the following example will prove.

My friend, Mr. BOWLES, an ingenious surgeon at Bristol, has transmitted to me the following account of *Mr. Bowles' case* the dissection of a man in whom a protrusion was discovered of a part of the abdominal viscera into the cavity of the chest. It differs from the foregoing case in the disease being placed on the right, instead of the left side, in the contents being free from strangulation, and in having been inclosed in a sac, instead of floating loosely in the cavity of the thorax.

He states, that in the month of October 1796, he opened the body of a man aged fifty years, who had died from excessive vomiting after the use of an emetic, and in whom the viscera of the cavity of the abdomen were found disposed in an unusual manner. Of the omentum only a small part could be seen; and the right extremity of the stomach, as well as the arch of the colon, had entirely disappeared.

On inspecting the thorax, a sac considerably larger than a tennis-ball was found in its right cavity, which contained the right extremity of the stomach, and beginning of the duodenum, a part of omentum, and the arch of the colon, which last was disposed in several convolutions.

The sac was formed by the united membranes of the pleura and peritoneum, and its orifice was placed at a small distance from the right side of the ensiform cartilage, where there appeared a deficiency of fibres in the larger muscles of the diaphragm corresponding to the size of the sac.

The parts which formed this hernia exhibited no marks of inflammation, were free from adhesion, either to each other, or to the sac, and could be returned without difficulty into the cavity of the abdomen.

The right lung was much smaller than usual, its anterior and inferior part having been compressed by the tumour. The other thoracic viscera appeared to be in a healthy state.

The stomach being next examined, was found to contain a number of peas, which he had taken in some broth just previous to his death, and a deep coloured mucus adhered to its inner surface, which, when removed, exhibited the internal membrane of the left extremity highly inflamed; an appearance which had probably arisen from the violent operation of the emetic, and appeared to be the immediate cause of his dissolution.

Mr. B. could learn nothing important of this man's history, but that he had, at various times, laboured under asthmatic complaints, which admit of an easy explanation from the appearances on dissection. No violence could be traced capable of producing so great a change of structure, and it seems therefore probable that it had arisen from original malconformation.

<small>Third cause.</small> A wound or laceration of the diaphragm is the third cause of protrusion of the viscera into the chest. Wounds with the small sword have been the most frequent causes of this disease; the opening made in the diaphragm being prevented from closing, by the pressure of the abdominal viscera, protrusions immediately occur, and gradually increase the size of the opening, so as at length to give passage to large portions of viscera. But in this country such weapons being scarcely worn, wounds of this kind hardly ever occur. The only accident I have known produce this species of hernia has been a laceration of the diaphragm, occasioned by the fracture of several of the ribs.

The following case will illustrate the nature of this disease.

CASE.

WILLIAM RATTLEY, aged 30 years, was admitted into Guy's Hospital Feb. 5, 1804. He had been a strong healthy man before this time, but in painting the mast of a ship he fell from the height of thirty-six feet, and pitching with his back on the edge of the pump, he broke six of the lowermost ribs of the right side. His symptoms were extraordinarily severe; he breathed with great difficulty, and complained of excessive pain in the right hypochondrium; and upon examining his back, a crepitus at the fractured ribs could be felt, and a slight emptrysema was observable. He was admitted at one o'clock in the afternoon, he vomited violently, and had frequent hiccough in the evening, and at eight o'clock on the following morning he expired.

DISSECTION.

Upon opening the cavity of the chest (which was done by my house-pupil, Mr. TRAVERS), no unnatural appearance of the lungs was observable, excepting some slight and recent adhesions of its surface to the pleura on the right side, and a small and partial wound at the lower and posterior part of the right lung. On pushing down the vault of the diaphragm, a fold of intestine of a livid colour was discovered, and upon extending the examination into the cavity of the abdomen, a portion of intestine, which proved to be ilium, was found proceeding upwards behind the liver into the cavity of the chest, through a large opening of the diaphragm. This opening, which appeared lacerated, was situated about two inches from the cordiform tendon, in the muscular portion of the diaphragm, and on its right side. The aperture was filled by the intestine, around which a very firm stricture existed. It had been strangulated by the muscle itself; and from the livid state of the intestine only nineteen hours after the accident, the strangulation seemed to have been unusually complete. The hole in the diaphragm had been occasioned by the broken pointof the tenth rib, which had penetrated the muscle when it was in a state of expiation, and the muscle had withdrawn itself from the point of the rib in inspiration, so as to leave the opening through which the intestine had protruded. The viscera in the cavity of the abdomen appeared little altered in any other respect, but about a quart of bloody serum had been extravasated into both cavities. See Plate.

OF THE MESENTERIC HERNIA.

<small>Mesentery formed of two layers.</small>   The Mesentery is composed of two layers of peritoneum, between which the blood-vessels, absorbents, and nerves are situated, which are distributed to the small intestines; and these layers are united together by a cellular membrane of a tender texture.

<small>Aperture in one of these.</small>   If in consequence of a blow upon the abdomen, one of these layers of peritoneum is torn, and the other remains in its natural state, the intestines will force themselves into the aperture, and form, according to my idea of the disease, a true hernia, since the intestine is protruded out of its proper cavity. Or if either of these layers is originally formed defectively, so as to leave an aperture in one of them, the same effect will ensue.

<small>Occasioned by malformation.</small>   Which of these circumstances is the cause of this disease, it is not in my power to determine; but I am disposed to believe, that it has its source in an originally defective structure, as in the case which I examined, there were no marks of preceding violence, but the parts had in all respects, excepting in the existence of this disease, their natural appearance. In whichever way the disease occurs, it shews strongly the degree of pressure which the bowels exert upon every point of the parietes of the cavity in which they are contained, for otherwise it would be impossible that all the small intestines should be forced out of their natural situation through a small opening in a moveable portion of membrane.

But when the protrusion has once began, there is no difficulty in conceiving how it will increase to the extent necessary to receive all the small intestines, as the cellular membrane which unites the two layers is not sufficiently strong to resist any considerable degree of pressure.

The Plate which I have given of this disease, was taken from a drawing made by Mr. Kavanagh, of Walthamstow, who was then a pupil at St. Thomas's and Guy's Hospitals.

The disease was found in a subject brought to Mr. Richard Pugh, of Gracechurch Street, for dissection at St. Thomas's Hospital, and the man had been a patient in Guy's Hospital under Mr. Forster, and had suffered the operation of amputation; he appeared to be about fifty-five years old.

<small>Situation of the tumour.</small>   When the abdomen was opened for demonstration, and the omentum and colon were raised, the small intestines did not appear, but in their stead, in the middle of the abdomen was found a tumour situated upon the lumbar vertebræ, and extending down to the basis of the sacrum. When this tumour was opened, it was found to be a sac containing all the small intestines, excepting the duodenum.

<small>Its contents.</small>   Mr. Pugh was so obliging as to give me the body for further examination. I found that the sac was formed by the peritoneum, which completely surrounded the intestines, excepting at the posterior part, where there was a small hole by which the intestines had entered. Tracing the intestine from the stomach towards the anus, the beginning of the jejunum was found passing into the sac at the posterior part, and by the same opening the ilium passed out on the right side, and descending to the right inguen, it entered the large intestines in the usual manner.

I injected the mesenteric vessels, and in the preparation they have been dried without dissection, but from their wanting their usual covering of peritoneum, they are as distinctly seen as they usually are after a minute dissection.

What effects, if any, this unusual position of the intestines had produced I could not ascertain. Every enquiry was made, but nothing had happened during the time the patient was in the Hospital which could lead to a suspicion of any disease having existed in the abdomen. However, from the confinement the intestines had suffered within the bag, I should naturally be induced to conclude, that the peristaltic motions of the bowels had been less free than usual, and that from this torpid state of intestine frequent constipations would have arisen; but if this was the effect, it had never gone so far as to produce inflammation, as the intestines did not appear thickened, and had not contracted any adhesions either to the sac or to each other.

OF THE MESOCOLIC HERNIA.

THE Plate of this disease is taken from a preparation which was made nine years ago, and which is deposited in the collection at St. Thomas's Hospital.

Seat of. On opening the abdomen of a subject brought there for dissection, the omentum and large intestines being turned aside, a large tumour was discovered on the left side of the abdomen, its upper part resting on the left kidney, whence it extended downwards to the brim of the pelvis, its lower part lying in the fold of the sigmoid flexure of the colon.

Contents. The large intestines took their usual course in the abdomen, excepting that the cæcum and beginning of the colon were placed nearer to its centre. On the left side the colon was placed between the tumour and abdominal muscles, and the swelling reached from the termination of its great arch to its sigmoid flexure.

The duodenum, a small part of the jejunum, and the termination of the ilium, were the only portions of the small intestines which were visible.

Upon examination of the tumour, it was found to contain all the small intestines which were not seen on first opening the abdomen, and the orifice, by which they had passed into the tumour, was situated on its right side. This orifice was more than sufficiently large to permit the passage of two folds of the intestines even in their most distended state, and through it all the small intestines were readily drawn from the bag.

Sac. The sac in which they were contained was formed between the laminæ of the peritoneum of the mesocolon, in the anterior layer of which on the right side, was placed the opening by which the intestines had entered. The bag was sufficiently large to be capable of containing all the small intestines in a half distended state. Two-thirds of the orifice of the sac were formed of peritoneum only, and one-third was covered by a branch of the inferior mesenteric artery. The peritoneum which formed the sac was somewhat thicker than that which was contiguous to the abdominal muscles, but, upon the whole, it had undergone less alteration in that respect, than the degree of pressure which it had sustained would have led me to expect.

No strangulation. When the intestines were very much distended with air or food, the opening into the sac was sufficiently large to allow of the escape of a part of them into the abdomen; but if the orifice had by pressure become thickened or contracted, the patient might have suffered the symptoms of strangulation.

These symptoms, however, in this species of hernia are not very likely to occur, for a contraction and thickening of a hernial sac, are generally produced by some pressure external to the sac resisting that from within, and thus therefore it happens, that the sac in inguinal hernia is sometimes contracted opposite to the two openings from the abdomen; but in this case there is nothing but the thin substance of the peritoneum to resist the pressure from within, and the orifice of the sac will yield so readily to the bowels, that no considerable compression of the contents would have been likely to occur. There was no appearance in this case which could lead to a belief that the symptoms of strangulation had ever occurred, nor was it probable that the person experienced so much torpor of bowels as in the case of mesenteric hernia which I have described in the preceding chapter, as the passage into the bag was much more free; but we had to lament in this case, as in the former, that no opportunity was given for ascertaining the symptoms which this disease had produced.

A posterior view of the colon is given in the Plate, as it was concealed by the tumour in an anterior view.

OF
STRANGULATION OF THE INTESTINE
WITHIN
THE ABDOMEN.

The intestines are sometimes found incarcerated within the abdomen, in consequence of the three following causes: Causes of.

First, From apertures in the omentum, mesentery, or mesocolon, through which the intestine protrudes.

Secondly, From adhesions having formed in consequence of inflammation, leaving an aperture, in which a portion of intestine becomes confined.

Thirdly, By membranous bands forming in the mouths of hernial sacs, which becoming elongated by the frequent protrusion and return of the viscera, surround the intestine so as to strangulate it within the abdomen, when it is returned from the hernial sac.

Of the first of these causes I have been favoured with the following account by Mr. Palmer, who was one of the most assiduous of our students.

DEAR SIR, Hereford, 1805.

I have at length, according to my promise, transmitted you the particulars of the strangulated intestine, the preparation of which I sent you during the last winter.

I am, &c.

HENRY JONES PALMER.

THE CASE.

"On the 22d of April 1804, *I was requested to attend Mrs. Ann Davis, who had been attacked the preceding day with bilious vomiting, which was immediately succeeded by an utter incapability of retaining any thing upon her stomach, either in a solid or liquid form: she complained of a slight pain in the epigastric region; her pulse was quick and small, the temperature of her skin was rather increased, and there was very considerable tension of the whole of the abdomen; she had not had any evacuation for several days: the primary object under these circumstances was, to obtain a speedy passage through the bowels, and with this view I ordered a laxative glyster to be administered, which operated in a very inconsiderable degree; I therefore prescribed a strong mercurial cathartic, and an aperient mixture; a given proportion of each was directed to be taken every four hours. Repeating my visit early in the following morning, I found my patient nearly in the same state as that in which I had left her; the belly was still tense and incompressible; the medicines had not operated, and she continued to reject every thing that she swallowed. In this stage of the case Dr. Blount was consulted, who recommended a continuance of the mercurial and aperient medicines, and an occasional repetition of the glysters; Castor oil alone, and combined with Senna and Julep, were also had recourse to, but not the least relief was obtained. The warm bath, saline draughts in a state of effervescence, conjoined with Opium, and blisters applied over the stomach, were each resorted to, and several times repeated, with a hope that they would tend to Mr. Palmer's case.

* The above case is collected from my Father's case-book.

diminish, if not entirely arrest the incessant vomitings: in this respect we were unfortunately disappointed; indeed every possible means we could devise, either to induce evacuation, or allay the extreme irritability of the stomach, proved equally ineffectual. In this lamentable state she remained, without experiencing scarcely a momentary intermission of these distressing symptoms, till the 30th, when an evident alteration for the worse took place: a considerable quantity of fæculent matter was now discharged in the act of vomiting; her pulse became quicker, hurried, and wirey, and her extremities cold; the parietes of the abdomen were more flabby and yielding. Though too well assured that this alarming change was the certain prelude to approaching dissolution, I considered it a duty incumbent upon me to do every thing in my power, whilst the vital spark existed; as a last and hopeless resource, therefore, some ætherial cordial was given, which however almost instantly returned, and in the course of four hours she expired.

"Upon inspecting the state of the abdomen, the immediate seat of the disease for some time eluded detection, owing to the collapsed state of the intestines; but upon a more accurate and minute examination an opening was found through the mysentery forming a stricture, inclosing the inferior portion of the ilium, and which decidedly and sufficiently accounted for the melancholy termination of the case."

In the plate the strangulated portion of intestine is engraved of a darker colour than it should have been, as the intestine was not much discoloured.

Dr. Monro, junior, gives an account of a similar case in his work on Crural Hernia.

Mr. Croakes's case.

Mr. Richard Croakes, Surgeon, of Barnsley, Yorkshire, sent me the following narrative of a case which he had attended and inspected.

"I was called up about one o'clock on Thursday morning (Feb. 23, 1804) to visit Mr. Wade (a farmer at Lewdon, about two miles from this town) aged eighty, of spare habit, and who had, previous to this attack, enjoyed a good state of health, and led a very active life. He complained of very acute pain in his abdomen, which he had had for three or four hours, chiefly about the umbilical region (unattended with sickness, or any degree of fever), which he supposed was occasioned by a little ham he had eaten for his dinner (about one o'clock) the preceding day, which was not sufficiently boiled; and I, not being able to discover any other existing cause at the time, coincided with him: but on further enquiry after death, was informed, that the day before, when attempting to mount his horse, he was thrown down, but did not complain of any inconvenience from this accident at that time. As he had no vomiting, I thought it best, on account of his age, not to give him an emetic (bleeding was also thought of, but omitted for the same reason), but I sent him a cathartic mixture; about noon I was again sent for, and the messenger informed me he had rejected every thing. I then gave him an emetic, but it only brought away the liquid he had taken with it; a glyster was then administered, which operated very well, but still the pain and sickness continued. He had then two grains of Opium, and I left him some pills, with four grains of Calomel in each, and ordered him to take one every two hours till they operated; but when I again saw him, whatever he had taken had been rejected, and I was again called up in the night, and Dr. Dow accompanied me, who had him put into a warm bath, and repeated the cathartic mixture, but with no better success than before: he had then his feet put into hot water, and the glyster repeated, Castor oil given, a large blister applied to the abdomen, and he was ordered effervescent mixtures. Our next resort was to quicksilver, of which he took a large quantity, but the vomiting still continued. On Saturday morning Dr. Dymond saw him, about which time he had become much easier, and it was apprehended mortification had taken place; he died that night (on the 25th) about eleven o'clock. Application being made with success to open the body, we found the omentum was much drawn towards the stomach, and a portion of the small intestines appeared in a state of sphacelus, which on farther examination was found to be occasioned by its protrusion through the omentum, by which the intestine was strangulated. The intestines were completely evacuated of hardened fæces, and in their natural state, except the strangulated portion. I also took out the quicksilver from above the stricture, not a particle having passed it."

Of the second cause of these strangulations I have been favoured with the following example from Mr. Hodson, a very excellent Surgeon at Lewes, in Sussex.

MY DEAR SIR,   Lewes, Feb. 13, 1807.

        AGREEABLY to my promise I send you the case, which I mentioned to you when I was at your house.

    A young man about twenty years of age had an attack of Interitis after going into the water to bathe while he was hot, in consequence of playing at cricket. The symptoms of Interitis were not violent, and soon gave way to the common remedies, and he appeared to be in a state of convalescence: under these circumstances he was attacked with vomiting soon after dinner, which he attributed to his having drank some porter with his dinner. The sickness continued in spite of every thing that could be done to relieve it, attended with a complete obstruction of the bowels, and he died in the course of a few days, under circumstances strikingly resembling those who die in consequence of incarcerated hernia. Upon examining the abdomen, it appeared that an adhesion had taken place between the omentum and peritoneum near Poupart's ligament, under which a portion of intestine had passed, and having become strangulated, it produced the obstruction in question.

                              I remain your very obedient servant,

                                                                    T. HODSON.

Case from Dr. Haighton. — Dr. HAIGHTON also informed me that he was requested by Mr. FEARON, Surgeon, in the Adelphi, to inspect the intestines of a person who had died with all the symptoms of incarcerated intestine. The Doctor found that the appendix cæci, which was longer than usual, had contracted an adhesion at its end to the surface of a portion of ilium which laid near it; and that it had formed a loop or doubling, into which a portion of intestine had passed, and become strangulated.

A membranous band forming the stricture. — With respect to membranous bands occasioning this strangulation, I have in my possession a most curious example, taken from the body of a patient of Mr. WESTON's in Shoreditch. See Plate XVII. The case is as follows:

    RICHARD SAXTON, aged 85 years, who lived in Workhouse-lane, Hoxton, was seized on Feb. 14, 1805, with pain in his bowels, from which he had often suffered before, although he thought this somewhat different to his former attacks. As the pain continued to increase, Mr. WESTON was sent for on the 15th, but he did not see him until the 16th, when he found him complaining of great pain in the abdomen, and vomiting frequently. The abdomen was also distended, and upon feeling in the right groin, Mr. W. discovered an hernia, which he pressed upon, and after a short time reduced. Purgative medicine was then ordered, and an enema injected, but without any good effect, for the symptoms still continued, and he died a few hours afterwards.

    I examined the body, and found that the intestine was returned, but with a membranous band embracing two of its convolutions, which were strangulated in the way which will be seen in the plate. The small intestines above the strangulated portion, which was ilium, were much inflated, and one portion of the strangulated part was very much discoloured. An irreducible omental hernia was found on the opposite side.

    In Plate XVII. a portion of intestine will be seen, which was given me by my friend Mr. HEADINGTON, Surgeon of the London Hospital, who favoured me with the following account of it.

DEAR SIR,

Communication from Mr. Headington. — OUR case-book having by some accident been misplaced, has prevented me from sending you the history of the preparation in your possession. I have only to regret that such a circumstance should have occasioned such an apparent remissness on my part.

                                    Believe me sincerely yours,

                                                             R. C. HEADINGTON.

    A. B. about fifty years of age, died in the London Hospital of general dropsy, under the care of Dr. FRAMPTON, and was examined at his request. Independently of a diseased state of the liver, and of a considerable quantity of fluid in the cavities of the thorax and abdomen, there was found an hernial sac through each of the abdominal rings, the one on the right side being of considerable extent; and a hernial sac under the left Poupart's ligament. In the course of the ilium an adhesion had taken place between many of the convolutions of that intestine, and which adherent portion had no doubt formed at one time the contents of a hernia. Above where this adhesion had taken place, along the greater part of the jejunum, a number of pouches were formed varying from the size of a pea to that of a walnut, chiefly situated between the layers of the mesentery. These pouches appear to have been the consequence of an obstruction in the alimentary canal, produced by the descent of the intestine, as they were all seated above the adherent portion we have mentioned. The intestine we may suppose had given way at that part where it was least supported. It appears likewise most probable, that the sacculi consist of the internal coat of the intestine only, resembling those pouches which are sometimes formed by a protrusion of the internal coat of the bladder between its muscular fibres. The sacculi were completely distended with flatus at the time of the removal of the jejunum, nor did they appear to contain any of the grosser contents of the intestine.

I have included in Plate XVII. a portion of the intestine of a Dog, in which, after having made a longitudinal incision, I brought the edges of the wound together by sutures, and cutting off the ligatures, returned the intestine into the cavity of the abdomen. The experiment is detailed in part the first of this work, page 37. The external view shews the omentum adhering to the intestine; the internal, the ligature separating into the intestine.

But I thought the experiment, to form a fair analogy with hernia, should be made upon an inflamed intestine, and I requested Mr. BOWEN (who attends my surgical lectures, and whose zealous pursuit of his profession merits the highest praise) to make the experiment, by first drawing the intestine from the abdomen, and suffering it to protrude until it inflamed, to cut away the inflamed part, and to bring the ends together. The following is his communication on the subject.

EXPERIMENT.

Division of the intestine. On Saturday, Feb. 14, I made a longitudinal incision into the cavity of the abdomen of a Dog, and took out a portion of the ilium, which I exposed to the atmospheric air for eight hours and a half; this produced that effect which the nature of the experiment required; the intestine was of a dark chocolate appearance, which part I completely detached (a preparation of which I have sent to you). I then brought the divided intestine together by means of five ligatures, one at the mesentery, the other four at equal distances from each other, using only a common sewing needle, with very small thread. The ligatures were cut as near as possible to the intestine, which was now returned into the cavity of the abdomen. In closing the external wound I made use of the interrupted suture, with small slips of sticking plaster. The following morning, the 15th, he appeared dull and heavy, and the abdomen tense. I opened both his jugular veins, and took from him about 20 ʒ of blood. The next morning, 16th, he appeared somewhat better, the tensity of the abdomen being diminished; had two evacuations the preceding day of natural consistence: the evening of this day I gave him a little broth, he would have taken more food, had I allowed him. 17th, the animal was sensibly better, more fæces had been discharged; I gave him a small quantity of broth. 18th, appeared more lively, craving for food, which was not refused him. 19th, the fifth day after the operation, I was desirous of seeing the external wound; accordingly I removed the dressings, and found that a complete union had taken place; the animal appeared so well, that I gave him a moderate quantity of food. The sixth day I found him perfectly recovered; he was lively and playful, and he ate every thing most greedily which was offered him, and continued in this manner till the eleventh day. On the twelfth day after the operation, I found that the dog had escaped from the place of his confinement.

Mr. ALLAN BURNS, of Glasgow, has kindly sent me the following communication respecting a congenital inguinal hernia in the female; and never having seen a similar example, I was anxious to introduce it into this work; also a dissection of a crural hernia, and his description of a fillet of fascia proceeding from the upper pillar of the abdominal ring. I am sorry I did not receive it sufficiently soon to allow me to place it amidst the crural herniæ; but the Engraving made from his drawing will be found in Plate XI. Fig. 4.

"The specimen of hernia, of which you now receive a drawing, was met with in the body of an aged female brought to the room last August for dissection. We were ignorant of the previous history of the woman, and have never been able to ascertain the immediate cause of death. On looking at the subject I perceived a slight fulness in each groin, and in the bend of both thighs. By pressing upon the abdomen, which contained a small quantity of fluid, I rendered these tumours much more distinct. This led me to examine the body carefully, when I discovered the person had inguinal and crural herniæ on both sides.

<small>Mr. Allan Burn's communication.</small>

"The inguinal herniæ were both of the congenite species, but still in their nature they were somewhat peculiar; for on both sides the inguinal canal was fully as large as it is usually met with in the male, and beside was so very short, that it presented when dissected almost the appearance of a mere aperture. The round ligament of the womb was enveloped in a distinct tunica vaginalis, and in this the gut lay, the ligament bearing the same relation to the intestine, that the spermatic cord does in the other sex. On the right side the herniary sac was about two inches in length, and in shape resembled a Florence flask, the bulbous extremity expanding from the lower orifice of the canal, was contained in the upper part of the thigh, lying more in the course of crural than of inguinal hernia. This direction of the tumour in inguinal hernia in females has been noticed by several authors. Dr. WILLIAM HAMILTON, the late ingenious Professor of Anatomy in this University, met with several cases of this kind; and Mr. ASTLEY COOPER mentions, in his work on Hernia, examples of a similar nature. By dissection we ascertained the cause of the deviation from the usual direction of the tumour to be a premature separation from each other of the external pillars of the inguinal canal. Where the inguinal canal is imperfectly formed, it is generally owing to the incomplete extension of the posterior or internal edge of the ring. When this happens, the internal orifice of the canal is brought nearer to the pubis than it ought to be; but when the imperfection is produced by a premature separation of the external pillars, then by dissection we find the internal orifice in its proper place, but the external outlet is removed from the pubis. In the first instance, when the herniary tumour protrudes, it lies just over the tubercle of the pubis, and follows the course of the spermatic cord into the scrotum, while in the latter it lies nearer to the spine of the ilium, is seated just over the crural foramen, and by extension descends along the thigh, counterfeiting the appearance of femoral rupture. By attention however it is readily distinguished from the latter by being felt lying over the crural arch, above the tubercle of the pubis.

"When describing figure 2d of the Sketches in the Edinburgh Medical Journal, I mentioned that a fillet originates from the upper pillar of the inguinal canal, which winds round the fascia of the adductor muscles of the thigh, incorporating itself with the fascia as it passes along, and reaching in some instances even to the gluteus tendon, to which it is finally attached. It is always intimately connected with the fascia, originating from the aponeurosis of the oblique muscle, and investing the tunica vaginalis. The action of this band upon the sac was clearly illustrated in the present case; for by its pressure an indentation was formed in the neck of the sac. Now this is a piece of anatomy which ought carefully to be studied with a reference to practice; for whoever is ignorant of the position and connection of this production from the upper pillar of the ring, must possess but a very confined notion of its action in disease. By a knowledge of the conformation of the pillars of the ring, we are led to an acquaintance with the effects of each other upon the spermatic cord, and are taught that, when by compression upon the abdomen we tend to dilate the aperture through which the cord passes, the pillars of the ring (in the fœtus or new born child) react upon the contained cord, embrace it closely, and thus effectually prevent the passage of any of the bowels. When however the force is still greater, when a portion of the gut does escape, then we know that we have it in our power in some degree to obviate the mechanical obstacles to the return of the bowel; for, by recollecting that the upper pillar sends off this fillet to decussate the insertion of the lower fascicules, and to course along the internal part of the thigh, it follows from this that the gut must be more acted on in one position of the limb than in another. By rolling the toes inward, if we at the same time extend the hip joint, this band comes to be very much put on the stretch, it is depressed, and thus to approach toward the lower pillar, and firmly to embrace whatever is placed between these columnæ. Of consequence, when any of the abdominal contents are displaced, its influence, if not contracted by the employment of artifice, tends to bind the protruded part firmly in its unnatural position; and thus we sometimes see one practitioner foiled in his attempts to reduce the hernia, and another afterward, by moving the limb in opposite direction, readily succeed. Every Surgeon ought to know this cause of difficulty, for it informs him that rolling the toes outward, and at the same time crossing the thigh of the affected side over the opposite, will, if genuflexion have been premised, remove as completely as possible all adventitious pressure from the protruded parts, and thus indirectly facilitate reduction.

" With regard to the crural hernia, we found a peculiar disposition of GIMBERNAT's duplicature; the formation was not however exactly alike on both sides. On the left of which I have sent a drawing, the crescentic duplicature was pushed out so as to form an enclose for the peritoneal herniary sac. In order to understand how this appearance was produced, we have to recollect that in some cases a septum is stretched across the crural aperture, being merely a small perforation in the centre. When pressure is applied to this septum, it is protruded, assumes the form of a capsule containing the herniary sac, and has a small opening in its extreme point. Over the upper and outer edge of the protruded duplicature lay the falciform process of the fascia vera; but in this instance it is obvious that the fascia might have been divided, without in any degree removing the cause of strangulation.

" On the right side the crescentic fold was also protruded; but here the lower cornu passed behind the femoral vein; the upper ran anterior to it. Afterward both horns attached themselves to the sheath of the femoral artery, or to that septum which separates the great artery from the vein. The falciform process on this side lay over the anterior horn of the protruded duplicature, and followed its course, consequently there was an appearance of two falciform processes, which is not uncommon, and both were in contact, and both must have been divided at once; and thus the arch must have been considerably relaxed, and the cause of strangulation removed."

PLATE I.

This Plate is intended to exhibit a view of the abdominal rings, and of the crural arch in the female. The fascia lata of the thigh, the crural sheath, and the passage of the round ligament of the uterus, from the internal to the external ring.

- *a.* Symphisis pubis.
- *b.* Tuberosity of the pubis.
- *c.* Anterior superior spinous process of the ilium.*
- *dd.* External oblique muscles.
- *e.* Linea alba.
- *f.* Linea semilunaris.
- *g.* Crural arch, or Poupart's ligament, extending from the spinous process of the ilium at *c*, beyond the tuberosity of the pubis at *b*.
- *h.* Tendonous fibres crossing the columns of tendon, of the external oblique: they proceed from the spinous process of the ilium, and the crural arch.
- *i.* The abdominal ring on the left side; its upper column inserted into the symphisis pubis, and the lower into the tuberosity, but afterwards extended forwards towards the symphisis.
- *k.* That part of the fascia lata of the thigh, which proceeds from the crural arch, and which covers the muscles on the outer part of the thigh, and femoral vessels.
- *l.* The other portion of the fascia lata covering the pectineus and triceps muscles, and united with the former portion of fascia behind the saphena major vein.
- *m.* Crural sheath cut open.

* I shall hereafter call this simply the spinous process of the ilium.

- *n.* Crural artery.
- *o.* Crural vein.
- *p.* Three absorbent vessels within the sheath, the first on the outer side of the artery, the second between the artery and vein, and the third on the inner side the vein, which last has the course of the crural hernia.
- *qq.* Saphena major vein.
- *rr.* Two absorbent glands sending forth the absorbent vessels of the sheath.
- *s.* Arteria circumflexa ilii.
- *t.* Epigastric artery.
- *u.* Tendon of the external oblique muscle laid open.
- *v.* Internal oblique muscle turned upwards.
- *w.* Transversalis muscle turned upwards.
- *x.* Fascia transversalis seen passing from the crural arch behind the transversalis muscle.
- *yyyy.* Round ligament of the uterus decending through the hole in the fascia, in the hollow above the crural arch, and through the abdominal ring, to be lost in the fat in the pubis.
- *z.* Course of the epigastric artery seen through the fascia transversalis.
- +   Absorbent vessels on the left side entering the crural sheath, at the part at which the crural hernia passes into the thigh.

PLATE 1.

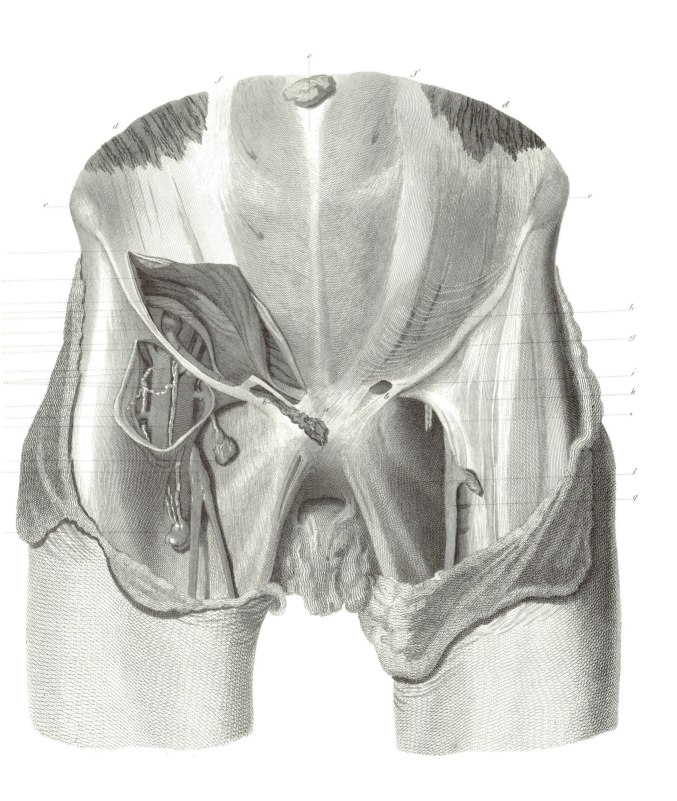

PLATE II.

CONTAINS sketches of the anatomy of the groin and upper part of the thigh in the female.

FIG. 1.
- a. Symphisis pubis.
- b. Spinous process of the ilium.
- c. Abdominal muscles.
- d. Abdominal ring.
- e. Crural arch.
- fff. Fascia lata of the thigh.
- gg. Semilunar edge of the fascia lata.
- h. Crural sheath or fascia enclosing the crural vessels.
- i. Saphæna major vein.
- k. Place at which the crural hernia descends.

FIG. 2. Shews the insertions of the external oblique muscle into the pubis and its ligament, and the fascia iliaca, or GIMBERNAT's fascia.
- a. Pubis.
- b. Spine of the ilium.
- c. Acetabulum.
- d. Thyroid foramen.
- e. Column of tendon. f. Another column. g. A third column, making together two apertures at the abdominal ring in the female, which is not uncommon.
- h. Anterior edge of the crural arch, or POUPART's ligament.
- i. Third insertion of the external oblique muscle.
- k. Ligament of the pubis, into which the external oblique i is inserted.
- l. Portion of fascia transversalis, and tendon of the rectus, passing behind the insertion of the external oblique.
- m. Fascia iliaca passing from the crural arch over the iliacus internus muscle.
- n. Orifice of the crural sheath, for the passage of the crural artery vein and absorbent vessels.

FIG. 3. Shews the crural sheath.
- a. Pubis.
- b. Ilium.
- c. Abdominal muscles drawn up.
- d. Transversalis muscle.
- e. Its tendon.
- f. Seat of the posterior edge of the crural arch.
- gg. Fascia transversalis.
- h. Inner portion of the same fascia.
- i. Fascia iliaca.
- k. Crural sheath.
- l. Crural artery,
- m. Crural vein.
- n. Saphæna major vein.
- o. Anterior crural nerve.
- p. Fascia lata turned back.
- q. Tendon of the external oblique muscle, drawn down.

FIG. 4. Posterior view of the place at which the crural hernia descends, as it appears when the peritoneum is first stripped off.
- a. Pubis.
- b. Abdominal muscles.
- c. Round ligament passing into the inner abdominal ring.
- d. Crural artery.
- e. Crural vein.
- f. Epigastric artery.
- g. Epigastric vein.
- h. Depression at which the crural hernia first descends.

FIG. 5. Posterior view, shewing the mode in which the abdomen is shut from the thigh. The peritoneum is removed.
- a. Pubis.
- b. Ilium.
- c. Abdominal muscles.
- d. Rectus.
- ff. Junction of the fascia iliaca and transversalis behind the crural arch.
- g. Round ligament passing from the abdomen through the fascia transversalis.
- h. A portion of fascia or tendon passing from the pubis to join the rectus.
- i. Fascia iliaca.
- k. Iliac artery.
- l. Iliac vein.
- m. Epigastric artery.
- n. Epigastric vein.
- o. Anterior crural nerve.
- p. Crural space, by which the crural hernia descends: it leads into the crural sheath.

FIG. 6. A similar view, but with a portion of the fascia transversalis raised.
- a. Pubis.
- b. Ilium.
- c. Iliacus internus.
- d. Psoas.
- e. Fascia iliaca.
- f. Rectus abdominis.
- g. Junction of the fascia iliaca and transversalis at the edge of the crural arch.
- h. Fascia transversalis.
- i. Ligamentum rotundum, passing from the abdomen through the fascia transversalis.
- k. Fascia transversalis, and portion of the tendon of the rectus raised.
- l. Inferior column of the tendon of the external oblique.
- m. The abdominal ring.
- n. The third insertion of the external oblique.
- o. Iliac artery.
- p. Iliac vein.
- q. Epigastric artery.
- r. Epigastric vein.
- s. Circumflexa ilii.
- t. Absorbent gland receiving the different crural absorbent vessels.
- v. Absorbent vessels passing through the crural space or ring which is seen situated between the third or semicircular insertion of the external oblique muscle.
- w. A part of the posterior edge of the crural arch which forms one of the seats of stricture in large crural hernia.

Fig. 5 and 6 were both drawn removed from the body as they appear in the plate, which accounts for the flatness of their appearance.

FIG. 7. Crural hernial sac removed to shew the hole by which it descends in the female.
- a. Seat of the pubis.
- b. Crural arch extending towards the ilium.
- cc. Abdominal muscles.
- d. Crural arch.
- ee. Fascia lata.
- f. Semilunar edge of the fascia lata.
- g. Third insertion of the external oblique.
- h. Crural artery.
- i. Crural vein.
- k. Crural sheath.
- l. Abdominal ring.
- m. The orifice by which the crural hernia descends formed on the outer side by the crural sheath, on the inner by the semicircular insertion of the tendon of the external oblique, and above in part by the crural sheath and in part by the semilunar edge of the fascia lata. The division in the crural hernia is made at the upper and inner part.

FIG. 8. Posterior view of the same preparation.
- a. Seat of the pubis.
- b. Abdominal muscles.
  Epigastric vein.
- d. Epigastric artery.
- e. Iliac vein.
- f. Peritoneum.
- g. Hernial sac drawn from the aperture.
- h. A fascia cut off which covers it.
- i. Third insertion of the external oblique muscle.
- k. Fascia on the inner side of the vein.
- l. Aperture by which the crural hernia descends.
- m. A line from this points out the posterior edge of the crural arch, which forms the posterior stricture of the crural hernia.

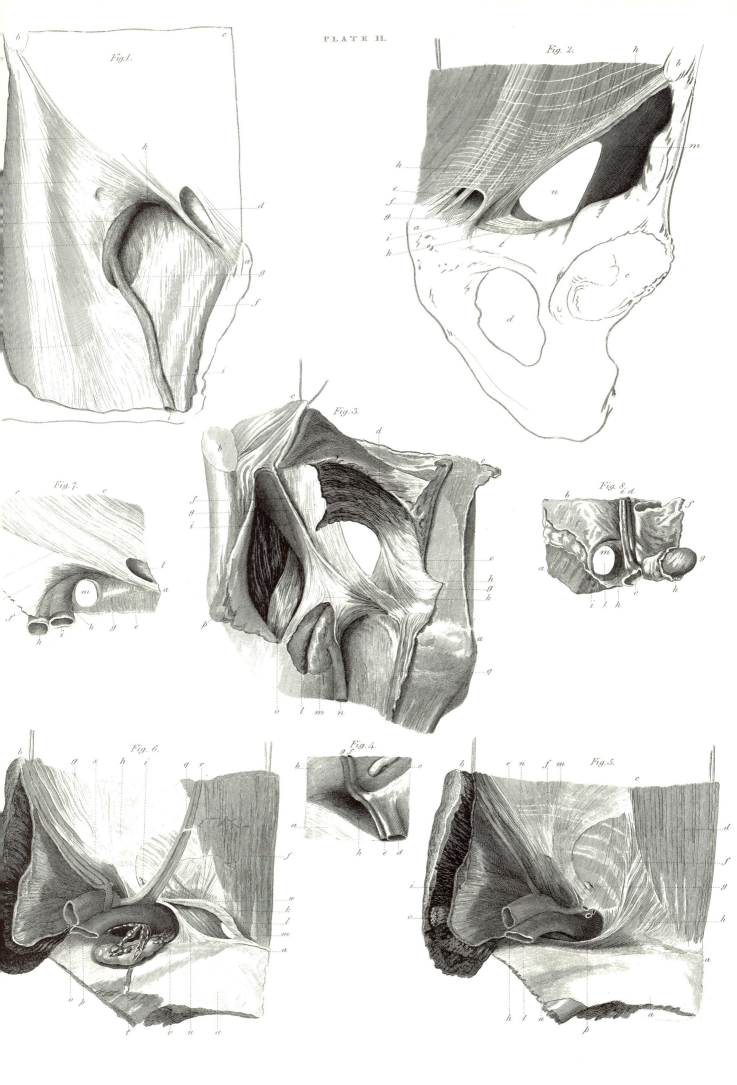

PLATE III.

SKETCHES of the parts in the groin of the male, intended to shew their anatomy.

FIG. 1. Posterior view of the external oblique muscle, of the external iliac artery and vein, and of the fascia iliaca.
- a. Symphisis pubis.
- b. Spinous process of the ilium.
- c. Pubis at the linea ileo pectinea.
- d. External oblique muscle and its tendon.
- e. Superior column of the tendon of the abdominal ring.
- f. Insertion of the inferior column of the ring into the tubercle of the pubis.
- g. The third insertion of the external oblique into the ligament of the pubis, from whence it is extended towards the symphisis.
- h. Abdominal ring.
- i. The fascia iliaca extending over the iliacus internus and psoas muscles.
- k. The junction of the fascia iliaca with the posterior edge of the crural arch, and it is seen extending near to the external iliac artery.
- l. External iliac artery.
- m. External iliac vein.
  [These vessels pass through an oval space, which is the beginning of the crural sheath, which is bounded internally by the third insertion of the external oblique muscle, externally by the fascia iliaca joining to the posterior edge of the crural arch, behind by the process of the same fascia, and before by the posterior edge of the crural arch.]
- n. Posterior edge of the crural arch extending from the pubis to the ilium. That part of it which is included between the two lines from n, forms the posterior stricture in large crural herniæ.
- o. Thyroideal foramen.

FIG. 2. A posterior view of the parts of the groin when the peritoneum is removed.
- a. Symphisis pubis.
- b. The seat of the spine of the ilium.
- c. Junction of the pubis and ilium.
- ddd. Abdominal muscles.
- e. Iliacus internus muscle covered by the fascia iliaca.
- f. Psoas muscle covered by a portion of the same fascia.
- ggg. Fascia transversalis lining the abdominal muscles, and descending to the crural arch.
- h. POUPART's ligament, or the crural arch, where the two fasciæ join.
- i. A process of fascia passing upon the iliac artery and vein, uniting them to the edge of the crural sheath.
- k. Internal abdominal ring, or upper aperture of the inguinal canal.
- l. Spermatic cord passing through that aperture.
- m. External iliac artery.
- n. External iliac vein.
- o. Epigastric artery and vein.
- p. Third insertion of the external oblique into the pubis, covered, however, by the fascia transversalis.
- q. The space by which the crural hernia descends, the finger having passed into it before the drawing was made to push down the fascia which extends over it.
- r. The obturator foramen.

FIG. 3. An anterior view of the groin.
- a. Symphisis pubis.
- b. Spine of the ilium.
- c. Tuberosity of the pubis.
- d. Crural arch, or POUPART's ligament.
- e. The place at which the crural hernia descends.
- f. Superior column of the abdominal ring.
- g. Inferior column.
- h. Abdominal ring.
- ii. Fascia lata.
- kk. Semilunar edge of the fascia lata, somewhat larger in this subject than usual.*
- ll. Crural sheath covering the crural artery and vein, at the inner and upper part of which at e the crural hernia descends.
- m. Saphæna major vein entering the sheath.
- n. A vein entering the saphæna major.

FIG. 4. Is intended to shew the crural sheath, and the insertions of the external oblique muscle.
- a. Pubis.
- b. Ilium.
- c. Superior column of the abdominal ring.
- d. Inferior column.
- e. Abdominal ring.
- f. Anterior edge of the crural arch, or POUPART's ligament.
- g. Fascia lata dissected from the crural arch and turned back.
- h. Third insertion of the external oblique into the ligament of the pubis; to see which the fascia lata and the origin of the pectineus muscle must be raised.
- i. Crural or femoral sheath covering the crural artery and vein.
- k. Saphæna major vein entering the sheath.
- l. Iliacus internus muscle.
- m. Pectineus muscle.

FIG. 5. Shews the connection of the crural sheath with the fascia transversalis.
- a. Pubis.
- b. Ilium.
- c. Abdominal muscles.
- dd. Transversalis muscle and tendon.
- e. Tendon of the external oblique muscle cut through and turned down.
- f. External portion of the fascia transversalis.
- g. Internal portion of the same fascia.
- h. Fascia lata turned back.
- i. Crural sheath covering the crural or femoral artery.
- k. Crural sheath covering the crural vein.
- l. Saphæna major vein.
- m. Some part of the semilunar edge of the fascia lata.
- n. Anterior crural nerve.
- o. Iliacus internus muscle.
- p. Seat of the crural arch to which the sheath adheres.
- q. Portion of the crural sheath passing behind the third insertion of the external oblique muscle into the pubis.
- r. Hole in the fascia transversalis for the passage of the spermatic cord.
- s. Two lines which include the spot at which the crural hernia descends, and which is situated at the inner and upper part of the crural sheath.†

FIG. 6. Shews the crural sheath cut open.
- a. Pubis.
- b. Ilium.
- cc. Transversalis muscle and tendon.
- d. Insertion of the external oblique turned down.
- ee. Fascia transversalis at its inner part, the epigastric artery and vein are seen.
- ff. Sheath cut open.—g. Crural artery.—h. Crural vein.—i. Saphæna major.—k. Epigastric artery and vein.—l. Circumflexa ilii.
- m. Internal abdominal opening for the spermatic cord.
- n. Space between the crural sheath and the crural or femoral vein, shewing the part at which the crural hernia descends.

FIG. 7. Artery and vein removed from the sheath.
- a. Pubis.—b. Ilium.—c. Fascia transversalis.—d. Aperture in it.—e. Fascia transversalis.—f. Anterior part of the crural sheath cut open.—g. Crural artery.—h. Crural vein.—i. Opening of the sheath from the abdomen.—k. Iliacus internus.—l. Fascia iliaca forming the posterior part of the crural sheath, and sending forwards a process between the crural artery and vein.

FIG. 8. Anterior view of the crural arch, a hernial sac having been removed from it to shew the orifice by which the crural hernia descends.
- a. Seat of the symphisis pubis.
- b. Crural arch.—cc. Fascia lata.
- d. Semilunar edge of the fascia lata.
- e. Crural sheath.—f. Abdominal ring.
- g. Spermatic cord.—h. Crural artery.
- i. Crural vein.
- k. Anterior column of the crural sheath, which requires division in the operation for the crural hernia.
- l. Lower column of the same opening.
- m. The hole in the side of the sheath by which the crural hernia descends.

FIG. 9. Posterior view of the same preparation.
- a. Symphisis pubis.—b. Ilium.—c. Pubis.
- d. Rectus muscle.—e. Other abdominal muscles.—f. Fascia transversalis.
- g. Spermatic artery and vein going through the internal abdominal ring.
- h. Crural artery.—i. Crural vein.
- k. Fascia between these vessels.
- l. Epigastric artery.
- m. The aperture by which the crural hernia quits the abdomen.
- n. The fascia forming the outer part of the stricture.
- o. That forming the inner.
- p. Fascia and posterior edge of the external oblique muscle forming that part of the stricture which requires division in the operation, if the division of the anterior column of the crural sheath k in the former figure is insufficient.

* To see this it is necessary to cut away some fibres covering the crural sheath.

† To make a similar preparation it is necessary that the semilunar edge of the fascia lata should be raised, and the finger be carried behind the edge of the crural arch.

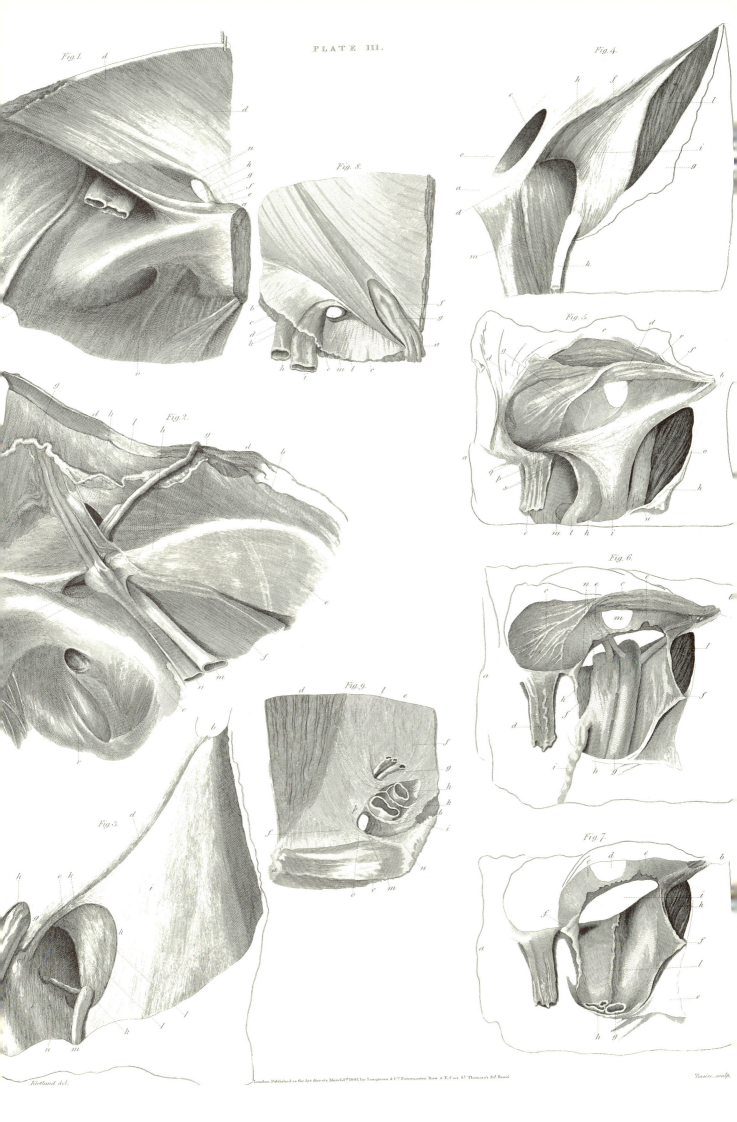

PLATE IV.

This Plate is intended to exhibit different views of crural herniæ in the female, in the order in which the parts appear in dissection.

Fig. 1. First dissection of the crural hernia.
- *a.* Symphisis pubis.
- *b.* Spinous process of the ilium.
- *c.* Situation of the crural arch, or Poupart's ligament.
- *dd.* Tendon of the external oblique muscle.
- *e.* Superficial fascia raised from the external oblique muscle.
- *fff.* Superficial fascia.
- *g.* Saphena major vein, the superficial fascia being cut away to shew it.
- *h.* A part of the superficial fascia attached to the crural arch.
- *i.* Abdominal ring and round ligament passing through it.
- *k.* Superficial fascia raised from the hernia.
- *ll.* Fascia propria raised from the hernial sac.
- *mm.* Hernial sac.
- *n.* Omentum within the hernial sac.
- *o.* Intestine within the hernial sac.

Fig. 2. Shews the form and contents of the hernial sac which has been removed from Figure 1.
- *aa.* Hernial sac.
- *b.* Neck of the hernial sac.
- *c.* Omentum within the hernia.
- *d.* Intestine within the hernia.
- *e.* Omentum at the mouth of the hernial sac.
- *f.* The intestine at the mouth of the sac.

Fig. 3. Shews the origin and appearance of the fascia propria.
- *a.* Seat of symphisis pubis.
- *b.* Spinous process of the ilium.
- *cc.* Abdominal muscles.
- *d.* Crural arch.
- *e.* Abdominal ring.
- *f.* Ligamentum rotundum uteri.
- *g.* Fascia lata.
- *h.* Portion of the fascia lata over the pectineus muscle.
- *ii.* Fascia propria, or protruded crural sheath, which covered the hernial sac after the sac in Fig. 2. had been removed.
- *k.* Attachment of the fascia propria to the sheath of the femoral vessels.
- *l.* A portion of the sheath covering the crural vessels, exposed by removing the semilunar edge of the fascia lata.
- *m.* The opening in the sheath through which the hernia had descended, above which is seen a dotted line, which marks the seat of the anterior stricture, and which is the part generally required to be divided.*

Fig. 4. A posterior view of the same preparation.
- *a.* Seat of symphisis pubis.
- *b.* Spinous process of the ilium
- *c.* Abdominal muscles.
- *d.* Rectus muscle.
- *ee.* Muscles of the thigh.
- *f.* Posterior edge of the crural arch.
- *g.* Fascia iliaca.
- *hh.* Fascia transversalis.
- *i.* Round ligament passing into the abdominal ring.
- *k.* External iliac artery.
- *l.* External iliac vein.
- *m.* Epigastric artery and vein.
- *n.* Obturator artery arising from the epigastric, and passing on the outer side of the crural opening.
- *o.* Meeting of the insertion of the external oblique into the ligament of the pubis, with the fascia iliaca.
- *p.* The crural orifice by which the hernial sac had descended, and a dotted line is extended from it, marking the situation of the posterior edge of the crural arch, covered by a fascia, which forms the posterior seat of the stricture.
- *q.* Fascia between the crural vein and mouth of the sac; this hole is, therefore, formed above by the posterior edge of the crural arch on the inner side by the semicircular insertion of the external oblique muscle, and externally by a fascia descending on the inner side of the crural vein, which is a process of the crural sheath.

Fig. 5. A small crural hernia dissected.
- *a.* Seat of symphisis pubis.
- *b.* Spinous process of the ilium.
- *c.* Tendon of external oblique muscle.
- *d.* Anterior edge of the crural arch.
- *e.* Abdominal ring.
- *f.* Superficial fascia turned from the external oblique.
- *g.* Superficial fascia upon the fascia lata.
- *h.* Crural vein.
- *i.* Absorbent gland thrust down by the hernia.
- *k.* Superficial fascia opened where it covered the hernia.
- *l.* Fascia propria of the hernial sac.
- *m.* Hernial sac unopened.

Fig. 6. The same preparation farther dissected.
- *a.* Seat of the symphisis pubis.
- *b.* Seat of the spinous process of the ilium.
- *c.* Tendon of the external oblique muscle.
- *d.* Internal oblique and transversalis.
- *e.* Fascia of the transversalis.
- *f.* Tendon of the transversalis.
- *g.* Inner portion of the fascia transversalis passing to unite itself with the tendon.
- *h.* The crural arch.
- *ii.* Round ligament.
- *k.* The round ligament passing into the abdomen.
- *l.* Crural artery.
- *m.* Crural vein.
- *n.* Origin of the epigastric artery.
- *o.* Course of the epigastric artery behind the round ligament.
- *p.* Crural nerve.
- *q.* Superficial fascia.
- *r.* Fascia propria of the crural hernia, the hernial sac having been drawn into the abdomen to shew this fascia distinctly.

Fig. 7. A small crural hernia in the female, shewing its passage through the crural sheath, and its distance from the crural arch.
- *a.* Seat of the symphisis pubis.
- *b.* Spinous process of the ilium.
- *c.* Crural arch.
- *d.* Abdominal ring.
- *e.* Fascia lata.
- *f.* Semilunar edge of the fascia lata.
- *g.* Portion of the crural sheath.
- *h.* Saphena major vein passing into the crural sheath.
- *i.* Hernial sac inclosed in its fascia, which is extremely dense, and is proportionably so as the hernia is small.
- *k.* The hole in the crural sheath through which the hernia passes.

Fig. 8. A small hernia in the male to shew the origin of the fascia propria.
- *a.* Seat of symphisis pubis.
- *b.* A portion of the crural arch.
- *c.* Insertion of the external oblique into the pubis.
- *d.* Portion of the fascia transversalis descending to unite itself to the crural vein.
- *e.* Portion of the crural vein.
- *ff.* Edge of the fascia lata cut from Poupart's ligament, and drawn downwards to expose the parts behind.
- *g.* Fascia lata wrinkled by its falling down.
- *h.* Semilunar edge of the fascia lata.
- *i.* Saphena major vein passing into the crural sheath.
- *k.* The portion of the crural sheath which covered the crural hernia, and forming the fascia propria, the hernial sac having been entirely removed, will be seen in Plate VIII.
- *ll.* The aperture by which the crural hernia had descended from the abdomen.
- *m.* A depression within the crural sheath, in which a process of the hernial sac was contained.

* This is the preparation on which for several years I have been in the habit of shewing the bag which encloses the hernial sac in my lecture on crural hernia.

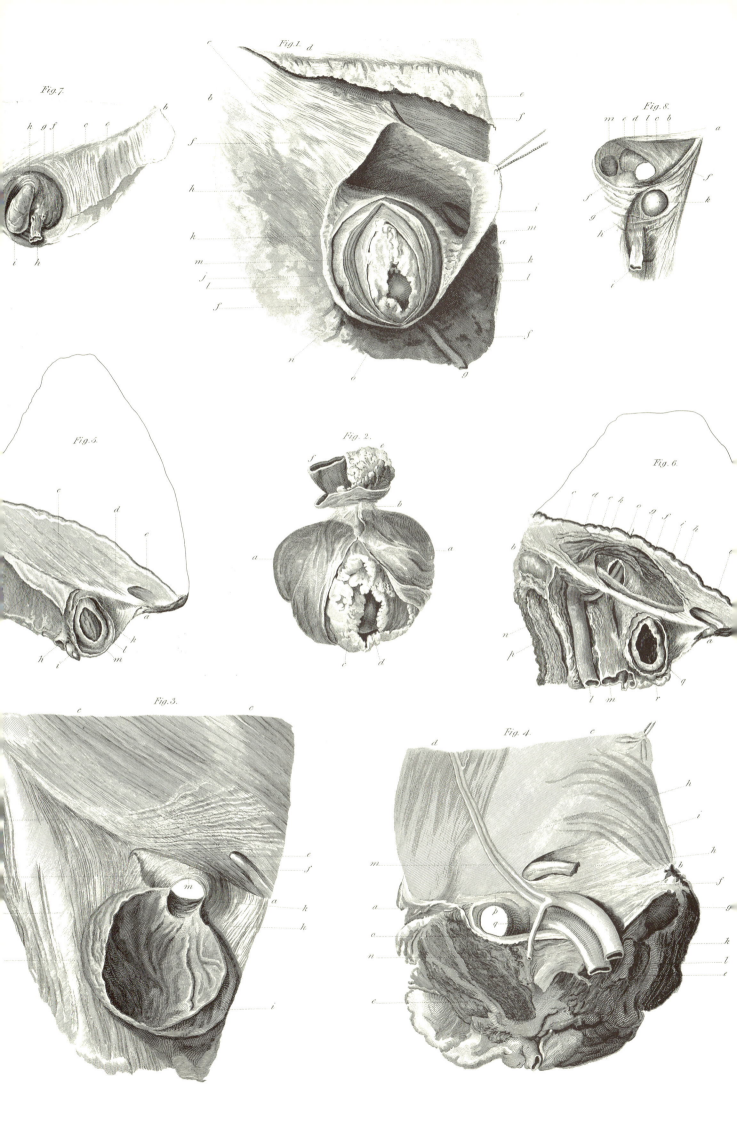

PLATE V.

This Plate exhibits three different views of the crural hernia in the male. Figure 1, is preserved in the collection at Guy's Hospital. Figure 2, is in my own possession.

Fig. 1. *a.* Symphisis pubis.
    b. Spinous process of the ilium.
    cc. Abdominal muscles.
    d. The crural arch, or Poupart's ligament.
    e. Semilunar edge of the fascia lata.
    f. Tendon of the external oblique cut open.
    g. Internal oblique and transversalis.
    h. External portion of the fascia transversalis.
    i. Internal portion of the same fascia.
    k. Internal abdominal ring.
    l. External abdominal ring.
    mmm. Spermatic cord passing through both apertures to the testis.
    n. Testis.
    o. Epigastric artery.
    p. Cremaster muscle.
    q. Crural hernia.
    r. The sac of the crural hernia.
    s. The fascia propria, or condensed cellular membrane, which covers the hernial sac.

Fig. 2.   Anterior view of another crural hernia.
    a. Symphisis pubis.
    b. Spinous process of the ilium.
    c. Abdominal muscles.
    d. Crural arch, or Poupart's ligament.
    e. Abdominal ring.
    f. Spermatic cord.
    g. Testis.
    h. Crural hernia.
    ii. Superficial fascia cut open and turned back.
    kk. Fascia propria of the sac laid open.
    ll. Hernial sac opened.
    m. Omentum seen within the sac.

Fig. 3.   Posterior view of Figure 1.
    a. Symphisis pubis.
    b. Spinous process of the ilium.
    c. Ilium cut through.
    ddd. Rectus and other abdominal muscles.
    e. Linea semilunaris.
    f. Posterior edge of the crural arch.
    g. Fascia iliaca.
    h. The iliacus internus muscle.
    ii. Fascia transversalis.
    k. Internal abdominal ring.
    l. Spermatic cord passing through the internal ring.
    m. External iliac artery.
    n. External iliac vein.
    o. Epigastric artery and vein.
    p. Sac of crural hernia.
    q. Mouth of the sac.
    r. Absorbent gland between the hernial sac and the iliac vein.

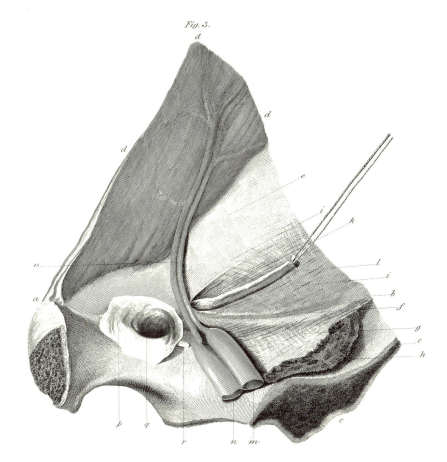
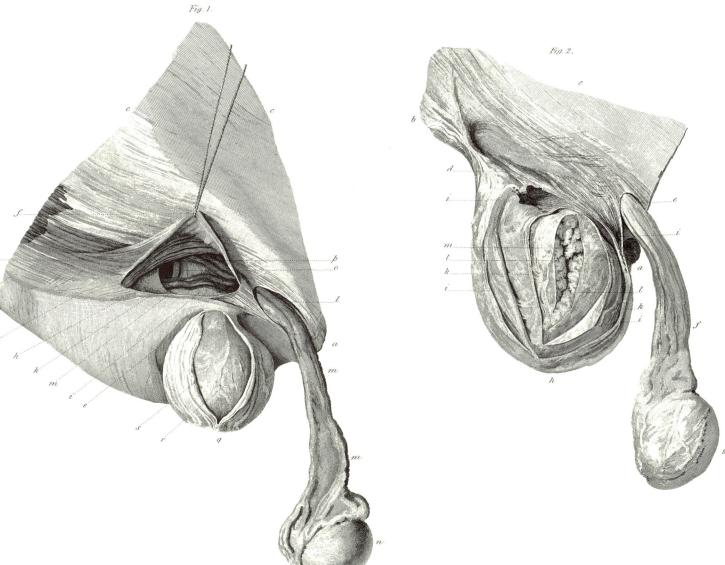

PLATE VI.

Exhibits an anterior and posterior view of two inguinal and a crural hernia in the same subject. Also views of the trusses which are required in large crural herniæ. The common inguinal truss may be applied for a small crural hernia; but in the larger, a truss which approaches the right angle is required, as the motions of the thigh displace the inguinal truss when put below the crural arch.

Fig. 1. Anterior view of a crural and two inguinal herniæ.
- a. Symphisis pubis.
- b. Spinous process of the ilium.
- cc. Crural arch sending off the fascia lata of the thigh.
- dd. Semilunar edge of the fascia lata.
- ee. Saphena major vein on each side.
- ff. Abdominal rings.
- g. Sac of the inguinal hernia on the left side.
- h. Its fascial covering.
- i. Inguinal hernial sac on the right side, its cavity obliterated by adhesion.
- k. Sac of crural hernia.
- m. Its orifice which had been dilated inwards in the operation for this hernia.

Fig. 2. Posterior view of the same preparation.
- aa. Seat of the spinous processes of the ilia, the upper *a* pointing to the abdominal muscles a little below the umbilicus.
- b. The bladder contracted.
- c. The uterus drawn to the right side towards the mouth of the hernial sac.
- dd. Ovaria.
- ee. Fallopian tubes.
- ff. Ligament arotunda.
- g. Orifice of the sac of the inguinal hernia on the left side.
- h. Orifice of the crural hernia.
- i. Sac of the right inguinal shut by adhesion.
- kk. Epigastric artery and vein.

Fig. 3.
- a. Inguinal truss.
- b. Crural truss.

Fig. 4.
- d. Truss for the large crural hernia.
- e. Upper abdominal opening.
- f. The place at which the crural hernia descends.
- g. Lower abdominal opening or ring.

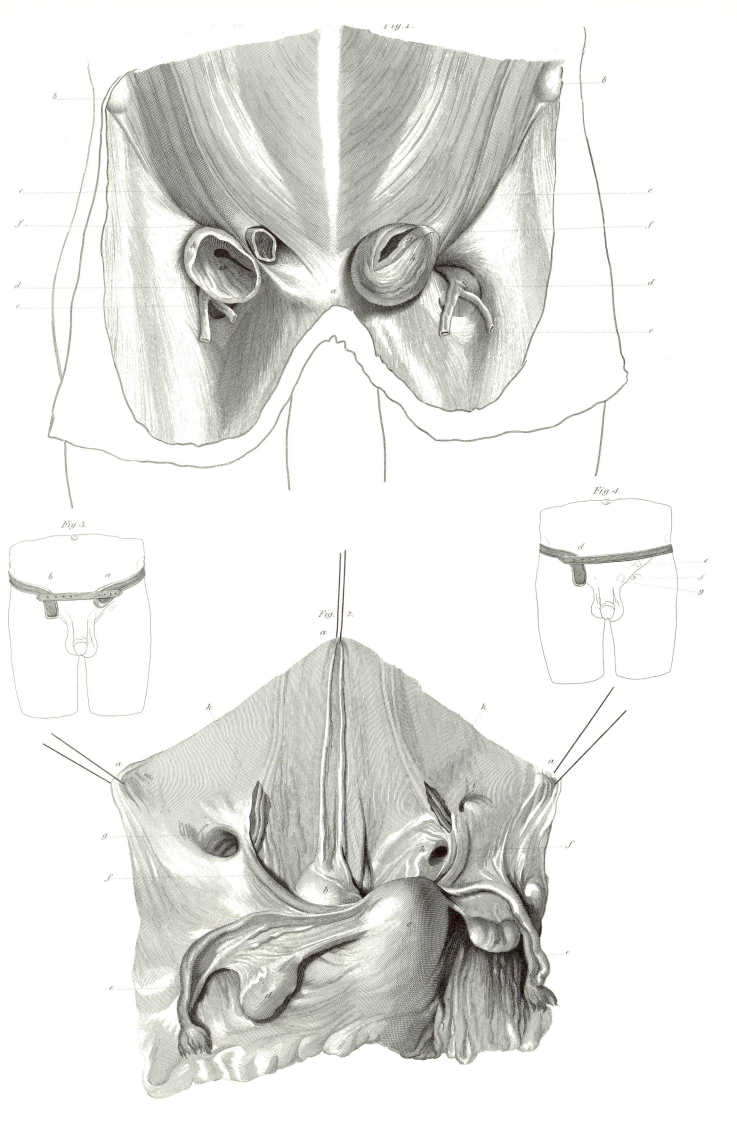

PLATE VII.

CONTAINING different views of Preparations made after the operation for the Crural Hernia.

FIG. 1. Anterior view of a crural hernia operated on by cutting directly inwards.
    a. Symphisis pubis.
    b. Spine of the ilium.
    cc. Abdominal muscles.
    d. Crural arch.
    e. Abdominal ring.
    f. Lower column of the ring inserted into the tubercle of the pubis.
    g. Fascia lata.
    h. Saphæna major vein.
    i. Fascia propria, or protruded crural sheath.
    k. Hernial sac included in the former.
    l. Insertion of the external oblique muscle into the ligament of the pubis, divided in the operation.

FIG. 2. Posterior view of the same.
    a. Symphisis pubis.
    b. Spine of the ilium.
    c. Ilium.
    d. Iliacus internus.
    e. Abdominal muscles.
    f. Rectus abdominis.
    g. Fascia iliaca.
    h. Fascia transversalis.
    i. Junction of the two fascia at the posterior edge of the crural arch.
    k. Internal abdominal ring, and the round ligament passing through it.
    l. Iliac artery.
    m. Iliac vein.
    n. Epigastric artery and vein.
    o. Obturator artery passing from the epigastric, but taking its course on the outer side of the hernial sac.
    p. Hernial sac.
    q. The insertion of the external oblique muscle, which had been divided in the operation inwards.

FIG. 3. A view of a preparation in which the intestine was divided by cutting inwards. See Cases.
    a. Seat of symphisis pubis.
    b. Crural arch.
    c. Abdominal muscles.
    d. Fascia lata.
    e. Crural artery.
    f. Crural vein.
    g. Hole in one fold of the intestine.
    h. Hole in the other fold.
    i. Hernial sac.

FIG. 4. Preparation of the hernial sac which had been returned into the abdomen unopened.
    a. Seat of symphisis pubis.
    b. Seat of the spine of the ilium.
    cc. Abdominal muscle.
    d. Muscles of the thigh.
    e. Muscles of the outer part of the thigh.
    f. Crural arch.
    g. Crural artery.
    h. Crural vein.
    i. Large hole at the crural arch, by which the hernia was pushed back.
    k. Fascia propria of the sac, which was also pushed into the abdomen.
    l. Hernial sac.
    mm. Peritoneum.
    n. Strangulated intestine.
    o. Intestine above the strangulated part.
    p. Stricture at the mouth of the sac remaining undivided.
    q. Mysentery.

FIG. 5. A large hernia which had been strangulated, and the operation was performed by cutting through the tendon of the external oblique muscle, drawing up the spermatic cord, and cutting the crural arch from the hernial sac. See Cases.
    a. Seat of the symphisis pubis.
    b. Spine of the ilium.
    cc. Abdominal muscles.
    d. Fascia lata.
    e. Crural arch.
    f. Abdominal ring.
    g. Crural artery.
    h. Crural vein.
    i. Testis.
    k. Spermatic cord.
    l. Fascia propria.
    m. Hernial sac.
    n. A hook put under the spermatic cord to draw it from the crural arch, whilst the arch was cut from the hernial sac.

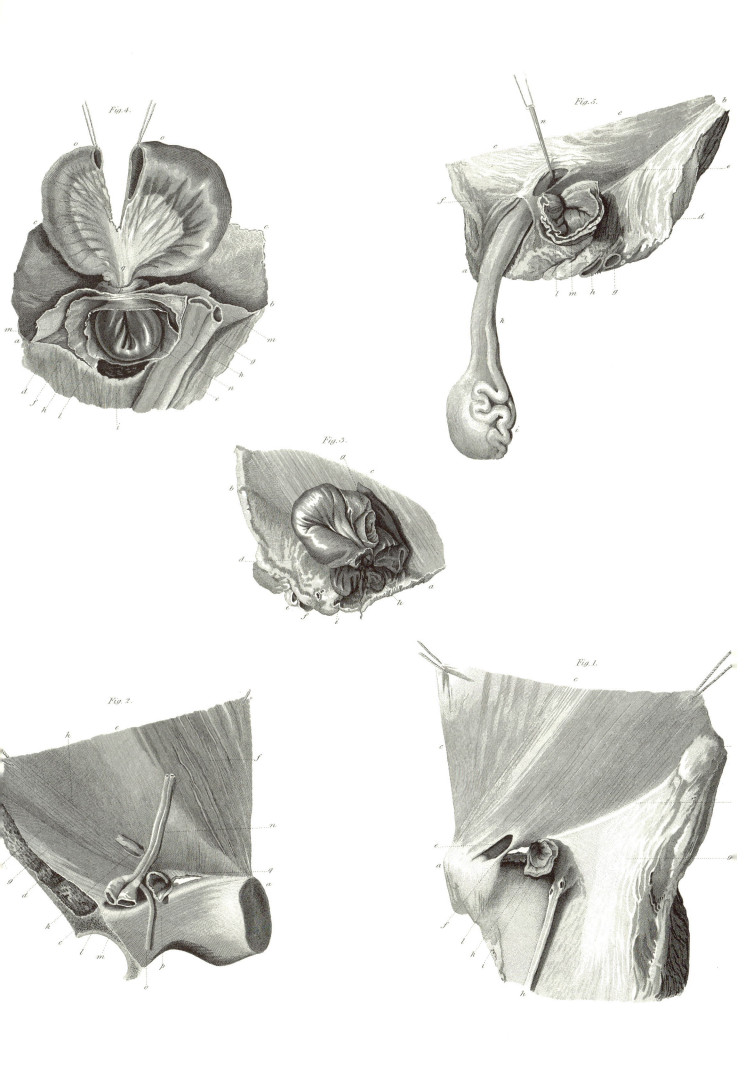

PLATE VIII.

CONTAINS some varieties of Crural Hernia, viz. a hernial sac, situated within the sheath of the crural vessels, which it had not protruded. A large hernia, having the remains of the umbilical artery placed on the outer part of the mouth of the sac. A hernial sac which had been contained in part in the sheath, and in part in the common situation. And lastly, the preparation with which I was kindly favoured, for the purpose of having an engraving made of it, by Dr. BARCLAY, Teacher of Anatomy in Edinburgh, shewing the obturator artery passing before the mouth of the hernial sac.

FIG. 1. Hernia within the crural sheath.
- *a.* Symphisis pubis.
- *b.* Spine of the ilium.
- *c.* External oblique muscle raised.
- *d.* Internal oblique muscle.
- *e.* Transversalis.
- *f.* Crural arch.
- *g.* Fascia transversalis passing from the crural arch under the transversalis muscle.
- *h.* Upper abdominal opening.
- *i.* Lower abdominal opening.
- *k.* Spermatic cord passing through both of these openings.
- *l.* Crural artery.
- *m.* Crural vein.
- *n.* Saphæna major vein.
- *oo.* Epigastric artery.
- *p.* Crural sheath opened and turned back.
- *q.* Hernial sac within the sheath.

FIG. 2. Large Hernia descending more inwards than usual, so as to have the umbilical artery on its outer side.
- *a.* Pubis.
- *b.* Spine of the ilium.
- *c.* Internal oblique muscle raised.
- *d.* Transversalis muscle raised.
- *ee.* Linea semilunaris.
- *f.* Rectus muscle.
- *g.* Abdominal ring.
- *h.* Fascia transversalis.
- *i* Inner part of the same fascia, with the tendon of the transversalis upon it.
- *kk.* Fascia lata.
- *mm.* Round ligament passing from the abdomen on the forepart of the mouth of the hernial sac.
- *n.* Crural arch.
- *o.* Obturator artery.
- *p.* Mouth of the hernial sac, which had the bladder much dilated resting upon it.
- *q.* Superficial fascia, and that of the hernia consolidated into one.
- *rr.* Hernial sac.
- *s.* Omentum adhering within the sac.

FIG. 3. A hernial sac, part within the sheath, and part in the usual situation.
- *a.* Peritoneum.
- *b.* Hernial sac, within the crural sheath.
- *c.* Hernial sac, which had protruded the sheath in the usual manner.
- *d.* Portion of the hernial sac which crossed the crural artery, and vein within the sheath.

FIG. 4. Dr. BARCLAY's Preparation.
- *a.* One of the lumbar vertebræ.
- *bb.* Spinous processes of the ilia.
- *c.* Abdominal muscles raised.
- *d.* Aorta.
- *e.* Bifurcation of the aorta.
- *f.* External iliac artery.
- *g.* Iliac artery of the left side.
- *hh.* Crural arteries.
- *i.* Arteria profunda.
- *k.* Epigastric artery on the left side, the rectus muscle being drawn down to shew it.
- *l.* Inferior cava.
- *m.* External iliac vein.
- *nn.* Crural veins.
- *o.* Peritoneum descending to form the hernial sac.
- *p.* The hernia.
- *q.* Common trunk of the epigastric and obturator arteries.
- *r.* Obturator artery passing before and on the inner side of the neck of the sac, in its course to the obturator foramen, and situated a little above the posterior edge of the external oblique muscle.
- *s.* Epigastric artery.

An Engraving of this Preparation has been published in an ingenious Thesis on Crural Hernia, by Dr. JAMES SANDERS. Edinburgh, 1805.

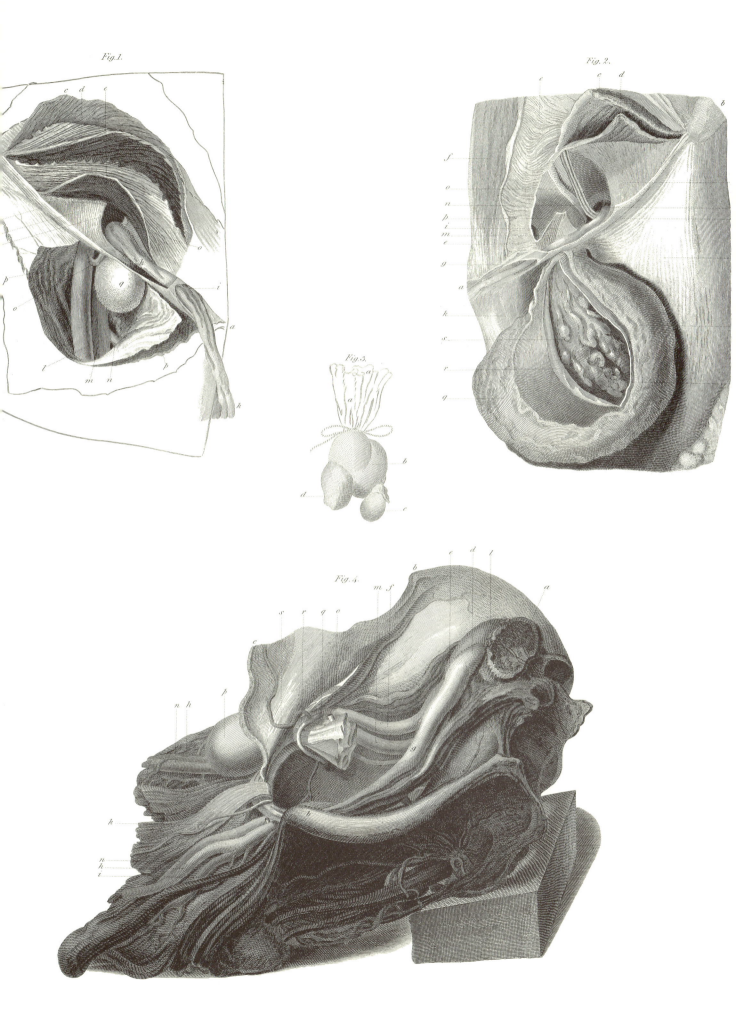

PLATE IX.

Shews three umbilical herniæ, one of which is curious, on account of two small omental herniæ being formed through orifices in the hernial sac. Also the trusses required in umbilical hernia, and two views of a ventral hernia. Fig. 2, and 3, were drawn by Mr. Cliff.

Fig. 1. The common appearance of umbilical hernia.
- *aaa.* Integuments.
- *bb.* Abdominal muscles.
- *ccc.* Peritoneum lining the abdominal muscles.
- *d.* Mouth of the hernial sac.
- *ee.* Hernial sac.
- *ff.* Termination of the linea alba around the mouth of the sac; also seen below at *b*.
- *g.* Fascia lining the integuments and covering the sac.

In this preparation some omentum adhered within the sac, which was not included in the drawing.

Fig. 2. Umbilical hernia in a very fat person.
- *aa.* The common integuments.
- *b.* The umbilicus.
- *cc.* Adeps between the integuments and abdominal muscles.
- *e.* Fascia over the sac.
- *f.* Hernial sac. The fascia, sac, and integuments adhering together at the umbilicus.
- *g.* Omentum adhering within the sac.
- *h.* Omentum descending to the sac.

Fig. 3. Umbilical hernia.
- *aa.* Integuments of the abdomen.
- *bb.* Integuments on the sac.
- *cccc.* Cicatrices from ulcers on the integuments.
- *dd.* Hernial sac.
- *eee.* Omentum within the sac, but a part of the sac absorbed so that it adheres to the skin from *l* almost to *k*.
- *ff.* Intestine ruptured by a fall. See case.
- *g.* An omental hernia.
- *h.* A smaller omental hernia.
- *i.* The hole in the sac through which the larger passed.
- *k.* The hole in the sac through which passed the smaller.
- *l.* Two other holes in the hernial sac.

Fig. 4. Truss for a small umbilical hernia; an ivory ball to be worn under it. If the person is corpulent he will require a belt similar to that in Fig. 6.

Fig. 5. Truss usually worn by corpulent women for the umbilical hernia.

Fig. 6. Improved truss by Mr. Marrison of Leeds.
- *a.* The pad.
- *b.* The spring added to the pad.
- *c.* An elastic band to assist the pressure of the pad.

The lower *b* points to the belt, which is added to keep this truss in its place in corpulent persons.

Fig. 7. Anterior view of the ventral hernia.
- *aaa.* Integuments.
- *bb.* Tendon of the external oblique, and rectus muscle behind it.
- *c.* Hernia.
- *d.* Fascia turned from the sac.
- *e.* Hernial sac.

Fig. 8. Posterior view of Fig. 7.
- *aa.* Peritoneum lining the abdominal muscles.
- *b.* The mouth of the hernial sac.
- *c.* The umbilical vein within the sac.

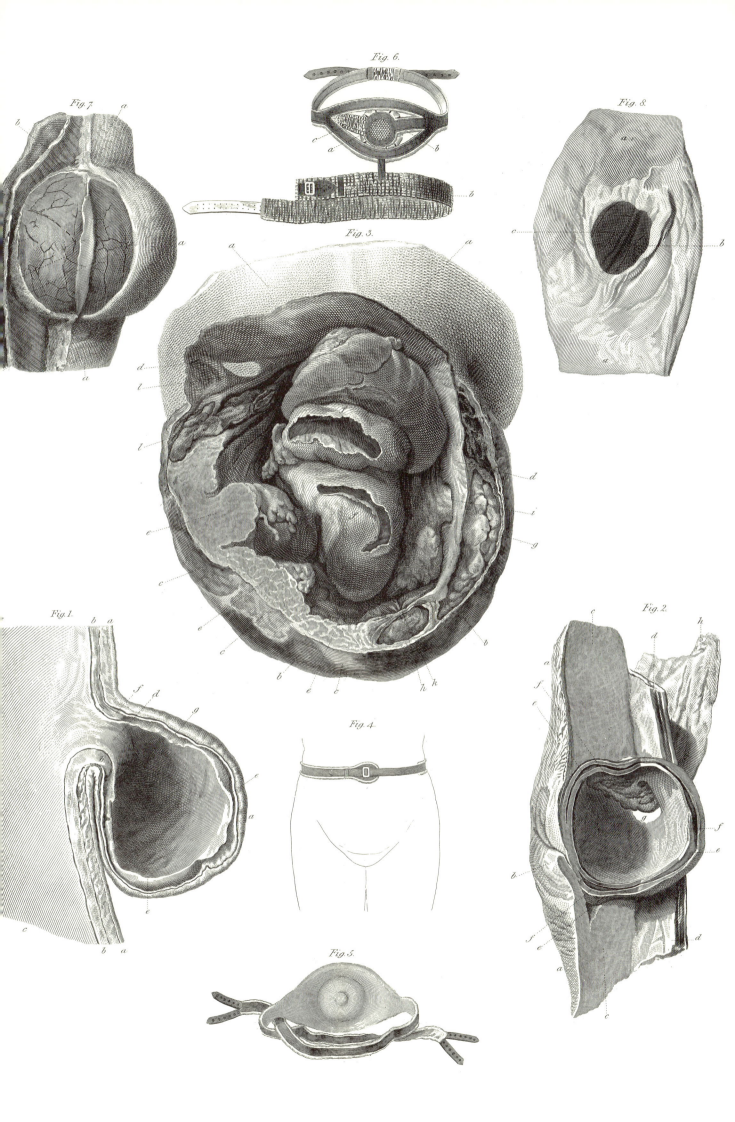

PLATE X.

CONTAINS an anterior and posterior view of a double umbilical hernia. Also anterior and posterior views of the umbilical hernia, shewing the danger of cutting the intestine within the abdomen. And two views of the ventral hernia, situated in the linea alba, about two inches above the umbilicus.

FIG. 1. Double umbilical hernia.
    aaa. Abdominal muscles.
    b. Linea alba.
    c. Large umbilical hernia. The sac opened. The skin adheres to it.
    d. Small umbilical hernia situated to the left side of the former, and the sac is opened.

FIG. 2. Posterior view of the same preparation.
    aaaa. Abdominal muscles.
    b. Linea alba.
    c. Orifice of the larger umbilical hernia.
    d. Orifice of the smaller hernia.
    e. A band of tendon situated between the two herniæ.

FIG. 3. Umbilical hernia—anterior view.
    aa. Linea alba.
    bbbb. Recti abdominis.
    cc. Lineæ transversales.
    d. Hernial sac within which the omentum is seen adhering.

FIG. 4. Posterior view of Fig. 3.
    aa. Recti abdominis.
    bb. Peritoneum.
    c. Remains of the umbilical vein.

    dd. Remains of the umbilical arteries.
    ee. Epigastric arteries.
    f. Linea alba.
    g. Intestine adhering to the orifice of the hernial sac.
    hh. The omentum glued to the mysentery and to the hernial sac, forming a pouch towards the abdomen.

FIG. 5. Anterior view of a ventral hernia.
    aa. Abdominal muscles.
    bb. Linea alba.
    c. Umbilicus.
    d. Fascia over this hernia.
    e. Hernial sac.
    f. Portions of fat between the fascia and the sac.

FIG. 6. Posterior view of Fig. 5.
    aa. Abdominal muscles.
    bb. Peritoneum.
    cc. Portions of adeps at the umbilicus.
    dd. Umbilical arteries.
    ee. Umbilical vein.
    f. Mouth of the ventral hernia.
    g. Fat adhering to the mouth of the hernial sac, into which the umbilical vein is seen to pass.

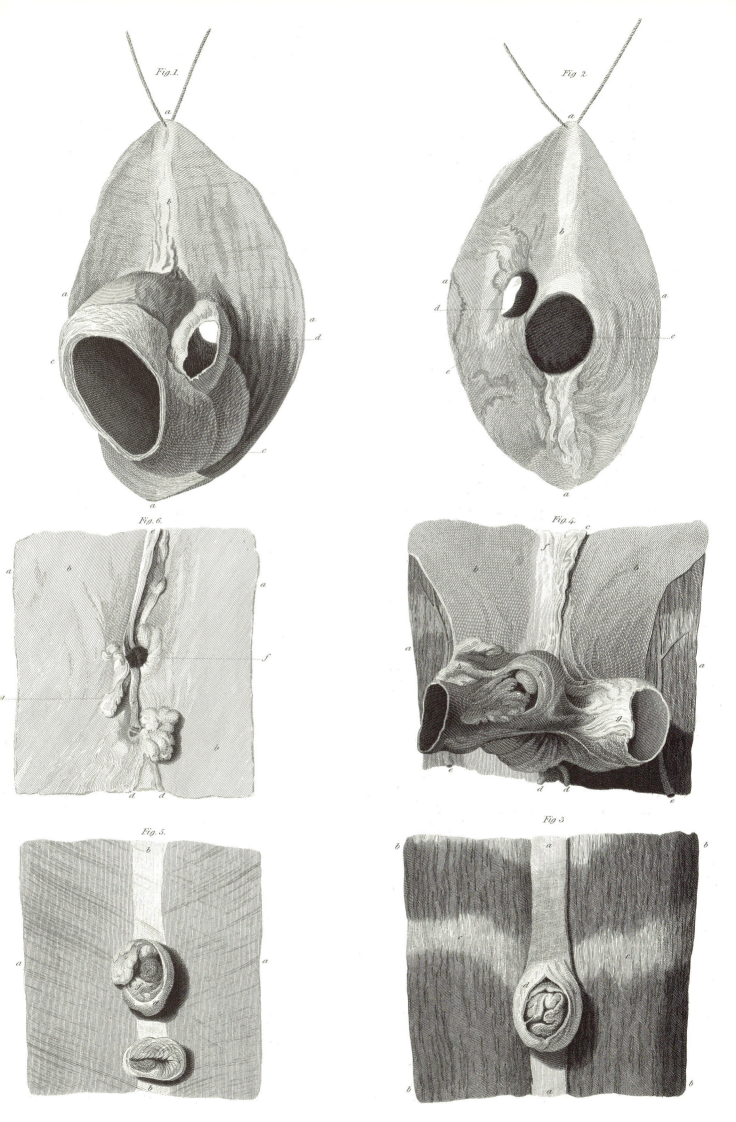

PLATE XI.

CONTAINS two views of a Thyroideal hernia (or hernia foramen ovalis). A view of a perineal hernia in the possession of Mr. CUTCLIFFE, of Barnstaple. Also a hernia congenita in the female, and a crural hernia sent me by Mr. ALLAN BURNS, Surgeon, of Glasgow.

FIG. 1. Thyroideal hernia.
- a. Symphisis pubis.
- b. Spine of the ilium.
- c. Abdominal muscles.
- d. Acetabulum
- e. Tuberosity of the ischium.
- f. Ligament of the obturator, or thyroid foramen.
- g. Crural artery.
- h. Artera cirumflexa ilii.
- i. Spermatic vein.
- k. Obturator artery.
- l. Inguinal hernia drawn aside.
- m. Thyroideal hernia situated just behind the pubis.

FIG. 2. Posterior view of the same preparation.
- a. Symphisis pubis.
- b. Tuberosity of the ischium.
- c. Sacro sciatic ligaments.
- d. Ligament of the thyroid foramen
- e. Abdominal muscles.
- f. External iliac artery.
- g. Epigastric.
- h. Circumflexa ilii
- i. Spermatic vein.
- k. Internal iliac artery.
- ll. Obturator, or thyroideal artery.
- mm. Internal pudendal artery.
- n. Mouth of the inguinal hernia.
- o. Mouth of the thyroideal hernia.

FIG. 3. Perineal hernia.
- a. The lumbar vertebræ.
- b. Spine of the ilium.
- c. Sacrum.
- d. Spinal marrow.
- e. Symphisis pubis.
- f. Erector penis.
- g. Accelerator urinæ.
- h. Bulb of the penis.
- i. Corpus cavernosum.
- k. Corpus spongiosum.
- l. The rectum.
- m. The bladder cut open, which it is not in the preparation.
- n. The urethra.
- o. Prostate gland.
- p. Vesicula seminalis.
- q. Anus.
- r. Mouth of the hernia.
- s. Body of the sac.
- t. Its fundus terminating nearly opposite the anus.

FIG. 4. From Mr. ALLAN BURNS.
1. The spine of the ilium.
2. The tubercle of the pubis.
3. The crural arch.
4. The abdominal muscles.
5. The inferior, or external orifice of the inguinal canal. The canal itself in this subject is very large and short, and contains
6. An incipient hernia congenita. The pillars of the canal are here seen to separate from each other fully an inch above the tubercle of the pubis, by which the herniary tumour appears much nearer to the spine of the ilium than it ought to do, and on the opposite side, where it protruded further, it lay more in the direction of the crural than of inguinal hernia.
7. The lower pillar of the canal inserted into the tubercle of the pubis.
8. The upper pillar, in part, inserted into the tubercle, but a production arising from it, which encircles the head of the gracilis and triceps muscles, reaching to the posterior part of the thigh, where it is lost. The healthy and morbid action of this fillet has been already explained.
9. GIMBERNAT's duplicature protruded so as to form an envelope of the herniary sac, which has been removed to shew the parts more distinctly.*
10. The opening which had been originally placed in the center of the septum stretched across the crural foramen.
11. The falciform process of the groin receiving a part of the protruded duplicature, and concealing from view the femoral vein.
12. The psoas aponeurosis covering the pectineus muscle, and rising up between the vena saphæna and deep-seated vein to join the falciform process.
13. The vena saphæna.
14. The (seat of the) femoral artery.

* I have called this the fascia propria of the hernial sac.

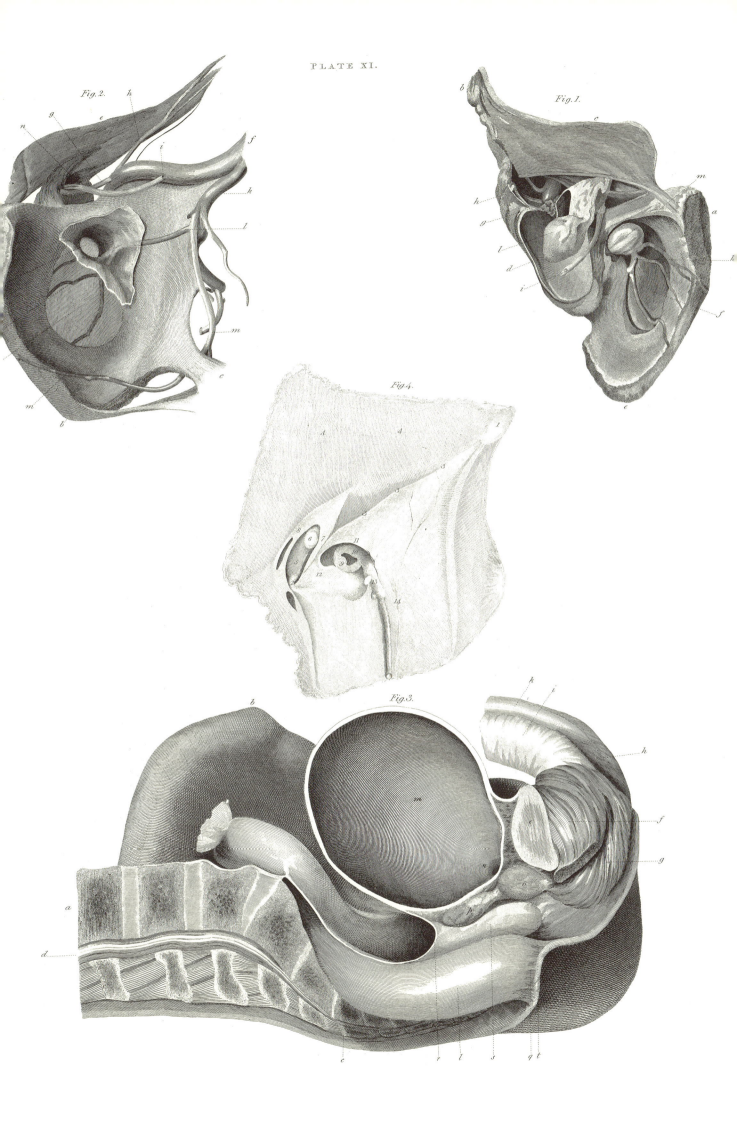

PLATE XI.

PLATE XII.

GIVES an internal view of the pelvis and of the Ischiatic hernia, from Dr. JONES's patient. The preparation is in the Anatomnial Collection at St. Thomas's Hospital.

- *a.* Section of the pubis.
- *b.* Spinous process of the ilium.
- *c.* Sacrum.
- *d.* Iliacus internus muscle.
- *e.* Psoas muscle.
- *f.* Pyriformis muscle.
- *g.* Coccygeus muscle.
- *h.* Termination of the external iliac artery in the crural.
- *i.* Beginning of the crural vein.
- *k.* Trunk of the common iliac artery.
- *l.* Internal iliac artery.
- *m.* Obturator artery, which may be traced before the sac as far as the obturator foramen.
- *n.* Internal iliac vein.
- *o.* Obturator vein passing behind the hernia to the obturator foramen, from which another vein *p.* is seen passing into the iliac vein.
- *q.* Hernial sac.
- *r.* Its orifice.

The artery was injected with red wax, the vein with yellow, which is the reason the artery is so much darker than the vein in the Plate.

PLATE XII.

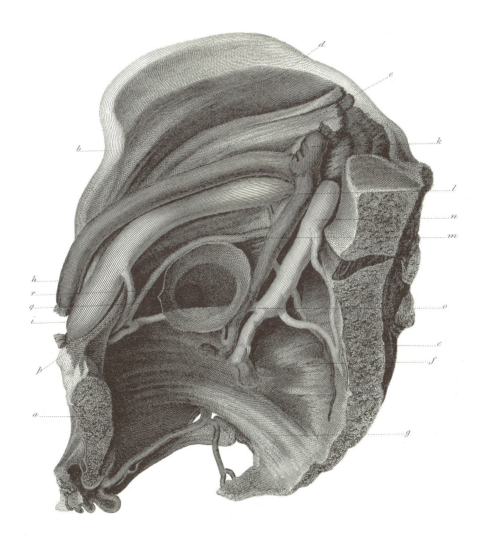

PLATE XIII.

A posterior view of the Ischiatic hernia.

a. Anterior superior spinous process of the ilium.
b. Crista of the ilium.
c. Sacrum.
d. Os Coxygis.
e. One of the sacro sciatic ligaments.

f. Acetabulum.
gg. Sciatic nerve.
h. Gluteal artery.
i. Ischiatic hernial sac situated between the artery and nerve.

PLATE XIII.

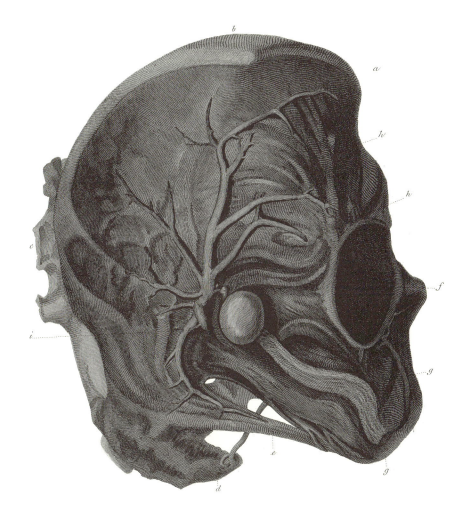

PLATE XIV.

Contains different views of the Phrenic Hernia.

Fig. 1. Phrenic Hernia, produced by fracture of the ribs.
- *aa.* Dorsal vertebræ.
- *bbb.* The ribs.
- *ccc.* The fractures of the ribs.
- *d.* The diaphragm.
- *e.* The intestine within the abdomen.
- *ff.* The intestine strangulated through a laceration of the diaphragm.

Fig. 2. Phrenic Hernia in the fœtus.
- *aa.* The liver.
- *b.* The stomach.
- *ccc.* The colon.
- *d.* The bladder.
- *eee.* The small intestines within the left cavity of the chest.
- *ff.* The diaphragm.
- *gg.* A bougie thrust through the aperture in the diaphragm, by which the intestines had passed into the chest.
- *h.* The heart.
- *i* The right lung.

Fig. 3. Phrenic Hernia in the adult strangulated. This plate is of a reduced size from the adult.
- *a.* The diaphragm.
- *b.* The omentum in the cavity of the abdomen.
- *c.* The small intestines.
- *d.* The colon, much smaller than usual.
- *e.* The left lung, much diminished by the pressure of the protruded parts.
- *f.* The heart.
- *g.* The strangulated omentum.
- *h.* The colon strangulated.
- *i.* A bougie introduced under the strangulated colon and omentum.

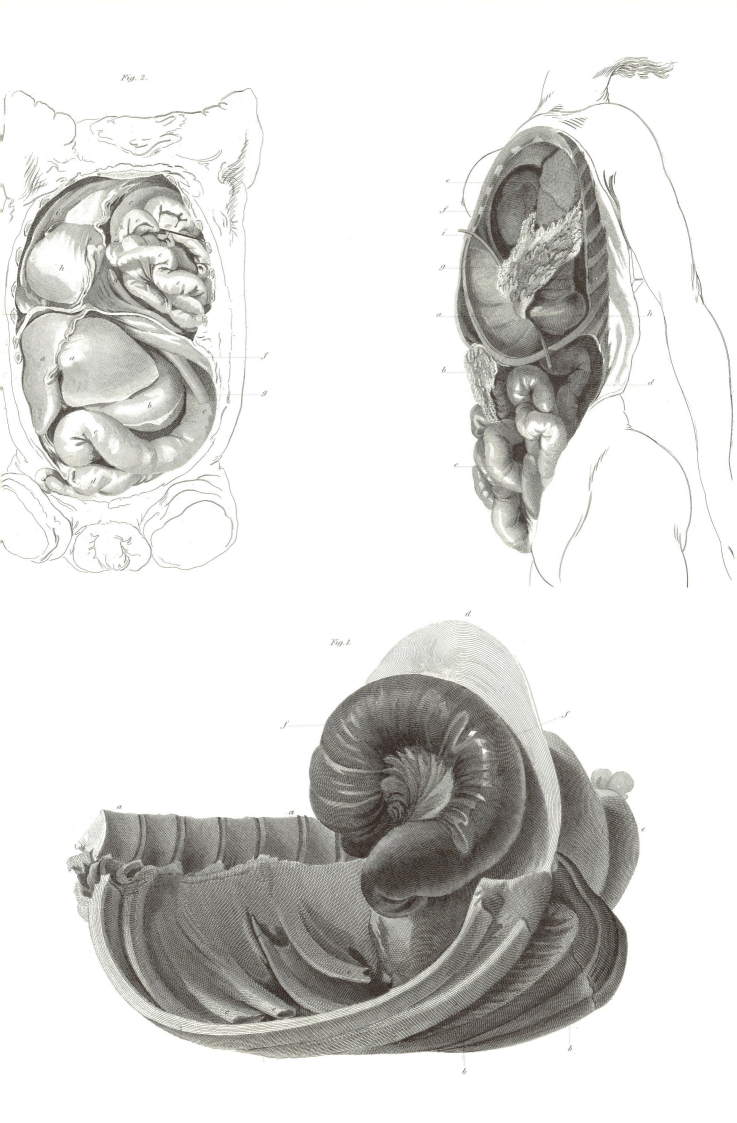

Fig. 2.

Fig. 1.

PLATE XV.

View of the mysenteric hernia taken from the body of a person opened by Mr. Richard Pugh, and preserved in the collection at St. Thomas's Hospital. The drawing was made by Mr. Kavanagh, one of our Students, from the recent subject.

aaa. The sternum and ribs.
bbb. The abdominal muscles turned back.
ccc. The great arch of the colon.
d. The omentum.
e. The upper *e* placed on the mesocolon.
e. The lower *e* placed on the bag formed by the mysentery.

f. The sac formed by the separation of the laminæ of the mysentery cut open.
gg. The small intestines within the bag.
h. The duodenum passing into the mysenteric sac.
i. The ileon passing from the sac to the cæcum.
kk. The thighs.

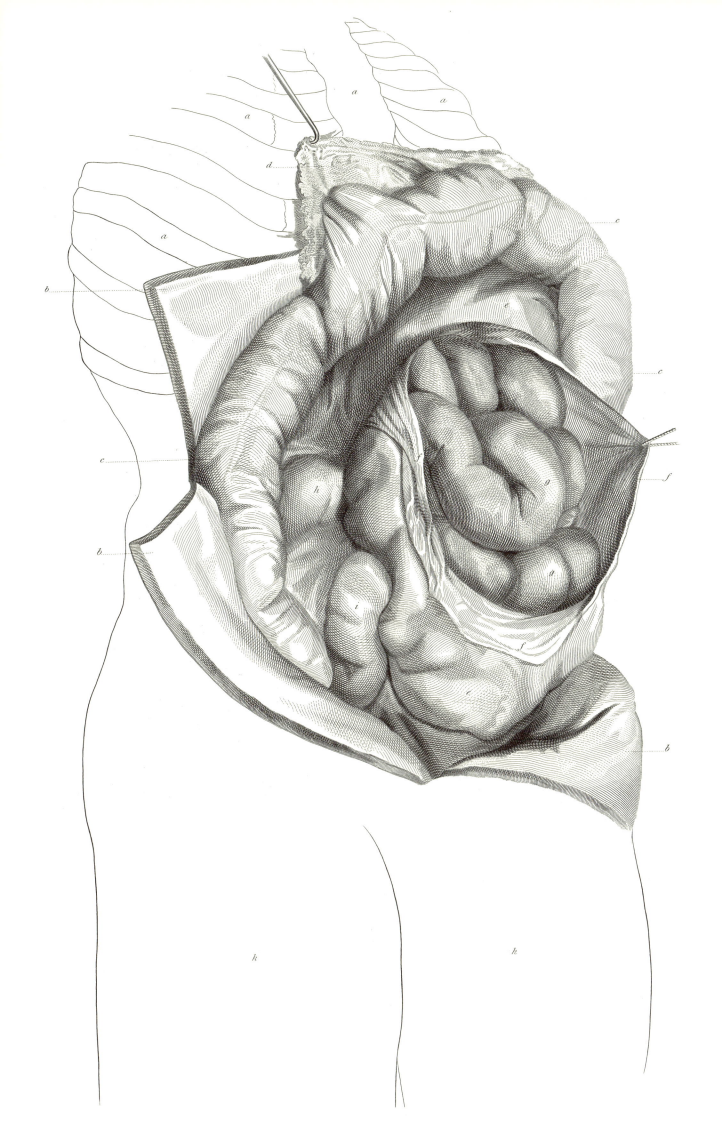

PLATE XVI.

View of a Mesocolic hernia. Taken from a preparation in the collection at St. Thomas's Hospital.

- *aa.* Posterior view of the colon from the left side.
- *b.* Sygmord flexure of the colon.
- *cc.* Arteria Colica.

- *d.* The sac formed by the separation of the laminæ of the mesocolon.
- *ee.* Small intestines passing into the sac.
- *ff.* The aperture by which the intestines entered the sac.

PLATE XVI.

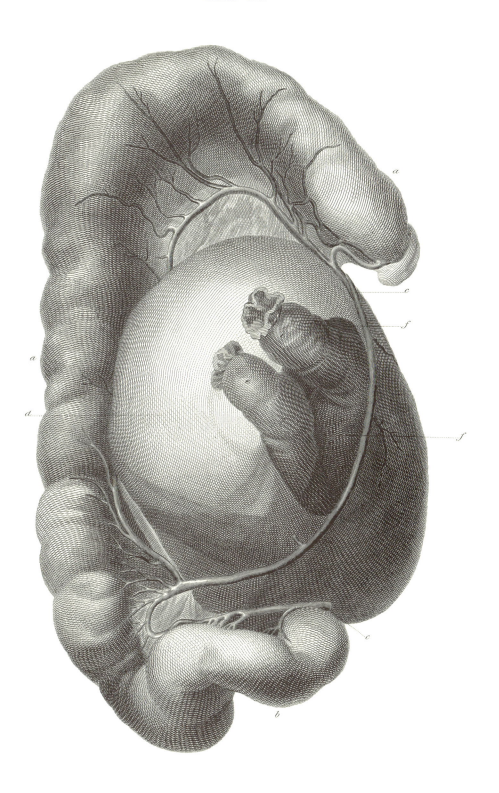

PLATE XVII.

This Plate shews a number of sacs found in an intestine, which was taken from the body of a person labouring under hernia, given me by Mr. HEADINGTON, Lecturer on Anatomy and Surgery, and Surgeon to the London Hospital. Also a View of an intestine strangulated through the mysentery, which was a present from Mr. PALMER, of Hereford, and two portions of intestine strangulated by a membranous band, which I took from a patient of Mr. WESTON's, of Shoreditch. The two other subjects are Views of the intestines of a dog, into which I made a longitudinal incision; the ligatures were cut off close to the intestine, and the intestine was returned into the cavity of the Abdomen. See Mr. THOMPSON's experiments, Part I.

FIG. 1. Intestine protruded through the mysentery.
    a. Portion of intestine.
    b. The other portion.
    c. The strangulated intestine.
    dd. The hole in the mysentery, through which the intestine had passed, and by which it was strangulated.

FIG. 2. Intestines strangulated by a membranous band.
    aa. Abdominal muscles (lined by the peritoneum) taken from the lower part of the abdomen.
    b. Hernia on the left side.
    e. Membranous band passing from the sac to the intestine.
    f. Membranous band returning to the sac from the intestine.
    g. The band passing around a part of the intestine.
    hh. The intestine strangulated by the band *g.*
    ii. Intestine strangulated in a less degree, by the portions of the membranous band *e,* and *f.*
    kk. The mysentery of each portion of the intestine.

FIG. 3. The same membranous band shewn without the intestine.

    ef. The band going from and towards the sac, including the intestine *ii.*
    g. The part which surrounded the intestine *hh.*

FIG. 4. Sacs on the intestine.
    aaaa. Intestine only in part engraved.
    bbb. The mysentery.
    cccc. Sacs communicating with the inner side of the intestine.

FIG. 5. *aa.* Intestine of a dog, into which an incision had been made.
    b. Its mysentery.
    c. The omentum.
    d. The omentum adhering at the part at which the incision had been made, and closing the aperture externally.

FIG. 6. Internal view of the same intestine.
    aa. Intestine.
    b. Ligature appearing within the intestine.
    d. The knot within the intestine.
    e. Omentum and intestine adhering.

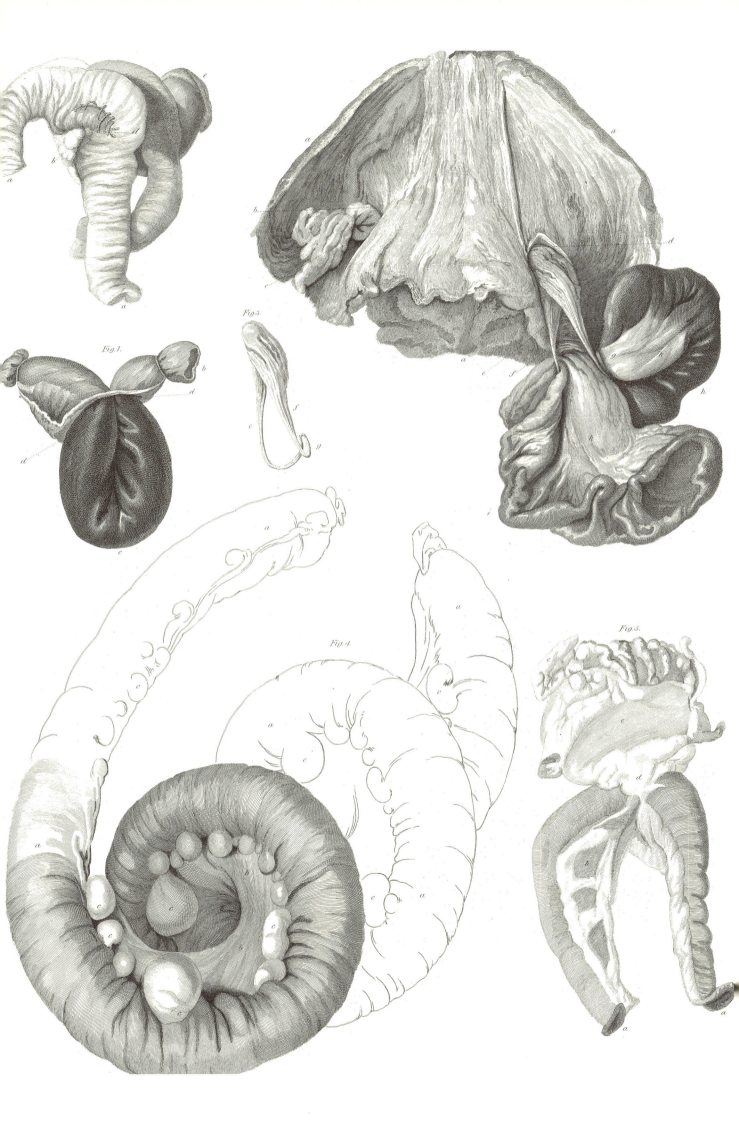